Case Studies in Systemic Sclerosis

Richard M. Silver • Christopher P. Denton
Editors

Case Studies in Systemic Sclerosis

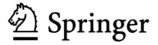 Springer

Editors

Richard M. Silver, M.D., FACP, FACR
Professor of Medicine & Pediatrics
Distinguished University Professor
Division of Rheumatology & Immunology
Department of Medicine
Medical University of South Carolina
Charleston, SC, USA

Christopher P. Denton, Ph.D., FRCP
Professor of Experimental Rheumatology
Centre for Rheumatology
Royal Free Hospital and UCL Medical School
Hampstead
London, UK

ISBN 978-0-85729-640-5   e-ISBN 978-0-85729-641-2
DOI 10.1007/978-0-85729-641-2
Springer New York Dordrecht Heidelberg London

British Library Cataloguing in Publication Data
A catalogue record for this book is available from the British Library

Library of Congress Control Number: 2011928402

Printed on acid-free paper

Springer is part of Springer Science+Business Media (www.springer.com)

We wish to dedicate this book to our mentors and close colleagues: Dr. Nortin Hadler, Dr. Barbara Ansell (deceased), Dr. Nathan J. Zvaifler, Dr. E. Carwile LeRoy (deceased), Dr. Joseph Korn (deceased), and Professor Dame Carol Black, for their wisdom and inspiration. We also dedicate this book to our families for their continued love and understanding.

Foreword

Systemic sclerosis is a rare and often complex disease. Its prevalence has been estimated to be about 240 cases per million adults, with an annual incidence of about 20 per million. Whether in its initial presentation, subsequent evolution, or coexistence with other often more common disorders, good care often depends on alertness to its clinical complexities and recognition of their nature. I can think of no better way to understand these complexities than by studying individual patient histories.

This book of case studies is drawn from experience worldwide. In thirty-five studies, it covers many of the clinical manifestations and complications of the disease. I suspect that even among specialists few will have experience of every clinical situation described in this book. Among the array of complex and therapeutically challenging situations described, there are experiences to be shared and insights gained even by the most practiced physician.

All who have encountered patients with systemic sclerosis and have taken responsibility for their treatment and care have known and remember instances – by no means rare in this specialist practice – where their therapies were of little avail and the disease ran its own unalterable course. The gathered experience contained in this book reminds us poignantly that always when we can do little to influence the disease there is a great deal to be done to help and care for the patient, relieving distress by the kindest and most effective means possible.

I am confident therefore that this book will quickly be seen as a thoughtful and valued source of reference, both to those training in this field and to experienced practitioners when they encounter unusual clinical features or therapeutic challenges in the patients who seek their help.

Dame Carol Black, M.D., FRCP, F.Med.Sci.

Preface

Sir William Osler liked to say, "To study the phenomena of disease without books is to sail an uncharted sea, while to study books without patients is not to go to sea at all."[1] Osler's admonition still rings true in today's world of rapid information retrieval but ever-increasing pressures on the time spent with patients. With the publication of *Case Studies in Systemic Sclerosis*, we aim to give our readers the two elements Osler deemed to be the essence of medicine: knowledge and devotion to patient care. Our goal is to convey knowledge of the many different manifestations of systemic sclerosis, presented in the context of real-life patient settings. Indeed, a case-based approach is in many ways an ideal format to illustrate and discuss the manifold and complex clinical issues encountered in the care of our patients. With each chapter, we present the clinical experiences and expertise of one or more specialists well versed in a particular facet of the disease. We have selected authors whose training and expertise provide both the breadth and the depth of knowledge required of those who manage such a complex disease as systemic sclerosis. It is our hope that *Case Studies in Systemic Sclerosis* will prove to be a useful resource, not only for students and trainees about to set sail on a lifelong voyage of the study of medicine, but also for practicing physicians challenged by the many complexities of the management of patients with systemic sclerosis.

Richard M. Silver, M.D., FACP, FACR
Christopher Denton, Ph.D., FRCP

[1]Osler W. *Aequanimitas, With Other Addresses to Medical Students, Nurses and Practitioners of Medicine*. 2nd ed. with three additional addresses. London: H.K. Lewis; 1920.

Acknowledgments

We gratefully acknowledge the contributions of the many authors of *Case Studies in Systemic Sclerosis*, whose expertise and dedication to people with scleroderma make a book such as this possible. We also express our appreciation for the expert team at Springer-Verlag London Limited, especially our developmental editor, Michael D. Sova, who managed to keep our international cast of authors on task and on time. Ultimately, a work such as this would not have been possible without the many patients through the years and from around the world, for whom we feel fortunate to have known and who have taught us so much.

Contents

1   **A 35-Year-Old Woman with Puffy Hands, Raynaud's
Phenomenon, and Positive Antinuclear Antibody Test** 1
Richard M. Silver

2   **A 30-Year-Old Woman with Puffy Hands, Raynaud's
Phenomenon, and Carpal Tunnel Syndrome.** 11
Christopher P. Denton

3   **A 22-Year-Old Woman with Raynaud's Phenomenon
but No Other Symptoms and No Abnormalities
on Examination** 23
Ariane L. Herrick

4   **A Young Adult with Localized Skin Sclerosis
and Positive ANA** 31
Elke M.G.J. de Jong and Frank H.J. van den Hoogen

5   **Localized Scleroderma in a Child** 39
Ronald M. Laxer, Elena Pope, and Christine O'Brien

6   **An 8-Year-Old Girl with Tight Skin, Digital Ulcers,
and Dysphagia** 53
Ivan Foeldvari

7   **A 60-Year-Old Woman with Skin Thickening,
Joint Contractures, and Peripheral Blood Eosinophilia** 63
Marcy B. Bolster

8   **A 35-Year-Old Man with Diffuse Scleroderma
and Chemical Exposure.** 73
László Czirják and Cecília Varjú

9   **A 65-Year-Old Woman with Hardened Skin,
Joint Contractures, and Yellow Scleral Plaques** 85
Jonathan Kay

10 **Painful Digital Ulcers in a Scleroderma Patient
    with Raynaud's Phenomenon** 95
    Fredrick M. Wigley and Peter K. Wung

11 **Rapidly Progressive Skin Disease in a Patient
    with Diffuse Systemic Sclerosis.** 107
    Elena Schiopu and James R. Seibold

12 **A 28-Year-Old Woman with Early Diffuse Scleroderma
    and Shortness of Breath** 115
    Otylia Kowal-Bielecka and Krzysztof Kowal

13 **Late Limited Systemic Sclerosis Patient Who Develops
    Shortness of Breath on Exertion.** 127
    Jérôme Le Pavec and Marc Humbert

14 **A Diffuse Scleroderma Patient Who Presents with
    Shortness of Breath and Enlarged Cardiac Silhouette.** 139
    Yannick Allanore and Christophe Meune

15 **A Patient with Systemic Sclerosis, Dyspnea on Exertion,
    Atypical Chest Pain, and Arrhythmia** 147
    André Kahan

16 **A Scleroderma Patient with Dysphagia and Reflux
    Who Experiences Worsening Cough** 155
    Romy Beatriz Christmann

17 **A Scleroderma Patient with Acute Drop in Hemoglobin
    and Occult Blood in Stool** 165
    Jayne Littlejohn and Chris T. Derk

18 **A 62-Year-Old Woman with Scleroderma and Severe
    Weight Loss.** 173
    Geneviève Gyger and Murray Baron

19 **A Patient with Diffuse Systemic Sclerosis
    with Hypertension and Acute Renal Failure** 185
    Ulf Müller-Ladner

20 **A 34-Year-Old Woman with Limited Cutaneous Scleroderma
    Who Develops Normotensive Renal Failure with Pulmonary
    Hemorrhage** 195
    Hirahito Endo

21 **A Scleroderma Patient Inquires About Pregnancy.** 203
    Virginia Steen

22 **A 38-Year-Old Man with Systemic Sclerosis and Erectile Dysfunction** 217
Edward V. Lally

23 **A Female Scleroderma Patient with Sexual Dysfunction** 221
Patricia E. Carreira

24 **A 38-Year-Old Woman with Elevated Muscle Enzymes, Raynaud's Phenomenon, and Positive Anti-Topoisomerase I Antibody: Is She Depressed?** 229
Lisa R. Jewett, Marie Hudson, and Brett D. Thombs

25 **A Scleroderma Patient with Swollen and Tender Joints of Both Hands** 239
Gabriele Valentini, Giovanna Cuomo, Virginia D'Abrosca, and Salvatore Cappabianca

26 **Two Scleroderma Patients with Differing Patterns of Muscle Disease** 251
Robyn T. Domsic and Thomas A. Medsger Jr.

27 **A Limited Cutaneous SSc Patient with Severe Calcinosis and Acro-osteolysis** 259
Francesco Porta and Marco Matucci-Cerinic

28 **A 54-Year Old Woman with Pain and Stiffness of Hands and Tendon Friction Rubs** 267
Dinesh Khanna and Puja P. Khanna

29 **A Young Diffuse Scleroderma Patient Having Difficulties with Activities of Daily Living** 273
Janet L. Poole

30 **A Middle-Aged Male Scleroderma Patient Who Can No Longer Perform His Occupation** 281
Janet Pope

31 **A Scleroderma Patient Presenting with Facial Pain** 293
David Launay, Hélène Zephir, and Pierre-Yves Hatron

32 **A Dentist Inquires About His Patient with Systemic Sclerosis** 299
Faye N. Hant and Michele C. Ravenel

33 **A Scleroderma Patient Complaining of Dry and Gritty Sensation of the Eyes** 317
Rajen Tailor and Vaneeta Sood

**34   A 34-Year-Old Woman with 2-Year History of Therapy-Resistant,
      Rapidly Progressive SSc Successfully Treated by
      Autologous Hematopoietic Stem Cell Transplantation**   331
      Alan G. Tyndall

**35   Sclerodactyly and Raynaud's Phenomenon in a Patient
      Who Has Primary Biliary Cirrhosis**   339
      Maureen D. Mayes and Shervin Assassi

Index   347

Contributors

Yannick Allanore, M.D. Department of Rheumatology A, Université Paris Descartes, Hôpital Cochin, Paris, France

Shervin Assassi, M.D. Department of Internal Medicine, The University of Texas-Houston Medical School, Rheumatology, Houston, TX, USA

Murray Baron, M.D. Department of Rheumatology, Jewish General Hospital, Montreal, QC, Canada

Marcy B. Bolster, M.D. Division of Rheumatology and Immunology, Medical University of South Carolina, Charleston, SC, USA

Salvatore Cappabianca, M.D. Departimento Di Internistica Clinica e Sperihentale "F. Magrassi-A. Lanzara" – Radiology Unit, Second University of Naples, Napoli, Italy

Patricia E. Carreira, M.D. Rheumatology Department, Hospital Universitario 12 de Octubre, Madrid, Spain

Romy Beatriz Christmann, M.D., Ph.D. Arthritis Center Rheumatology Division, University of Sao Paulo/Boston University School of Medicine, Boston, MA, USA

Giovanna Cuomo, M.D. Departimento Di Internistica Clinica e Sperimentale "F Magrassi-A. Lanzara" – Rheumatology Unit, Second University of Naples, Napoli, Italy

László Czirják, M.D. Department of Rheumatology and Immunology, University of Pécs, Medical Center, Pécs, Hungary

Virginia D'Abrosca, M.D. Departimento Di Internistica Clinica e Sperimentale "F Magrassi-A. Lanzara" – Rheumatology Unit, Second University of Naples, Napoli, Italy

Elke M. G. J. de Jong, M.D., Ph.D. Department of Dermatology, Radboud University Nijmegen Medical Centre, Nijmegen, The Netherlands

Christopher P. Denton, Ph.D., FRCP. Centre for Rheumatology, Royal Free Hospital and UCL Medical School, Hampsted, London, UK

Chris T. Derk, M.D., M.Sc. Department of Rheumatology, Thomas Jefferson University, Philadelphia, PA, USA

Alan G. Tyndall, M.D., FRACP, FMH. Rheumatology & Internal Medicine Department of Rheumatology, University Clinic, Felix Platter Spital Basel (Hospital), Basel, Switzerland

Robyn T. Domsic, M.D., MPH. Department of Medicine & Rheumatology, University of Pittsburgh, Pittsburgh, PA, USA

Hirahito Endo, M.D., Ph.D. Division of Rheumatology, Department of Internal Medicine, Toho University School of Medicine, Tokyo, Japan

Ivan Foeldvari, M.D. Hamburger Zentrum Fuër Kinder- und Jugendrheumatologie, Schön Klinik Eilbek, Hamburg, Germany

Geneviève Gyger, M.D. Department of Rheumatology, Jewish General Hospital, Montreal, QC, Canada

Faye N. Hant, D.O., MSCR. Department of Medicine, Rheumatology & Immunology, Medical University of South Carolina, Charleston, SC, USA

Pierre-Yves Hatron, M.D. Department of Internal Medicine, Claude-Huriez Hospital, Lille, France

Ariane L. Herrick, M.D., FRCP. Manchester Academic Health Science Centre, The University of Manchester, Salford Royal NHS Foundation Trust, Salford, UK

Marie Hudson, M.D., MPH. Department of Medicine, McGill University & Lady Davis Institute of Medical Research of Jewish General Hospital, Montreal, QC, Canada

Marc Humbert, M.D., Ph.D. Department of Respiratory Medicine, Antoine Béclère, Assistance Publique, Hôpitaux de Paris, Clamart, France

Lisa R. Jewett, B.A. Department of Psychiatry, McGill University & Lady Davis Institute of Medical Research of Jewish General Hospital, Montreal, QC, Canada

André Kahan, M.D., Ph.D. Paris Descartes University, Department of Rheumatology A, Hôpital Cochin, Paris, France

Jonathan Kay, M.D. Rheumatology Division, Department of Medicine, UMass Memorial Medical Center, University of Massachusetts Medical School, Worcester, MA, USA

Dinesh Khanna, M.D., M.S. University of Michigan, Ann Arbor, MI, USA

Puja P. Khanna, M.D., MPH. University of Michigan, Ann Arbor, MI, USA

Krzysztof Kowal, M.D., Ph.D. Department of Allergology and Internal Medicine, Medical University of Bialystok, Bialystok, Poland

Otylia Kowal-Bielecka, M.D., Ph.D. Department of Rheumatology and Internal Medicine, Medical University of Bialystok, Bialystok, Poland

Edward V. Lally, M.D. Department of Medicine, Rhode Island Hospital, The Warren Alpert Medical School of Brown University, Providence, RI, USA

David Launay, M.D., Ph.D. Department of Internal Medicine, Claude-Huriez Hospital, Lille, France

Ronald M. Laxer, M.D.C.M., FRCPC. Division of Rheumatology, Department of Paediatrics, University of Toronto, The Hospital for Sick Children, Toronto, ON, Canada

Jérôme Le Pavec, M.D., Ph.D. Department of Service de Pneumologie, AH-HP, Centre National de Référence de l'Histiocytose Langerhansienne, Hôpital Saint Louis, Paris, France

Jayne Littlejohn, M.D. Department of Rheumatology, Thomas Jefferson University, Philadelphia, PA, USA

Marco Matucci-Cerinic, M.D., Ph.D. Department of Medicine, University of Florence, Azienda Ospedaliero-Universitaria Careggi, Florence, Italy

Maureen D. Mayes, M.D., MPH. Department of Internal Medicine, The University of Texas-Houston Medical School, Rheumatology, Houston, TX, USA

Thomas A. Medsger Jr., M.D. Division of Rheumatology & Clinical Immunology, Department of Medicine, University of Pittsburgh Medical Center, Pittsburgh, PA, USA

Christophe Meune, M.D., Ph.D. Cardiology Department, Paris Descartes University, Cochin Hôpital, APHP, Paris, France

Ulf Müller-Ladner, M.D. Department of Rheumatology & Clinical Immunology, Kerckhoff-Clinic, Justus-Liebig-University Giessen, Bad Nauheim, Germany

Christine O'Brien, M.Sc., B.Sc. Occupational Therapy Department of Rehabilitation Services, The Hospital for Sick Children, Toronto, ON, Canada

Janet L. Poole, Ph.D., O.T.R/L. Department of Occupational Therapy Graduate Program, Pediatrics, University of New Mexico, Albuquerque, NM, USA

Elena Pope, M.D., M.Sc. Section of Dermatology, Department of Paediatrics, The Hospital for Sick Children, Toronto, ON, Canada

Janet Pope, M.D., MPH, FRCPC. Division of Rheumatology, Department of Medicine, St. Joseph's Health Care, Schulich School of Medicine & Dentistry, University of Western Ontario, London, ON, Canada

Francesco Porta, M.D. Azienda Ospedaliero-Universitaria Careggi, Florence, Italy and Department of Medicine, University of Florence, Florence, Italy

Michele C. Ravenel, DMD, MSCR. Department of Stomatology, Medical
University of South Carolina, College of Dental Medicine, Charleston, SC, USA

Elena Schiopu, M.D. Scleroderma Program, Division of Rheumatology,
University of Michigan, Ann Harbor, MI, USA

James R. Seibold, M.D. Division of Rheumatology, University of Connecticut
Health Center, Scleroderma Research Consultants, LLC, Avon, CT, USA

Richard M. Silver, M.D., FACP, FACR. Division of Rheumatology &
Immunology, Department of Medicine, Medical University of South Carolina,
Charleston, SC, USA

Vaneeta Sood, MRC.Ophth, M.B.B.S., B.Sc (Hons). Department of Ophthalmology, Birmingham & Midland Eye Centre, Birmingham, West Midlands, UK

Virginia Steen, M.D. Department of Rheumatology & Clinical Immunology,
Georgetown University, Washington, DC, USA

Rajen Tailor, B.Sc (hons), M.B.B.S., MRCP, MRC.Ophth. Department of
Ophthalmology, Birmingham & Midlands Eye Centre, City Hospital,
Birmingham, West Midlands, UK

Brett D. Thombs, Ph.D. Lady Davis Institute for Medical Research,
Jewish General Hospital, Montreal, QC, Canada

Gabriele Valentini, M.D. Dipartimento di Internistica Clinica e Sperimentale
"F Magrassi-A. Lanzara" – Rheumatology Unit, Second University of Naples,
Naples, Italy

Frank H.J. van den Hoogen, M.D., Ph.D. Rheumatology Centre,
Sint Maartensklinick Nijmegen (Hospital), Nijmegen, Gelderland,
The Netherlands

Cecília Varjú, M.D., Ph.D. Department of Rheumatology and Immunology,
University of Pécs, Medical Center, Pécs, Hungary

Fredrick M. Wigley, M.D. Department of Medicine, Division of Rheumatology,
Johns Hopkins University School of Medicine, Baltimore, MD, USA

Peter K. Wung, M.D., MHS. Department of Medicine, Johns Hopkins Medical
Institutions, Lutherville, MD, USA

Hélène Zephir, M.D., Ph.D. Department of Neurology, Roger-Salengro Hospital,
Lille, France

Chapter 1
A 35-Year-Old Woman with Puffy Hands, Raynaud's Phenomenon, and Positive Antinuclear Antibody Test

Richard M. Silver

Keywords Limited cutaneous systemic sclerosis • Sclerodactyly • Telangiectasias • ANA • Nailfold capillary morphology • Raynaud's phenomenon

Case Study

A 35-year-old woman presented with a 6-month history of bilateral hand stiffness and swelling. Initially she noted puffy hands with paresthesia of all fingers except the fifth, and she was frequently awakened from sleep with bilateral hand pain. She underwent carpal tunnel release with improvement of paresthesia; however, she continued to have puffy, stiff hands, and lost ability to make a full fist.

The patient had a 15-year history of Raynaud's phenomenon with blanching and cyanosis of the fingertips on cold exposure, and recalls having been told a blood test for antinuclear antibody (ANA) had tested positive. In the beginning her cold-induced vasospasm caused few problems but as the years went by digital ischemia became more pronounced and she began to develop painful sores on several finger-pads. These digital lesions were slow to heal, and at times white chalky material would extrude from the ulcers. She also complained of dysphagia and heartburn and was found on barium swallow to have esophageal dysmotility with gastroesophageal reflux. Her primary care provider prescribed proton-pump inhibitor therapy which improved her gastrointestinal symptoms. When serological studies confirmed a positive ANA, she was referred to a rheumatologist.

R.M. Silver
Division of Rheumatology & Immunology, Department of Medicine,
Medical University of South Carolina, 96 Jonathan Lucas Street,
Suite 912, Charleston, SC 29425, USA

R.M. Silver and C.P. Denton (eds.), *Case Studies in Systemic Sclerosis*,
DOI: 10.1007/978-0-85729-641-2_1, © Springer-Verlag London Limited 2011

Physical Examination

Temperature 36.6°C; pulse 80 bpm; respirations 14 per min; blood pressure 120/80 mmHg. Skin: puffy fingers with loss of skin creases over dorsum of distal fingers; shallow digital pitted scars on several fingerpads, some with ulceration and chalky white exudate; periungual erythema and telangiectasias on fingers, hands and face; normal skin texture of the proximal arms and legs, chest, and abdomen. HEENT: perioral skin furrowing with reduced oral aperture. Chest: no adventitial breath sounds. Cardiac: regular rate and rhythm with normal S1 and S2 heart sounds. Abdomen: nondistended and nontender. Extremities: no edema. Neurologic: negative Tinel's sign over both wrists. Musculoskeletal: mild flexion contractures of the fingers with inability to flatten hand; no joint tenderness or swelling. Firm, nontender subcutaneous nodules overlying each elbow. Nailfold capillary microscopy revealed dilated capillary loops with few capillary hemorrhages and rare capillary dropout.

Laboratory Findings

Complete blood count (CBC), serum chemistry panel, and urinalysis: normal. ANA by IIF positive (titer 1:1280; centromere pattern). Hand radiographs: focal, dense well-defined calcifications in the soft tissues of multiple distal fingertips; no joint erosions. Chest radiograph: clear lung fields, and normal cardiac size. PFTs: FVC 2.10 L (80% predicted); FEV1 1.76 L (89% predicted); DLco 14.5 (70% predicted). Echocardiogram: normal LV ejection fraction, normal RA and RV dimensions, no tricuspid regurgitation present so estimate of RVSP not possible.

Course

A diagnosis of limited cutaneous systemic sclerosis (lSSc) was made based on the following clinical and laboratory findings: Raynaud's phenomenon with digital pitted scars, sclerodactyly, telangiectasias, calcinosis, and esophageal dysmotility. Also supporting the diagnosis was the positive ANA with a centromere pattern and the "slow" pattern on nailfold capillary microscopy. Baseline investigation revealed no evidence for lung involvement; that is, there was nothing to suggest interstitial lung disease or pulmonary arterial hypertension. Raynaud's phenomenon was managed with calcium-channel blocker therapy and cold avoidance. Proton pump inhibitor therapy was continued to manage gastroesophageal reflux. Physical therapy hand exercises were prescribed. Annual assessment including pulmonary function tests and echocardiogram with Doppler flow study was recommended.

Table 1.1 Preliminary criteria for classification of systemic sclerosis (scleroderma)

A. Major criterion

    Proximal scleroderma: Symmetric thickening, tightening, and induration of the skin of the fingers and the skin proximal to the metacarpophalangeal or metatarsophalangeal joints. The changes may affect the entire extremity, face, neck, and trunk (thorax and abdomen)

B. Minor criteria

    1. Sclerodactyly: Above-indicated skin changes limited to fingers

    2. Digital pitting scars or loss of substance from the finger pad: Depressed areas: At tips of fingers or loss of digital pad tissue as a result of ischemia

    3. Bibasilar pulmonary fibrosis: Bilateral reticular pattern of linear or lineonodular densities most pronounced in basilar portions of the lungs on standard chest roentgenogram; may assume appearance of diffuse mottling or "honeycomb lung." These changes should not be attributable to primary lung disease

(Reprinted from Masi[2] with permission from John Wiley and Sons Inc)

Discussion

Scleroderma (systemic sclerosis, SSc) is currently classified based on the extent of skin involvement, that is, limited cutaneous SSc versus diffuse cutaneous SSc; the presence of digital pitted scars; and radiographic signs of bibasilar pulmonary fibrosis. Limited cutaneous involvement is defined as skin tightness distal to the elbows and knees, and the face.[1] Diffuse cutaneous involvement is defined as skin tightness of the trunk and/or proximal extremities, as well as more acral areas and the face.[1] The American College of Rheumatology (ACR, formerly American Rheumatism Association) preliminary classification of SSc (Table 1.1), which requires either the major criterion or two of three minor criteria for the classification of SSc, was formulated over three decades ago.[2] Since then its limitations have been noted, particularly the relatively low sensitivity for the diagnosis of limited cutaneous SSc. For example, in the above case study, the criteria for classification would not have been fulfilled for 15 years following the onset of Raynaud's phenomenon with positive ANA. Revised classification criteria are now being considered so that patients with earlier features consistent with SSc would be included. Newer proposals incorporate the use of nailfold capillary microscopy, ACA testing and telangiectasias, as well as the extent of skin involvement, for classification (Table 1.2).[1,3,4]

    Patients such as in the one in this case study, who are classified as having limited cutaneous SSc, often share one or more of the following characteristics: a long history of Raynaud's phenomenon, which usually is the initial symptom and often precedes the onset of other symptoms by years or even decades; induration affecting only distal (acral) and facial skin; dilated capillary loops with little or no dropout observed by nailfold capillary microscopy; ACA being the most frequently detected autoantibody (30–90% depending on the patient population).[5]

    The subset of limited cutaneous SSc was formerly denoted by the acronym *CREST* syndrome, standing for *C*alcinosis, *R*aynaud's phenomenon, *E*sophageal dysmotility, *S*clerodactyly, and *T*elangiectasia. All of the CREST features need not

Table 1.2 Subsets of systemic sclerosis (SSc)

Diffuse cutaneous SSc (dSSc)[a]
- Onset of Raynaud's phenomenon within 1 year of onset of skin changes (puffy or hidebound)
- Truncal and acral skin involvement
- Presence of tendon friction rubs
- Early and significant incidence of interstitial lung disease, oliguric renal failure, diffuse GI disease, and myocardial involvement
- Absence of anticentromere antibodies (ACA)
- Nailfold capillary dilatation and capillary destruction[b]
- Anti-topoisomerase (Scl-70) antibodies (30% of patients)

Limited cutaneous SSc (lSSc)
- Raynaud's phenomenon for years (occasionally decades)
- Skin involvement limited to the hands, face, feet, and forearms (acral) or absent
- A significant late incidence of pulmonary hypertension, with or without interstitial lung disease, trigeminal neuralgia, skin calcifications, telangiectasia
- A high incidence of ACA (70–80%)
- Dilated nailfold capillary loops, usually without capillary dropout

(Reprinted from Leroy et al.[1] with permission from the Journal of Rheumatology Publishing Co.)
[a]Experienced observers note some patients with dSSc who do not develop organ insufficiency and suggest the term chronic dSSc for these patients
[b]Nailfold capillary dilatation and destruction may also be seen in patients with dermatomyositis, overlap syndromes, and undifferentiated connective tissue disease. These syndromes may be considered as part of the spectrum of scleroderma-associated disorders

necessarily be present in a given patient classified as limited cutaneous SSc and, conversely, many patients with diffuse cutaneous SSc often have one or more CREST features.

In the patient who presents with cold-induced digital vasospasm, there are a number of clinical and laboratory features useful for distinguishing primary Raynaud's phenomenon from that associated with SSc. The presence of digital pitted scars, telangiectasias, abnormal nailfold capillary morphology, and/or antinuclear antibodies should lead the clinician to suspect a diagnosis of SSc. Some of these features may precede the onset of skin induration by years or even decades and, in some cases, the skin is apparently spared from induration (systemic sclerosis *sine* sclerosis).

Digital pitted scars are one of the minor criteria for the classification of SSc. These digital pits represent areas of ischemic injury to the distal fingertip (Fig. 1.1). Such digital pitted scars are never seen in subjects with primary Raynaud's phenomenon. The presence of digital pitted scars, even in the absence of skin thickening, should raise concern for the diagnosis of SSc, that is, systemic sclerosis *sine* scleroderma. Digital ulcers may occur at sites of trauma or may manifest solely as a result of the vascular insufficiency, a hallmark of scleroderma. Severe digital ischemia can result in digital ulcers which, in some cases, may progress to gangrene. Treatment of digital ulcers can be challenging and involves protection from cold exposure and trauma, as well as a variety of different vasodilators (discussed in more detail in Chap. 10).

Fig. 1.1 Digital pitted scars on the fingertip (3rd) of a patient with limited cutaneous systemic sclerosis (lSSc)

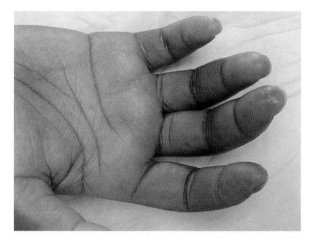

Calcinosis is usually a late manifestation of SSc and is seen more frequently in patients with the limited cutaneous form than in those with diffuse cutaneous SSc. It consists of calcium hydroxyapatite deposits in the fingertips (*calcinosis circumscripta*) (Fig. 1.2); larger deposits in subcutaneous tissues around joints and even in the spine (*tumoral calcinosis*); or sheets of dystrophic calcifications in muscles (*calcinosis universalis*), which usually is seen in patients with an overlap syndrome of SSc with dermatomyositis. Calcinosis most commonly is found over areas of trauma such as the extensor surfaces of the forearms and of the fingers. The calcifications may remain subcutaneous or may ulcerate, drain from the skin surface, and become infected (discussed in more detail in Chap. 27).

Vascular features useful for diagnosing and classifying SSc may be observed at the edge of the nailfold by the use of widefield, low-powered microscopy.[6,7] In normal subjects and in subjects with primary Raynaud's phenomenon, nailfold capillaroscopy reveals a regular disposition of capillary loops (Fig. 1.3a). The presence of microvascular abnormalities such as dilated or giant capillary loops, hemorrhage, loss of capillaries or areas of avascularity strongly suggests the presence of an underlying connective tissue disease, usually SSc. Dilated or giant capillary loops, as seen in this case study, appear as periungual erythema on physical examination and are consistent with limited cutaneous SSc (Fig. 1.3b); in contrast, patients with diffuse cutaneous SSc often will show areas of capillary dropout in addition to dilated capillary loops and cuticular hemorrhage (Fig. 1.3c).

Telangiectasias are dilated capillaries most commonly present on the face (Fig. 1.4), mucosal membranes, chest, and hands. Telangiectasias may also occur in visceral organs, most notably the gastrointestinal tract where they may hemorrhage leading to iron-deficiency anemia.[8] Increased numbers of telangiectases have been shown to be associated with the presence of pulmonary vascular disease.[9]

Although skin involvement is by definition limited in this subset, some degree of internal organ involvement is nearly always present; in some cases, visceral organ diseases may actually be the presenting manifestation of SSc. The most common

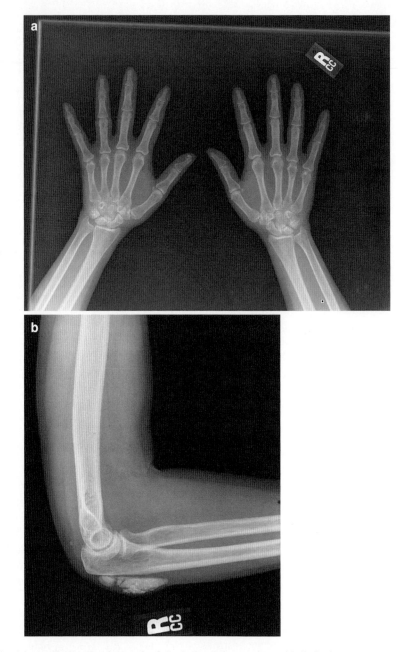

Fig. 1.2 (**a**) Calcinosis of the tuft of the L thumb in a patient with limited cutaneous systemic sclerosis. (**b**) Calcinosis of the olecranon and triceps tendon

Fig. 1.3 Nailfold capillaroscopy using a widefield microscope demonstrating (**a**) normal nailfold capillary morphology, (**b**) "slow" phase capillaries most commonly seen in limited cutaneous systemic sclerosis characterized by capillary dilatation, and (**c**) "active" phase nailfold capillaries typical of diffuse cutaneous systemic sclerosis with capillary dilatation and avascular areas. (This article was published in *Rheumatology*, 4th ed. Hochberg et al. Mosby Elsevier. pp. 1377. © Elsevier 2008)

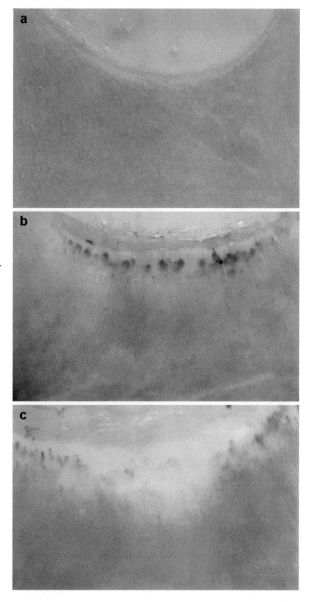

symptoms of visceral organ involvement usually include dysphagia and gastroesophageal reflux and, as the disease progresses, intestinal and anorectal involvement may lead to significant functional impairment with reduced quality of life.[10,11] Even in the absence of symptoms, abnormal gastrointestinal motility is usually present on functional testing. Treatment to prevent or minimize acid reflux should be prescribed in all patients. Dysmotility may lead in some cases to bacterial overgrowth with resultant diarrhea and malabsorption. If suspected, bacterial overgrowth is

Fig. 1.4 Facial telangiectasias. Extensive facial telangiectasias in a female patient with limited cutaneous systemic sclerosis

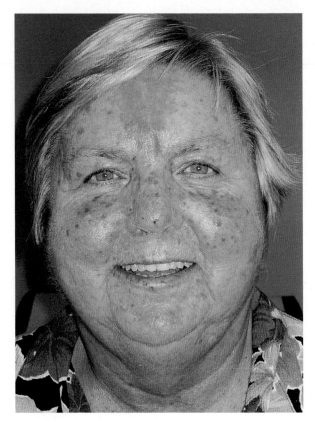

treated with rotating courses of antibiotics and promotility agents (discussed in more detail in Chap. 18).

As opposed to patients who have diffuse cutaneous disease, scleroderma renal crisis rarely occurs in those with limited cutaneous SSc.[12] And, although interstitial lung disease (ILD) occurs less frequently and tends to be less severe than in the diffuse subset, patients with limited cutaneous SSc may develop dyspnea and cough secondary to ILD. Approximately 40% of the subjects fulfilling entry criteria for the Scleroderma Lung Study had limited cutaneous SSc with evidence for significant ILD.[13] Others will experience dyspnea in the absence of ILD. Dyspnea and reduced DLco in a patient with limited cutaneous SSc should raise concern for pulmonary arterial hypertension (PAH), a major complication which requires investigation with echocardiogram and, if strongly suspected, right heart catheterization for definitive confirmation[14] (see Chap. 13).

In summary, one should consider the diagnosis of limited cutaneous systemic sclerosis in any patient who has a history of Raynaud's phenomenon with one or more of the following clinical features: sclerodactyly, digital pitted scars, telangiectasias, calcinosis, antinuclear antibodies (particularly, ACA), abnormal nailfold capillary morphology, and signs or symptoms of internal organ disease. Such patients usually have a slower pace of disease, but various complications, for example, digital ulcers, pulmonary arterial hypertension, and gastrointestinal complications, may contribute to significant morbidity and mortality. Proper diagnosis is essential since early ascertainment of internal organ involvement leads to better outcomes.[15]

References

1. Leroy EC, Medsger TA Jr, et al. Scleroderma (systemic sclerosis): classification, subsets and pathogenesis. *J Rheumatol*. 1988;15:202-205.
2. Masi AT, Subcommittee for Scleroderma Criteria of the American Rheumatism Association Diagnostic and Therapeutic Criteria Committee. Preliminary criteria for the classification of systemic sclerosis (scleroderma). *Arthritis Rheum*. 1980;23:581-590.
3. Maricq HR, Valter I. A working classification of scleroderma spectrum disorders: a proposal and the results of testing on a sample of patients. *Clin Exp Rheumatol*. 2004;22(3 suppl 33):S5-S13.
4. Hudson M, Fritzler MJ, Baron M, Canadian Scleroderma Research Group (CSRG). Systemic sclerosis: establishing diagnostic criteria. *Medicine (Baltimore)*. 2010;89:159-165.
5. Steen VD. Epidemiology and classification of scleroderma. In: Hochberg MC, Silman AJ, Smolen JS, Weinblatt ME, Weisman MH, eds. *Rheumatology*. 4th ed. Amsterdam: Mosby Elsevier; 2008:1361-1368.
6. Gitzelmann MM, Koppensteiner R, Amann-Vesti BR. Predictive value of nailfold capillaroscopy in patients with Raynaud's phenomenon. *Clin Rheumatol*. 2006;25:153-158.
7. Murray AK, Moore TL, Manning JB, Taylor C, Griffiths CE, Herrick AL. Noninvasive imaging techniques in the assessment of scleroderma spectrum disorders. *Arthritis Rheum*. 2009;61:1103-1111.
8. Duchini A, Sessoms SL. Gastrointestinal hemorrhage in patients with systemic sclerosis and CREST syndrome. *Am J Gastroenterol*. 1998;93:1453-1456.
9. Shah AA, Wigley FM, Hummers LK. Telangiectases in scleroderma: a potential clinical marker of pulmonary arterial hypertension. *J Rheumatol*. 2010;37:98-104.
10. Forbes A, Marie I. Gastrointestinal complications: the most frequent internal complications of systemic sclerosis. *Rheumatology (Oxford)*. 2009;48(Suppl 3):iii36-iii39.
11. Franck-Larsson K, Graf W, Rönnblom A. Lower gastrointestinal symptoms and quality of life in patients with systemic sclerosis: a population-based study. *Eur J Gastroenterol Hepatol*. 2009;21:176-182.
12. Sugimoto T, Soumura M, Danno K, et al. Scleroderma renal crisis in a patient with anticentromere antibody-positive limited cutaneous systemic sclerosis. *Mod Rheumatol*. 2006;16:309-311.
13. Tashkin DP, Elashoff R, Clements PJ, et al. Cyclophosphamide versus placebo in scleroderma lung disease. *N Engl J Med*. 2006;354:2655-2666.
14. McLaughlin V, Humbert M, Coghlan G, Nash P, Steen V. Pulmonary arterial hypertension: the most devastating vascular complication of systemic sclerosis. *Rheumatology (Oxford)*. 2009;48(Suppl 3):iii25-iii31.
15. Nihtyanova SI, Tang EC, Coghlan JG, Wells AU, Black CM, Denton CP. Improved survival in systemic sclerosis is associated with better ascertainment of internal organ disease: a retrospective cohort study. *QJM*. 2010;103:109-115.

Chapter 2
A 30-Year-Old Woman with Puffy Hands, Raynaud's Phenomenon, and Carpal Tunnel Syndrome

Christopher P. Denton

Keywords Diffuse scleroderma • Pregnancy • Raynaud's phenomenon • Anti-RNA polymerase autoantibodies

Case Study

A 30-year-old woman presented with a 9-month history of general fatigue, bilateral hand stiffness, and swelling of her fingers that had led her to remove her wedding ring. She had felt tired and generally unwell over the previous 12 months but had attributed this in part to looking after twin baby girls who were born 18 months before her presentation. She had been closely monitored in pregnancy with no hypertension or other complications. Delivery was by elective caesarian section at 36 weeks due to severe pruritus gravidarum that resolved immediately post-partum. She reported pain in the hands and wrists, worse at night, and affecting especially the thumb, index and middle finger. The symptoms were similar to those of carpal tunnel syndrome that she had described in pregnancy and that had been treated with local corticosteroid injection of the wrists. In the 4 weeks prior to presentation she had developed swelling of both ankles, pain in her feet, generalized itching of the skin over her chest wall, abdomen, and upper thighs aggravated by clothing. She described intermittent blanching of her fingers, triggered by going to the refrigerator, that had started 12 weeks prior to presentation. This was similar to her mother's symptoms of Raynaud's phenomenon. She described increased heartburn at night similar to symptoms she had noticed during pregnancy.

C.P. Denton
Professor of Experimental Rheumatology, Centre for Rheumatology,
Royal Free Hospital and UCL Medical School,
Pond Street, Hampstead, London NW3 2QG, UK

R.M. Silver and C.P. Denton (eds.), *Case Studies in Systemic Sclerosis*,
DOI: 10.1007/978-0-85729-641-2_2, © Springer-Verlag London Limited 2011

Physical Examination

Temperature 36.9°C; pulse 60 bpm; respirations 16/min; blood pressure 140/90 mmHg. Skin: puffy hands and wrists with loss of skin creases over dorsum of fingers and periungual pallor. Puffy skin around ankles to mid-calf. Indurated, tight, and diffusely erythematous skin over chest and abdomen, especially around the belt line and inner aspects of both thighs. Scratch marks over lower back. Modified Rodnan skin score was 19/51. HEENT: Mask-like facial features with reduced oral aperture. Chest: fine crackles at left lung base clearing with coughing. Cardiac: regular rate and rhythm with normal S1 and S2 heart sounds. Abdomen: non-distended and non-tender. Extremities: no edema. Neurologic: Tinel's sign negative at each wrist. Musculoskeletal: puffy fingers with inability to completely flatten hand on table; diffuse tenderness and swelling of dorsum of both hands and wrists. Ten-degree limitation of full elbow extension. Tendon-friction rubs were present anteriorly at both knees. She had difficulty sitting up from lying supine on examination table without using her arms. Nailfold capillary microscopy revealed cuticles that were widened and marked capillary loop drop out with three areas of hemorrhage.

Laboratory Findings

CBC: mild microcytic anemia with hemoglobin 10.5 g/dL and MCV 72 fL. Serum chemistry: CK just above normal. CRP: 14 mg/L (normal less than 5 mg/L). Urinalysis: trace of protein and no blood. ANA (antinuclear antibody) positive at 1:640, fine speckled pattern with nucleolar staining. RF and anti-CCP (cyclic citrullinated peptide) antibodies: negative. Hand radiographs: soft tissue swelling around both wrists with no joint erosions. Chest radiograph: clear lung fields and normal cardiac size. PFTs (pulmonary function tests): FVC 2.60 L (82% predicted); FEV1 2.22 L (75% predicted); DLco 12.1 mL/min/mmHg (77% predicted). Echocardiogram: normal LV ejection fraction, normal RA and RV dimensions, tricuspid regurgitant velocity 2.4 m/s with estimate of RVSP 22 mmHg plus RA pressure.

Course

A diagnosis of diffuse cutaneous systemic sclerosis (dSSc) was made based on the presence of proximal scleroderma in the context of new onset Raynaud's phenomenon and positive ANA with nucleolar staining pattern. She was classified to the diffuse subset (dSSc) based upon the involvement of skin proximal to the knees and over her chest and lower abdomen. Additional supportive features typical of dSSc included marked constitutional symptoms, abrupt new onset Raynaud's phenomenon that had developed after other features of the disease, and prominent pruritus and swelling of the lower limbs. Furthermore, she had tendon friction rubs typical of dSSc. She received advice on exercises and skin care and information about her disease together with contact details for patient support groups. Vasodilator therapy was prescribed for Raynaud's phenomenon. She had previously tried nifedipine and had developed a severe headache, so losartan was prescribed. HRCT was normal with no lung fibrosis. She was given advice about regular blood pressure monitoring and planned to buy a machine and check BP three times a week together with attendance for urinalysis monthly. Information about immunosuppression using mycophenolate mofetil (MMF) was provided and it was suggested that she might start this at the next follow-up appointment in 6 weeks. PPI was provided for heartburn and antihistamine prescribed for skin itching. She was advised not to consider becoming pregnant in the near future. Regular assessment including PFTs, initially every 6 months, annual echocardiogram and every 3-month clinical follow-up in the rheumatology clinic was recommended.

Discussion

This case illustrates a typical presentation of the diffuse subtype of systemic sclerosis. Scleroderma (systemic sclerosis, SSc) is currently classified based on the extent of skin involvement. Diffuse cutaneous involvement is defined as skin tightness of the trunk and/or proximal extremities, as well as more acral areas and the face.[1] The American College of Rheumatology (ACR) preliminary classification of SSc (Fig. 2.1)[2] requires only the major criterion for the classification of SSc (see Chap. 1). However, the two subsets, limited and diffuse, of SSc are markedly different in many ways and several cardinal features are illustrated by this case. First, there is objective proximal skin involvement. This is not just proximal to the MCP or MTP joints, which is specified in the ACR preliminary criteria, but also proximal to the knees and elbows, and involves the abdominal and chest wall skin. These proximal territories and truncal changes mandate diffuse cutaneous classification (dSSc). Additional frequent features of dSSc include the prominent constitutional and inflammatory symptoms, diffuse lower limb edema likely reflecting microvascular permeability, and widespread pruritus. Moreover, the onset of Raynaud's phenomenon concurrent with or even slightly after the onset of skin and other features is typical and is a major discriminator from the limited cutaneous subset (lSSc) as described in Chap. 1 Finally, tendon fiction rubs are mostly observed in dSSc and have been associated with the active phase of the disease (see Chap. 28). Carpal tunnel syndrome symptoms are commonly observed early in the course of patients with dSSc and are usually transient. Initiation of immune suppressive therapy is often associated with improvement of median nerve neuropathy; surgery is rarely required although often performed prior to diagnosis of SSc being made.

Features of the major subsets of SSc

dSSc

- 30-40% of cases of SSc
- Truncal or proximal limb skin sclerosis
- MRSS over 18 within 12 months of onset
- Prominent pruritis and inflammatory skin changes
- Raynaud's onset within 12 months of skin changes which may precede vascular symptoms
- Tendon friction rubs common
- High frequency of significant lung fibrosis and high risk of SRC
- Scl-70 and anti-RNA pol III antibodies more frequent

lSSc

- 60-70% of cases of SSc
- Distal limbs face and neck only sites of skin sclerosis
- Low skin score
- Long pre-existing Raynaud's history
- Prominent telangiectasis and calcinosis at diagnosis
- ACA commonest autoantibody but any SSc related reactivity can occur and associated organ based complications risk as in dSSc

Shaded area shows maximal extent of dSSc skin involvement

Shaded area shows maximal extent of lSSc skin involvement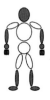

Fig. 2.1 Clinical and laboratory hallmarks of the two major scleroderma subsets. Although subset classification is determined by the extent of skin involvement in SSc, there are clear differences in other clinical and laboratory features between the two major subsets and this means that patients can be robustly classified and this permits a subset-specific approach to management and follow-up. Very early diffuse disease may have a low skin score but other clinical features aid classification of such cases

Differential Diagnosis

The presentation of this case is typical of early diffuse cutaneous SSc (dSSc) and over the first 12 months of the disease a clear pattern of clinical and laboratory features emerges that makes the diagnosis. Earlier in the natural history, matters are much less clear as illustrated in this case. Thus, the later onset of Raynaud's phenomenon symptoms may obscure the diagnosis. Likewise, ANA positivity is often weak initially and may be missed if the defined reactivity is not identified. HEp-2 cell line IIF screening is much more reliable than ELISA methods. Constitutional symptoms of fatigue and musculoskeletal pain can make diagnosis difficult and not infrequently a diagnosis of fibromyalgia or depression may be given in the very early stages of disease. Important differential diagnoses are within the scleroderma spectrum – undifferentiated connective tissue disease, limited cutaneous SSc or overlap syndromes within the scleroderma spectrum such as mixed connective tissue disease. The presence of mildly elevated CK and axial skeletal muscle weakness is typical of dSSc and does not necessarily imply myositis overlap. Weakness that is more generalized with MRC power of less than three out of five or CK more than four times the upper normal laboratory range is used in our unit to define overlap myositis and prompt investigation by EMG and, if clearly abnormal, a muscle biopsy examination (see Chap. 26). It is important to clarify diagnosis if high-dose oral corticosteroid is contemplated due to the risk of renal crisis in the setting of dSSc (see below). Other conditions to consider include generalized morphea, but this would not generally be associated with dyspepsia or acral involvement, and skin changes are typical and spare key sites such as periareolar skin of the breast. In morphea and other forms of localized scleroderma, ANA is present less commonly and Raynaud's phenomenon would only be present coincidentally (see Chap. 4). Diffuse fasciitis with eosinophilia (DFE or eosinophilic fasciitis) could present with the inflammatory and musculoskeletal manifestations, although tendon friction rubs are less likely and limb pain and swelling together with restricted limb movement and a groove sign together with woody texture to forearms would be expected clinically (see Chap. 7). Finally, the hand and wrist symptoms could lead to a diagnosis of inflammatory polyarthritis, for example, rheumatoid arthritis.

Skin Score

The cornerstone of assessment of skin involvement in SSc is the modified Rodnan skin score (MRSS). This was first proposed as a way of quantifying the extent and severity of SSc and is much more applicable to patients with the diffuse subset (dSSc) than to patients with the limited subset (lSSc). In addition, it appears to be most meaningful in the early stages of dSSc when the score has been shown to be associated with outcome and risk of internal organ complications.[3] The MRSS is generally determined by assessing the skin at 17 sites and grading 0–3 based on the assessment of skin thickness, not tethering or tightness. This is important as skin often becomes less thick in later stage disease even though it remains tethered. The maximum skin score is 51 and dSSc usually has a score at diagnosis of at least 15. However, it can be less either because the skin is in evolution and involvement not widespread or because even though many sites are involved it is mild and scores only 1 or 2 in each territory. Skin score has been used as the primary outcome measure in clinical trials and has been useful in demonstrating change in disease severity over time and for the ascertainment of clinically meaningful changes in other disease variables, such as HAQ-DI. As a validated outcome measure the MRSS has limitations, the most important being that improvement can occur spontaneously in a substantial number of cases. This has confounded many clinical trials of drugs studied for the treatment of SSc. Detailed analysis of skin score trajectory in early dSSc has confirmed the poor prognosis for cases that are severe and fail to improve. Immunosuppressive therapy with MTX or oral cyclophosphamide has been demonstrated to improve MRSS compared with placebo, and there are encouraging case series and uncontrolled data emerging for MMF,

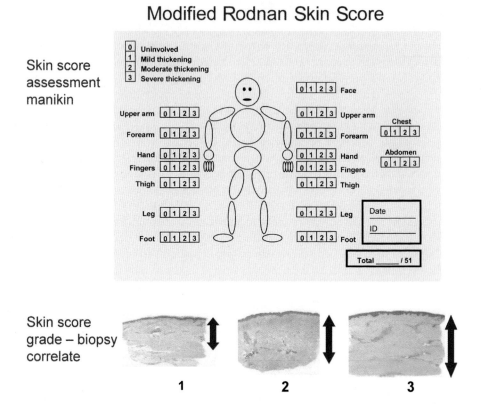

Fig. 2.2 Determination of the 17-site modified Rodnan skin score (MRSS). The most widely used assessment tool for skin sclerosis is the MRSS. Seventeen sites are assessed with a range from 0, defined as normal skin thickness, to 3, defined as severe skin thickening, compared to a healthy individual at each site. Thickness is assessed by palpation and rolling a fold of skin between thumb and forefinger. Assessment can be difficult in established disease when skin may be tethered to deeper structures. Forearm skin biopsy studies confirm that each score reflects different skin thickness (Histology kindly provided by Korsa Khan, Royal Free Hospital)

a drug which has become a first line treatment in early dSSc when there is no major lung fibrosis.[4] Sites of assessment are indicated in the figure below together with histological correlates of each skin grade (Fig. 2.2).

Renal Crisis

There are several features in this case that should raise concern for an increased risk of scleroderma renal crisis (SRC). First, patients with diffuse SSc are much more likely to develop SRC. In addition, the duration of disease, assessed from the first definite non-Raynaud's phenomenon manifestation of SSc, is less than 12 months; over 60% of SRC cases occur within this time frame.[5] Also, this patient has an ANA staining pattern compatible with the presence of anti-RNA polymerase III autoantibody (see below), which is very strongly associated with an increased risk of SRC. Additional risk factors include a history of rapidly worsening skin disease, which is less obvious in this case, and the presence of tendon friction rubs. Of much greater concern is the elevated blood pressure – which could be significantly higher than the expected baseline blood pressure in this case in which there was documentation of low-normal blood pressure throughout her closely monitored twin pregnancy. In addition, trace proteinuria is present although hematuria would be of more concern. Together, these factors make vigilant monitoring of BP the highest priority in this patient with dSSc (see Chap. 19). Home monitoring is advocated and we provide all patients with a warning card containing BP parameters for which emergency medical care must be sought. Corticosteroid therapy should be avoided but if required should be kept below a target of 10 mg prednisolone equivalent per day.[6] There is no evidence that angiotensin converting enzyme inhibitor (ACEi) drugs have value for prophylaxis of SRC, but these are essential treatment for new onset hypertension and full dose therapy should be given if there is sustained hypertension above 130/90 mmHg or 10 mmHg above documented baseline.

Immunosuppression

There is an emerging evidence base to support the use of broad spectrum immunosuppression at diagnosis of dSSc. Our current practice is to treat early dSSc patients with immunosuppression, and MMF is our first choice agent. We have compared outcome with other immunosuppressive strategies in a retrospective cohort analysis from our center[4] and as part of a prospective UK observational study.[7] Alternative approaches include use of cyclophosphamide, which was shown to be superior to placebo in the dSSc cases included in the Scleroderma Lung Study (SLS).[8] Our practice is to consider cyclophosphamide for progressive skin disease (rising MRSS) despite MMF therapy, or if there is lung fibrosis with high risk of progression (see below). MTX can be considered and may be used in cases where there is significant overlap of musculoskeletal inflammation and is used first line in some centers. A second observational study is underway in Europe to compare these different standard treatments for dSSc. In addition, for dSSc with moderate internal organ disease high-dose cyclophosphamide with autologous peripheral stem cell rescue may be considered. This is being compared with intravenous cyclophosphamide in two large clinical trials (ASTIS and SCOT).[9] Data from cohort studies support efficacy for skin disease (see Chap. 34).

Monitoring Lungs

In addition to SRC, another major concern in early dSSc patients is the development of lung fibrosis. In our large cohort, 38% of SSc patients develop significant pulmonary fibrosis at 5 years. Lung fibrosis is common and we recommend a baseline HRCT chest scan to define the extent and severity of parenchymal lung disease in dSSc and in any case of SSc with lung function impairment. There is minor restrictive physiology on PFTs in this case, but lungs are normal on HRCT and so chest wall skin tightness may explain the PFT abnormality (extrinsic restriction). Whenever pulmonary fibrosis is detected we stage disease as mild or extensive using the published UK-RSA staging system that integrates global HRCT evaluation together with FVC (% predicted) with a threshold of 70% defining disease likely to progress provided it is not trivial on HRCT scan.[10] Such patients would be offered therapy with intravenous cyclophosphamide. Lung function should be monitored every 6 months in the initial 3 years and then yearly. HRCT scans are not used for monitoring but may be repeated if there is concern about progression and when PFTs are equivocal.

ANA Pattern

ANA is almost always positive in SSc and is a very important investigation for diagnosis. Many cases of SSc have one of the hallmark scleroderma-specific ANA reactivities for which there exist defined clinical associations summarized in Fig. 2.3. IIF screening with HEp-2 cell substrate is widely used and ELISA is often employed for screening. It should be remembered that important reactivities such as anti-U3RNP or anti-RNA polymerase III are not usually identified using commercial ENA screens. Line blot assays and other new methods are proving more sensitive. In this case, the fine speckled ANA with nucleolar pattern is strongly suggestive of anti-RNA polymerase III reactivity and this was later confirmed by ELISA testing. As reactivities are mutually exclusive, negative anti-topoisomerase 1 (Scl-70) reactivity in this clinical context raises immediate suspicion for the presence of anti-RNA polymerase III antibody which has an 11-fold increased risk for SRC compared to patients without this reactivity. It is, however, associated with overall good survival.[11]

Risk Stratification and Prognosis

There has been a substantial improvement in survival for patients with dSSc over the past 20 years. This is probably a result of better treatment of organ-based disease, and there is clear demonstration of SRC being a less common cause of death. Survival for patients who have pulmonary arterial hypertension (PAH) also seems to be improving. Interestingly, improved survival is associated with greater ascertainment of moderate to severe organ-based disease which suggests that the condition is not being diagnosed in milder forms, that is, improved survival is not attributable to ascertainment bias.[12] In SSc, the subset, stage, and ANA profile can be used to predict outcome. The patient in this case study has features pointing to high risk of SRC. Also, elevated acute phase markers, for example, CRP and ESR, have been associated with worse survival. However, overall 5-year survival at our center is in excess of 90% for patients with dSSc and anti-RNA polymerase III positivity.

Clinical associations of autoantigen specificity for hallmark ANA reactivities in SSc

- Centromere
  - ISSc, isolated PAH, bad gut disease
- Topoisomerase-1
  - interstitial lung disease
  - dSSc, renal crisis
- RNApol I, III
  - renal crisis
  - dSSc
- Fibrillarin
  - pulmonary hypertension, myositis
- PM-Scl
  - Myositis
- Th/To
  - ISSc with respiratory involvement

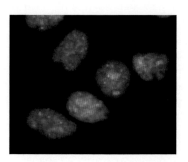

Typical immunofluorescence pattern for anti-RNApolymerase III

Fig. 2.3 Clinical associations of the major scleroderma-associated antinuclear autoantibodies. The majority of systemic sclerosis cases demonstrate a positive ANA and in many cases there is a scleroderma-associated specificity. ANA patterns are generally mutually exclusive when assessed by immunofluorescence. Each pattern is associated with particular clinical features and these associations are helpful for management. The associations are summarized together with representative immunofluorescence staining pattern for anti-RNA polymerase III as demonstrated in the clinical case described (Immunofluorescence image kindly provided by Dr Chris Bunn, Royal Free Hospital)

All cases receive careful education and support from our nursing staff, and patient organizations perform invaluable work supporting patients and their families through a disease that most have never heard of when the diagnosis is made. For the majority of patients with dSSc, the disease reaches a plateau with a fall in skin score and improvement of constitutional and musculoskeletal manifestations within 3–5 years of disease onset. Overall, peak in skin tightening (MRSS) occurs at 18 months in patients with dSSc.[3] Other long-term morbidity such as Raynaud's phenomenon, digital ulcers, and gut disease do not usually plateau or improve. Calcinosis and telangiectasias can be prominent features of late stage dSSc after 5 years.

Importance of Early Diagnosis

There has been much recent interest in early detection and diagnosis of SSc, the concept of pre-scleroderma and very early dSSc. An initiative has been commenced to try to make the diagnosis as early as possible and to collect clinical and biological samples that can be used to better understand the development of SSc. One such study, termed VEDOSS (Very Early Diagnosis of Systemic Sclerosis), is now underway and will underpin future work looking to diagnose and intervene as early as possible in the natural history of scleroderma.[13] However, when SSc starts in earnest with the diffuse pattern of skin involvement there is nothing subtle about the development and progress of the disease. This is a challenging time for the patient, the medical team, and the family. Often the events occur with startling rapidity and this is a very traumatic time when the risk of certain major complications developing are especially high and when there can be rapid and frightening progression of symptoms. This case illustrates many of these points and discusses key aspects about the diagnosis and detection of complications and the general approach to such cases that are fortunately relatively uncommon.

Relationship to Pregnancy

Although the topic of pregnancy in scleroderma is dealt with in detail elsewhere (see Chap. 21), the present case is worthy of more discussion in this respect. First, the patient presented within 2 years of a pregnancy which is not uncommon given the demographic typically affected by SSc, but is outside the window associated with pregnancy-induced SSc (during pregnancy or within 6 months of delivery). Nevertheless, it does give us a clear idea that baseline BP is normal (see above) and is relevant in that further pregnancy within the first 3 years of dSSc is not advisable due to reported association with worsening disease and potential impact of organ-based complications such as cardiac, renal, and pulmonary disease that may develop especially in early stage dSSc. In addition, immunosuppression with MTX, MMF, or cyclophosphamide is contraindicated, and important drugs such as ACEi for hypertension would not be safe for the developing fetus.

Concluding Remarks

This case illustrates that early stage dSSc often presents in quite a nonspecific manner but that typical skin and vascular symptoms together with ANA positivity make diagnosis quite straightforward by the time most cases are seen in referral centers. The goal of VEDOSS and other initiatives is to hasten referral to specialized scleroderma centers. The disease is treatable but vigilant monitoring is the mainstay of management.

References

1. Khanna D, Denton CP. Evidence-based management of rapidly progressing systemic sclerosis. *Best Pract Res Clin Rheumatol.* 2010;24:387-400.
2. LeRoy EC, Black C, Fleischmajer R, et al. Scleroderma (systemic sclerosis): classification, subsets and pathogenesis. *J Rheumatol.* 1988;15(2):202-205.
3. Shand L, Lunt M, Nihtyanova S, et al. Relationship between change in skin score and disease outcome in diffuse cutaneous systemic sclerosis: application of a latent linear trajectory model. *Arthritis Rheum.* 2007;56:2422-2431.
4. Nihtyanova SI, Brough GM, Black CM, Denton CP. Mycophenolate mofetil in diffuse cutaneous systemic sclerosis–a retrospective analysis. *Rheumatology.* 2007;46:442-445.
5. Penn H, Howie AJ, Kingdon EJ, et al. Scleroderma renal crisis: patient characteristics and long-term outcomes. *QJM.* 2007;100:485-494.
6. Steen VD, Medsger TA Jr. Case-control study of corticosteroids and other drugs that either precipitate or protect from the development of scleroderma renal crisis. *Arthritis Rheum.* 1998;41:1613-1619.
7. Herrick AL, Lunt M, Whidby N, et al. Observational study of treatment outcome in early diffuse cutaneous systemic sclerosis. *J Rheumatol.* 2010;37:116-124.
8. Tashkin DP, Elashoff R, Clements PJ, Scleroderma Lung Study Research Group, et al. Effects of 1-year treatment with cyclophosphamide on outcomes at 2 years in scleroderma lung disease. *Am J Respir Crit Care Med.* 2007;176:1026-1034.
9. Nash RA, McSweeney PA, Crofford LJ, et al. High-dose immunosuppressive therapy and autologous hematopoietic cell transplantation for severe systemic sclerosis: long-term follow-up of the US multicenter pilot study. *Blood.* 2007;110(4):1388-1396.
10. Goh NS, Desai SR, Veeraraghavan S, et al. Interstitial lung disease in systemic sclerosis: a simple staging system. *Am J Respir Crit Care Med.* 2008;177:1248-1254.
11. Nihtyanova SI, Denton CP. Autoantibodies as predictive tools in systemic sclerosis. *Nat Rev Rheumatol.* 2010;6:112-116.
12. Nihtyanova SI, Tang EC, Coghlan JG, Wells AU, Black CM, Denton CP. Improved survival in systemic sclerosis is associated with better ascertainment of internal organ disease: a retrospective cohort study. *QJM.* 2010;103:109-115.
13. Matucci-Cerinic M, Allanore Y, Czirják L, et al. The challenge of early systemic sclerosis for the EULAR Scleroderma Trial and Research group (EUSTAR) community. It is time to cut the Gordian knot and develop a prevention or rescue strategy. *Ann Rheum Dis.* 2009;68: 1377-1380.

Chapter 3
A 22-Year-Old Woman with Raynaud's Phenomenon but No Other Symptoms and No Abnormalities on Examination

Ariane L. Herrick

Keywords Primary Raynaud's phenomenon • ANA • Nailfold capillaroscopy • Calcium channel blockers

History

A 22-year-old woman presented with a 5-year history of Raynaud's phenomenon. For as long as she could remember her hands had been sensitive to the cold, but for 5 years her fingers had turned white in the cold then blue, often with a mottled appearance. On rewarming her fingers turned red and were painful. Initially she was not particularly anxious about this, as her mother's fingers also changed color in the cold and she thought it was nothing to worry about. However, she was a keen swimmer and she found that in the cool water of the swimming pool, the Raynaud's phenomenon was becoming a major problem. Sometimes coming out of the pool her hands were so cold that she was no longer able to grip things properly, and on several occasions she had problems turning the key of the locker door. For this reason she sought medical advice.

Otherwise she was well (other than occasional migraine headaches) and during the summer months she had no problems. Her Raynaud's phenomenon had not progressed over the previous 3 years, but she had become more aware of it because of its impact on her leisure activities. Her feet were also affected, but were much less of a problem than her hands. She had had no finger ulcers. Specifically, she denied any history of rashes, mouth ulcers, or sicca symptoms and she had no problems with swallowing and no heartburn. She was a nonsmoker.

A.L. Herrick
Manchester Academic Health Science Centre,
The University of Manchester, Salford Royal NHS Foundation Trust,
Stott Lane, M68HD Salford, UK

R.M. Silver and C.P. Denton (eds.), *Case Studies in Systemic Sclerosis*,
DOI: 10.1007/978-0-85729-641-2_3, © Springer-Verlag London Limited 2011

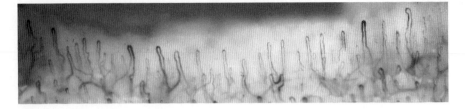

Fig. 3.1 Normal nailfold capillaries. The capillary architecture is normal with no capillary enlargement, loop drop-out, or hemorrhages (×300 magnification)

Her primary care provider prescribed nifedipine 5 mg three times daily, but this caused headaches and so she discontinued this. Because of her ongoing troublesome symptoms, she was referred to a rheumatologist.

Physical Examination

On examination she looked well. Her temperature was 36.5°C. Heart rate 70 bpm, blood pressure 108/74 mmHg. Skin: hands were cool to touch, but were otherwise normal. Specifically, there was no sclerodactyly and no digital pitting, and the nailfold margins looked normal to the naked eye. Cardiac and peripheral vascular: heart rate was regular, heart sounds normal, no edema, all distal pulses easily palpable. Chest: no adventitial breath sounds. Abdomen: soft and non-tender, no masses palpable. Neurological: negative Tinel's sign over both median nerves. Musculoskeletal: no abnormalities.

Laboratory Findings

Complete blood count, erythrocyte sedimentation rate (ESR), biochemical profile and urinalysis: all normal. ANA testing was negative. Chest radiograph: normal, specifically there was no evidence of unilateral or bilateral cervical ribs. Nailfold capillaroscopy (Fig. 3.1) showed normal appearances: capillary architecture was normal with no capillary enlargement, no areas of avascularity and no hemorrhages. The rheumatologist to whom she was referred had a special interest in Raynaud's phenomenon, and thermography was performed (this is available only in some specialist centers). Thermograms at a baseline room temperature of 23°C confirmed that the fingers were cold, but on heating the room to 30°C the fingers rewarmed so that there were no persisting temperature gradients (fingers cooler) along any of the fingers.

Fig. 3.2 Cyanotic fingers in a patient with Raynaud's phenomenon. This is the "blue/purple" (deoxygenation) phase. (Copyright Salford Royal NHS Foundation Trust)

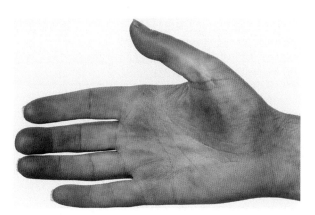

Course

A diagnosis of primary Raynaud's phenomenon (PRP) was made based on the following clinical and laboratory findings: cold-induced vasospasm which was entirely reversible (no evidence of digital ulceration or scarring), strong and symmetrical peripheral pulses, a normal full blood count and ESR, a negative ANA, and normal nailfold capillaroscopy. The fact that the Raynaud's phenomenon had begun in her late teens and had not changed recently was further supportive of the diagnosis of PRP.

She was reassured that she had no serious underlying disease to account for her Raynaud's phenomenon, but that this was primary (idiopathic). Advice was given about keeping warm and minimizing the impact of changes in temperature. Given that her hobby was swimming, her doctor suggested that she ask the pool attendant if she could keep a towel and bathing robe near the pool side, to avoid becoming cold walking to the changing rooms. She was commenced on a sustained release calcium channel blocker, which she tolerated in low dosage and which she found beneficial.

Discussion

Raynaud's is a *phenomenon*: it is not a disease per se but a symptom complex which requires explanation. Essentially it represents an exaggerated vasospastic response to cold or emotion. Classically the digits turn white (ischemia), then blue (deoxygenation) (Fig. 3.2), and then red (reperfusion). Not all patients report the classic triphasic color change. There are several possible causes of Raynaud's phenomenon (Table 3.1), and the key point for the clinician is to separate out primary (idiopathic) Raynaud's phenomenon, which is believed to be purely vasospastic and which does

Table 3.1 "Causes" of Raynaud's phenomenon

Idiopathic (primary Raynaud's phenomenon)
Connective tissue disease (especially systemic sclerosis [SSc]-spectrum disorders)
Hand-arm-vibration syndrome
Extrinsic vascular compression (e.g., cervical rib)
"Intravascular" causes (e.g., paraproteinemia, polycythemia)
Endocrine causes (e.g., hypothyroidism)
Chemicals and drugs (e.g., polyvinyl chloride, beta blockers)

not progress to irreversible tissue injury, from secondary Raynaud's phenomenon associated with some underlying condition/disease which may require specific treatment. Conditions associated with Raynaud's phenomenon include connective tissue disease (most characteristically systemic sclerosis [SSc]-spectrum disorders), extrinsic vascular compression (as with a cervical rib), hand-arm-vibration syndrome, conditions associated with increased blood viscosity (e.g., paraproteinemias), and certain drugs/chemicals (e.g., beta blockers, polyvinyl chloride).[1,2]

In the past the terminology has been confusing: PRP was previously termed "Raynaud's disease," and secondary Raynaud's phenomenon "Raynaud's syndrome." However, the preferred terms are now "primary Raynaud's phenomenon" and "secondary Raynaud's phenomenon."

PRP is common. Reported prevalence rates of Raynaud's phenomenon vary, reflecting at least, in part, different definitions, with one study reporting prevalence in France as high as 20% in females and 14% in males.[3] Young women are most commonly affected by PRP, and prevalence is increased in family members.[4] Probably the mother of the case described above also had PRP. Allen and Brown in 1932[5] discussed criteria for what was then termed "Raynaud's disease," and more recently LeRoy and Medsger[6] proposed the prerequisites for Raynaud's phenomenon to be primary: there should be no clinical features of any underlying connective tissue disease or of any other condition associated with Raynaud's phenomenon, the peripheral pulses should be strong and symmetrical, there should be no signs of irreversible tissue injury (digital ulceration, pitting, or gangrene), the ESR should be normal, the ANA negative (titer < 1/100), and the nailfold capillary morphology should be normal. All these criteria are fulfilled in the case described.

Therefore, in approaching such a case, the key points in the history are whether or not there are any features suggestive of underlying connective tissue disease and whether there have been any digital ulcers: if so, then the Raynaud's phenomenon is not primary. When examining the patient, the physician must look for any signs of underlying connective tissue disease, paying special attention to the fingers and face (looking for any skin thickening, digital pitting, telangiectases, or calcinosis – any of which would be suggestive of SSc) and remembering to check for the peripheral pulses. Regarding investigations, anemia, a high ESR, or a positive ANA (titer > 1/100), all raise the suspicion of an underlying connective tissue disease. Especially in those in whom Raynaud's phenomenon is confined to the upper limbs, a chest or thoracic outlet radiograph should be requested to look for a cervical rib.

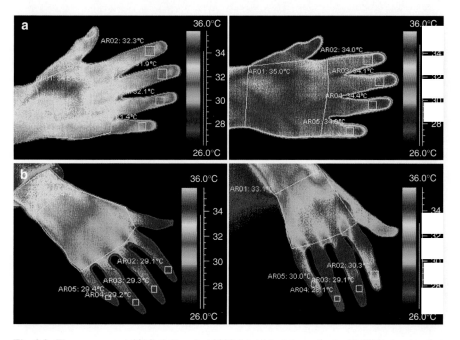

Fig. 3.3 Thermograms at 23°C (*left*) and at 30°C (*right*) in (**a**) a patient with PRP, showing that although the fingertips are very cold at 23°C this gradient normalizes at 30°C, and (**b**) a patient with SSc, in whom the temperature gradient persists even at a room temperature of 30°C

Abnormal nailfold capillaroscopy, reflecting structural microvascular change, is highly predictive of an underlying SSc-spectrum disorder[7,8]: this is reflected in proposed criteria for early SSc which have suggested that Raynaud's phenomenon and abnormal nailfold capillaroscopy are sufficient for the diagnosis.[9] Recent criteria (yet to be validated) proposed by the European League Against Rheumatism (EULAR) Scleroderma Trial and Research Group[10] require one other abnormal clinical or laboratory feature for a diagnosis of early SSc in the patient with Raynaud's and abnormal capillaroscopy. In the case described, the normality of the nailfold capillaries was reassuring. Recently, Koenig et al.[11] have highlighted how in the patient presenting with Raynaud's phenomenon, abnormal nailfold capillaroscopy and SSc-specific autoantibodies are independently predictive of progression to SSc.

The patient described underwent thermography, which measures skin temperature as an indirect measure of blood flow. This is not a routine test in the assessment of Raynaud's phenomenon, but is useful in discriminating between primary and SSc-related Raynaud's phenomenon: if a temperature gradient of greater than 1°C between any fingertip and the dorsum of the hand persists at a room temperature of 30°C (Fig. 3.3), then this is highly predictive of an underlying SSc-spectrum disorder.[12] Several investigators have used the rewarming response after a cold challenge test in the assessment of Raynaud's phenomenon.[13]

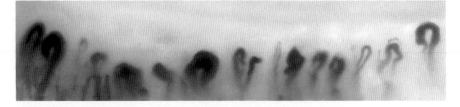

Fig. 3.4 Abnormal, grossly enlarged capillaries in a patient with SSc. Capillary density is lower than in Fig. 3.1 (×300 magnification)

Table 3.2 Drugs used in the treatment of Raynaud's phenomenon

Calcium channel blockers (these are first line, e.g., nifedipine, amlodipine)
Alpha-adrenergic blockers (e.g., prazosin)
Angiotensin converting enzyme inhibitors (seldom used – very little evidence base)
Angiotensin II receptor antagonists (e.g., losartan)
Serotonin reuptake inhibitors (e.g., fluoxetine)
Phosphodiesterase inhibitors (e.g., sildenafil)
Topical nitrate therapy (at present seldom used, can cause both systemic and local vasodilation)
Intravenous prostanoids (e.g., iloprost, epoprostenol: but seldom used in patients with *primary* Raynaud's phenomenon)

A key point is that, contrary to the situation in SSc, PRP does not progress to tissue injury. This most likely reflects the differing pathophysiologies of the two conditions.[14] PRP is thought to be purely vasospastic. In contrast, in SSc, structural vascular abnormalities occur and intravascular factors (including increased platelet activation and oxidative stress) also contribute to pathogenesis. The microvascular structural change of SSc is well demonstrated on nailfold capillaroscopy (Fig. 3.4).

Many patients with PRP do not require drug treatment, but can be effectively managed with "non-drug" treatment. Patient education is a key aspect of management: patients should be advised to minimize the effects of temperature changes by dressing warmly including wearing warm gloves, socks, and hats, and to avoid exposure to cigarette smoke. For those patients whose symptoms remain troublesome and who therefore require drug treatment, calcium channel blockers[15] are usually the first choice, but can cause vasodilatory side effects. Sustained release preparations, such as sustained release nifedipine or amlodipine, are often better tolerated than shorter-acting formulations. There is very little evidence base for other vasodilators, but for those patients who do not respond to calcium channel blockers, or who are intolerant of them, other options are alpha-adrenergic blockers, angiotensin-converting enzyme inhibitors, or angiotensin II receptor antagonists (Table 3.2). Newer treatments are being investigated, including phosphodiesterase inhibitors and topical nitroglycerine.[16]

In summary, most patients with Raynaud's phenomenon have PRP. However, it is always important to consider the possibility of a secondary cause requiring specific treatment, and therefore a careful history should always be taken and a physical examination always performed, supplemented by a small number of investigations (full blood count, ESR, antinuclear antibody, and nailfold capillaroscopy). Many patients are reassured by being told that they have PRP without an underlying disorder, and do not require drug treatment. For those who do, sustained release calcium channel blockers are first line.

References

1. Block JA, Sequeira W. Raynaud's phenomenon. *Lancet*. 2001;357:2042-2048.
2. Wigley FM. Clinical practice: Raynaud's phenomenon. *N Engl J Med*. 2002;347:1001-1008.
3. Maricq HR, Carpertier PH, Weinrich MC, et al. Geographic variation in the prevalence of Raynaud's phenomenon: Charleston, SC, USA, vs Tarentaise, Savoie, France. *J Rheumatol*. 1993;20:70-76.
4. Freedman RR, Mayes MD. Familial aggregation of primary Raynaud's disease. *Arthritis Rheum*. 1996;39:1189-1191.
5. Allen EV, Brown GE. Raynaud's disease: a critical review of minimal requisites for diagnosis. *Am J Med Sci*. 1932;183:187-200.
6. LeRoy EC, Medsger TA. Raynaud's phenomenon: a proposal for classification. *Clin Exp Rheumatol*. 1992;10:485-488.
7. Maricq HR, LeRoy EC. Patterns of finger capillary abnormalities in connective tissue disease by 'wide-field' microscopy. *Arthritis Rheum*. 1973;16:619-628.
8. Herrick AL, Cutolo M. Clinical implications from capillaroscopic analysis in patients with Raynaud's phenomenon and systemic sclerosis. *Arthritis Rheum*. 2010;62:2595-2604.
9. LeRoy EC, Medsger TA. Criteria for the classification of early systemic sclerosis. *J Rheumatol*. 2001;28:1573-1576.
10. Matucci-Cerinic M, Allanore Y, Czirják L, et al. The challenge of early systemic sclerosis for the EULAR Scleroderma Trial and Research Group (EUSTAR) community: it is time to cut the Gordian knot and develop a prevention or rescue strategy. *Ann Rheum Dis*. 2009;68:1377-1380.
11. Koenig M, Joyal F, Fritzler MJ, et al. Autoantibodies and microvascular damage are independent predictive factors for the progression of Raynaud's phenomenon to systemic sclerosis: a twenty-year prospective study of 586 patients, with validation of proposed criteria for early systemic sclerosis. *Arthritis Rheum*. 2008;58:3902-3912.
12. Anderson ME, Moore TL, Lunt M, Herrick AL. The 'distal-dorsal difference': a thermographic parameter by which to differentiate between primary and secondary Raynaud's phenomenon. *Rheumatology*. 2007;46:533-538.
13. Foerster J, Wittstock S, Fleischanderl S, et al. Infrared-monitored cold response in the assessment of Raynaud's phenomenon. *Clin Exp Dermatol*. 2005;31:6-12.
14. Herrick AL. Pathogenesis of Raynaud's phenomenon. *Rheumatology (Oxford)*. 2005;44:587-596.
15. Thompson AE, Pope JE. Calcium channel blockers for primary Raynaud's phenomenon: a meta-analysis. *Rheumatology (Oxford)*. 2005;44:145-150.
16. Chung L, Shapiro L, Fiorentino D, et al. MQX-503, a novel formulation of nitroglycerin, improves the severity of Raynaud's phenomenon. *Arthritis Rheum*. 2009;60:870-877.

Chapter 4
A Young Adult with Localized Skin Sclerosis and Positive ANA

Elke M.G.J. de Jong and Frank H.J. van den Hoogen

Keywords Localized scleroderma • Morphea • Methotrexate • UV-light • Phototherapy

Case Study

A 19-year-old woman presented with a 1-year history of itching erythematous lesions on her right leg. During the past 3 months the lesions gradually increased and became sclerotic and painful. Within the lesions hyperpigmented and hypopigmented areas developed. Initially she was treated with topical corticosteroids, but without success. At the moment of presentation she reported recent extension of the lesions to the right part of the abdomen, the right groin, the right upper and lower leg. She did not report skin thickening of the fingers, nor Raynaud's phenomenon, dyspnea, or dysphagia; she could not recall a tick bite. Several months before she was diagnosed with hypothyroidism. Thyroxine replacement therapy was the only medication she used. Her family history was unremarkable.

Physical Examination

General physical examination showed now abnormalities, especially no sclerodactyly, telangiectasis, nailfold capillary changes on nailfold capillaroscopy, acrocyanosis on cold provocation or pitting scars were present. The flexion of the right hip

F.H.J. van den Hoogen (✉)
Rheumatology Centre, Sint Maartensklinick Nijmegen (Hospital),
Hengstdal 3, P.O. Box 9011, 6500 GM Nijmegen, Gelderland, The Netherlands

R.M. Silver and C.P. Denton (eds.), *Case Studies in Systemic Sclerosis,*
DOI: 10.1007/978-0-85729-641-2_4, © Springer-Verlag London Limited 2011

Fig. 4.1 Hyperpigmented
and partly hypopigmented
sclerotic lesion with
erythematous border on the
right abdomen

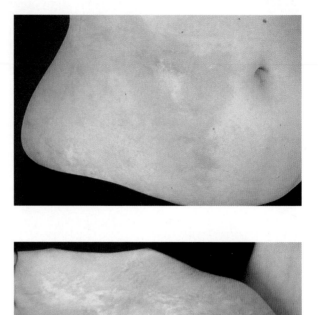

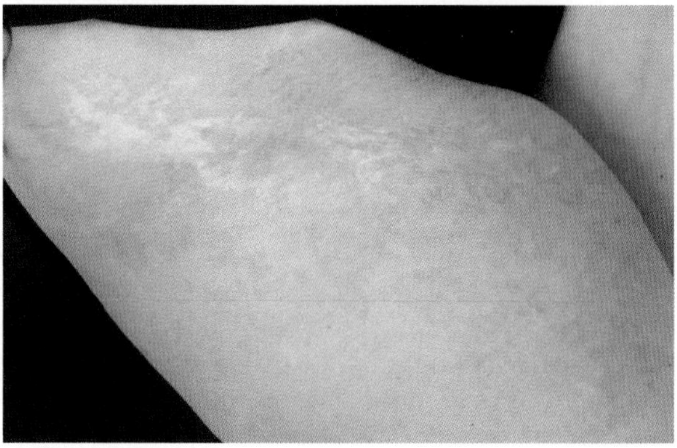

Fig. 4.2 Hyperpigmented
and partly hypopigmented
sclerotic lesions with
erythematous border and a
cobble stone appearance on
the right groin and upper leg

joint, knee, and ankle was slightly reduced. Examination of the skin revealed hyper-pigmented and partly hypopigmented sclerotic lesions with erythematous borders and a cobble stone appearance on the right belly, groin, upper and lower leg (Figs. 4.1 and 4.2).

Laboratory Findings

Complete blood cell count, chemistry panel, and urinalysis were within normal limits. The percentage of eosinophils in the leukocyte differentiat and absolute counts of eosinophils were normal. TSH was within the normal range and serology against *Borrelia burgdorferi* was negative. Antinuclear autoantibodies could be detected on immunofluorescence, with a homogeneous pattern. Further examination revealed no disease-specific autoantibodies. X-rays of chest, pelvis, knees, and ankles showed no abnormalities. A biopsy was performed containing skin, muscle, and muscle fascia of a lesion on the right upper leg.

On histopathologial examination the skin showed a partly normal, partly atrophic epidermis. The dermis was broadened with horizontally oriented collagen bundles and deep lying sweat glands. A sparse inflammatory cell infiltrate consisting of lymphocytes was present. Fibrosis was present deep in the dermal compartment. The muscle fascia showed no inflammation. No eosinophils were present.

Course

A diagnosis of deep linear localized scleroderma, in combination with plaque type morphea, was made. Treatment was initiated with methotrexate in a dosage of 15 mg/week in combination with folic acid 10 mg/week 24 h after methotrexate intake. Topical treatment with emollients was given. Methotrexate was increased to 20 mg/week after 4 weeks. Eight weeks thereafter a clear improvement was seen. After 9 months of treatment, the skin sclerosis had resolved 50% and restriction of mobility of her right hip, knee and ankle was restored to normal. She had mild complaints of nausea the day after ingestion of methotrexate. Methotrexate was reduced to 15 mg weekly. No further reduction of skin sclerosis was achieved in the following year, and methotrexate was discontinued 2 years after installment. Since then, with a 3 year follow-up, no extension of the lesions has been observed.

Discussion

The scleroderma spectrum of diseases is characterized by skin induration and can be divided into three main categories: systemic sclerosis, localized scleroderma, and scleroderma variants. The clinical presentation of localized scleroderma and scleroderma variants differs from systemic sclerosis in skin distribution, the absence of Raynaud's phenomenon, and internal organ involvement. Localized scleroderma, also called morphea, is an uncommon disease, with an incidence of 2.7 per 100,000 population and a prevalence of 2 per 1,000 population.[1] It is more common in females than males (ratio 2.6:1), with the exception of linear scleroderma, which has an equal sex distribution. The mean age at onset for children is 9 years, and for adults 44 years.[2] Based upon 50% resolution of skin softening, the disease has an active phase ranging from 3 (plaque morphea) to 6 years (deep morphea). The typical initial lesion starts with a wide patch of erythema, reflecting inflammation, followed by an induration with a yellowish white shine of the center of the lesion. Later on, an ivory white central area surrounded by a sclerotic hyperpigmented plaque can be seen. A violet ring, often called the lilac ring, borders the colored hardened region. This sclerotic area is usually permanent, but over many years the lesion becomes atrophic, though a depigmented or hyperpigmented area will persist.

Table 4.1 Classification of localized scleroderma

1. Plaque morphea
Guttate
Generalized
Keloidal (nodular)
Atrophoderma of Pasini and Pierini
Overlap with lichen sclerosis (et atrophicans)
2. Bullous morphea
3. Linear morphea
En coup de sabre
Progressive facial hemiatrophy (Parry–Romberg syndrome)
4. Deep morphea
Subcutaneous
Morphea profunda
Disabling pansclerotic morphea

Adapted from Peterson et al.[5]

The etiology of localized scleroderma is unknown. The association of several autoimmune diseases such as type I diabetes mellitus, Hashimoto thyroiditis, vitiligo, systemic lupus erythematosus, psoriasis, and multiple sclerosis with localized scleroderma suggests an autoimmune mechanism. This association is more present in adult patients with generalized morphea. Children with morphea are relatively spared of concomitant autoimmune disease.[2] More support for an autoimmune pathogenesis is derived from the occurrence of autoantibodies. In up to 80% of patients, ANA can be detected, as well as antibodies to single-stranded DNA, histone, fibrillin, mitochondria, and topoisomerase II. Seldom autoantibodies specific for systemic sclerosis (anti-topoisomerase I, anti-centromere, U3RNP) can be found.[3] Morphea has occurred after BCG vaccination and at the site of radiotherapy for breast cancer. Because of a resemblance between morphea and acrodermatitis chronica atrophicans, an association with Lyme disease has been suggested. Additionally, repetitive stress or implantation of silicone transplantation for breast augmentation has been reported as causes for localized scleroderma. Localized scleroderma can be classified according to Chung et al.[4] into four groups with several subtypes (Table 4.1).

Plaque morphea consists of one or more circumscript patches of affected skin. Plaque morphea is the most common subtype of localized scleroderma, comprising more than 50% of cases.[1,4] These patches are mostly located on the trunk. Guttate morphea consists of multiple plaques, less than 10 mm in diameter, usually on the shoulders and chest. Generalized morphea is a confluence of multiple plaques, accounting for 13% of patients with morphea[1] and can progress to involve widespread areas of the body. Keloid or nodular morphea is characterized by indurated plaques, several centimeters in diameter, that resemble post-traumatic scars. Atrophoderma of Pasini and Pierini resembles plaque morphea, but the lesions usually lack inflammation or induration. This subtype usually involves the trunk, especially the buttocks and lower parts of the back. An association between lichen sclerosis (et atrophicans, LSA) and morphea is still in debate. Some consider LSA as pseudoscleroderma. In contrast to morphea, LSA lesions show follicular plugging and a lichenoid infiltrate. Clinically, these lesions are characterized by white, sclerotic plaques. Morphea and lesions of LSA can coexist in one patient.[4] Bullous morphea consists of tense subepidermal bullae that occur in the plaques of morphea. Linear morphea is a single, linear, and unilateral band of skin fibrosis and may extend to the subcutaneous tissue, causing atrophy and sclerosis of subjacent fat, muscle, and bone. This type of morphea accounts for approximately 20% of morphea and is the most common form in children and adolescents.[1] It is usually located on an extremity and causes contractures when crossing a joint. When bone is affected in childhood, a typical radiological cortical hyperostosis of the long bones (called melorheostosis) can be seen. A disturbed bone growth and consequently leg-length discrepancy may be the result. Morphea en coup de sabre is a subtype of linear scleroderma and affects the face and scalp.[5] Progressive facial hemiatrophy or Parry–Romberg syndrome is considered to be a severe outcome of en coup de sabre and affects the subcutis, muscle, and bone of face and scalp resulting in hemifacial atrophy. Ocular complications, such as eyelid retraction or glaucoma, and neurologic complications, such as seizures, oculomotor nerve palsies, uveitis, and dental abnormalities, are more common in progressive facial hemiatrophy than in coup de sabre.[6] Deep morphea involves the deeper layers of the skin and subcutaneous tissues (fascia and muscles). In subcutaneous morphea, the primary site of involvement is the panniculus or subcutaneous tissue. The onset of sclerosis is rapid over a period of several months. In morphea profunda, the skin has a bumpy, depressed surface and sclerosis is present in the septae of the subcuts and the underlying fascia. Disabling pansclerotic morphea is a rare but extremely severe subtype characterized by generalized full-thickness skin involvement of the trunk, extremities, face, and scalp, sparing fingertips and toes. It occurs predominantly in children and causes joint contractures and scarring deformities on the trunk and face.[7]

The diagnosis of linear scleroderma is mainly based on clinical findings. Histopathological examination is sometimes necessary for confirmation or to exclude scleroderma variants. In localized scleroderma, three discriminative histopathological features can be found: mononuclear cell infiltration, increased deposition of collagen in the dermis and subcutis, and vascular changes. The early lesions are characterized by a dense inflammatory cell infiltrate, consisting of lymphocytes, macrophages, some plasma cells, and occasional mast cells and eosinophils.[4] The infiltrate is predominantly present around blood vessels, but also more diffusely throughout the lower dermis and subcutis,[8] most notably at the border of active lesions. The fibrotic phase is characterized by an increased thickened dermis and composed of broad sclerotic collagen bundles. Collagen also replaces fat around the sweat glands and extends into the subcutis. Eccrine glands are often situated at a relatively high level in the dermis due to collagen deposition below them. The vascular changes are thickening of the walls of small blood vessels, thereby narrowing the lumen.

There are no laboratory tests that are specific for localized scleroderma. Laboratory abnormalities that can be detected in patients with morphea are antinuclear antibodies in up to 80%[9], with antihistone specificity. Also rheumatoid factor, antibodies to mitochondria, nucleosome, single-stranded DNA, anti-topoisomerase II[3], polyclonal hypergammaglobulinemia, and eosinophilia may be found.

The course of localized scleroderma is unpredictable. Sometimes progression of deep scleroderma can be seen despite clinical improvement of the superficial layers, leading to substantial loss of function.[10] Treatment is mainly based on findings reported in case reports or pilot studies although some placebo-controlled studies are avaliable.[11] The rarity and different phenotypes of the disease, the difficult evaluation, the possibility of spontaneous resolution of sclerotic skin lesions, and the absence of life-threatening internal organ involvement preclude randomized controlled trials. Treatment is indicated for progressive skin lesions and in linear lesions crossing joints. In early or slowly progressive lesions, treatment can consist of topical application of corticosteroids, calcipotriene, tacrolimus ointment, or imiquimod cream. After some favorable outcomes in uncontrolled studies, topical and oral calcitriol appeared to be ineffective in a double-blind, placebo controlled trial.[12] Reports on antimalarials in the treatment of localized scleroderma are scarce and contradictory. In rapidly progressive lesions, methotrexate, alone or combined with oral corticosteroids, have been advocated.[13,14] In a recent randomized, double-blind placebo-controlled trial in children with localized scleroderma (linear, generalized, or deep subtypes) oral methotrexate (15 mg/m^2, with a maximum of 20 mg/week), for 12 months or until flare of the disease was compared to placebo. Oral prednisone, 1 mg/kg/day, with a maximum of 50 mg/day for 3 months and then tapered down until stopping in 1 month, was added to both groups. After an initial response, methotrexate was superior to placebo in reduction of skin score rate and preventing disease relapse.[15] The use of ultraviolet light (phototherapy) has been reported to be beneficial in the treatment of morphea. Ultraviolet light leads to the induction of collagenases.[16] Several studies demonstrated the initial clinical effectiveness of UVA-1; furthermore, broadband ultraviolet A treatment with or without 8-methoxypsoralen (oral or topical) has also resulted in skin softening in several studies. Most of the studies are uncontrolled and with insufficient numbers to provide solid results. The optimal dose, frequency, and duration of phototherapy need to be further examined.[17]

References

1. Peterson LS, Nelson AM, Su WP, Mason T, O'Fallon WM, Gabriel SE. The epidemiology of morphea (localized scleroderma) in Olmsted County 1960–1993. *J Rheumatol.* 1997;24: 73-80.
2. Leitenberger JJ, Cayce RL, Haley RW, Adams-Huet B, Bergstresser PR, Jacobe HT. Distinct autoimmune syndromes in morphea: a review of 245 adult and pediatric cases. *Arch Dermatol.* 2009;145:545-550.
3. Takehara K, Sato S. localized scleroderma is an autoimmune disorder. *Rheumatology (Oxford).* 2005;44:274-279.

4. Chung L, Lin J, Furst DE, Fiorentino D. Systemic and Localized scleroderma. *Clin Dermatol.* 2006;24:374-392.
5. Petterson LS, Nelson AM, Su WP. Classification of morphea (localized scleroderma). *Mayo Clin Proc.* 1995;70:1068-1076.
6. Appenzeller S, Montenegro MA, Dertkigil SS, et al. Neuroimaging findings in scleroderma en coup de sabre. *Neurology.* 2004;62:585-589.
7. Wollina U, Looks A, Uhlemann C, Wollina K. Pansclerotic morphea of childhood-follow-up over 6 years. *Pediatr Dermatol.* 1999;16:245-247.
8. Torres JE, Sánchez JL. Histopathologic differentiation between localized and systemic scleroderma. *Am J Dermatopathol.* 1998;20:242-245.
9. Sato S, Fujimoto M, Ihn H, Kikuchi K, Takehara K. Antigen specificity of antihistone antibodies in localized scleroderma. *Arch Dermatol.* 1994;130:1273-1277.
10. Voermans NC, Pillen S, de Jong EM, Creemers MC, Lammens M, van Alfen N. Morphea profunda presenting as a neuromuscular mimic. *J Clin Neuromuscul Dis.* 2008;9:407-414.
11. Kroft EB, Groeneveld TJ, Seyger MM, de Jong EM. Efficacy of topical tacrolimus 0.1% in active plaque morphea: randomized, double-blind, emollient-controlled pilot study. *Am J Clin Dermatol.* 2009;10(3):181-187.
12. Hulshof MM, Pavel S, Breedveld FC, Dijkmans BA, Vermeer BJ. Oral calcitriol as a new therapeutic modality for generalized morphea. *Arch Dermatol.* 1994;130:1290-1293.
13. Seyger MM, van den Hoogen FH, de Boo T, de Jong EM. Low-dose methotrexate in the treatment of widespread morphea. *J Am Acad Dermatol.* 1998;39:220-225.
14. Kroft EB, Creemers MC, van den Hoogen FH, Boezeman JB, de Jong EM. Effectiveness, side-effects and period of remission after treatment with methotrexate in localized scleroderma and related sclerotic skin diseases: an inception cohort study. *Br J Dermatol.* 2009;160:1075-1082.
15. Zulian F, Vallongo C, Martini G, et al. Methotrexate in children with juvenile localized scleroderma: a randomized, double-blind, placebo-controlled trial. *Arthritis Rheum.* 2010;62 (Supplement 599).
16. Fisher GJ, Kang S. Phototherapy for scleroderma: biologic rationale, results, and promise. *Curr Opin Rheumatol.* 2002;14:723-726.
17. El-Mofty M, Mostafa W, El-Darouty M, et al. Different low doses of broad-band UVA in the treatment of morphea and systemic sclerosis. *Photodermatol Photoimmunol Photomed.* 2004;20:148-156.

Chapter 5
Localized Scleroderma in a Child

Ronald M. Laxer, Elena Pope, and Christine O'Brien

Keywords Morphea • Localized scleroderma • Methotrexate • Corticosteroids • Childhood

A 13-year-old white girl was referred to the combined Dermatology-Rheumatology-Morphea Clinic at The Hospital for Sick Children with an 8-month history of skin lesions involving her left flank and leg. Its onset was with "scar-like" plaques on the left side of the abdomen, which rapidly spread to the left thigh and down the medial aspect of the left leg. It was described as yellow in color with a purplish border. The patient complained of some dryness with a rough feel to the lesion, local pruritus, and left knee pain. Topical vitamin E cream did not help. The patient had received hepatitis B vaccination 1 month prior to the onset of the illness, but otherwise there was no preceding trauma, infection, or recent travel.

The past medical history was unremarkable. The mother had a history of Raynaud's phenomenon. There was no other family history of rheumatic disease.

The general physical examination was normal. Other than mild joint line tenderness of the left knee, the musculoskeletal examination was normal as well. Skin examination revealed two thickened and white "porcelain" discolored plaques on the left side of the abdomen, approximately 5 cm in diameter, one anterior and the other lateral near the midaxillary line. In addition, there was a large linear lesion extending from the left lateral thigh progressing down the anterior aspect of the leg to the medial aspect of the thigh, which then continued below the knee along the lateral aspect of the leg (Fig. 5.1). It shared similar thickening with the abdominal plaques,

R.M. Laxer (✉)
Division of Rheumatology, Department of Paediatrics,
University of Toronto, The Hospital for Sick Children,
555 University Ave, Toronto, ON, Canada M5G 1X8

R.M. Silver and C.P. Denton (eds.), *Case Studies in Systemic Sclerosis,*
DOI: 10.1007/978-0-85729-641-2_5, © Springer-Verlag London Limited 2011

Fig. 5.1 Pretreatment appearance of a large linear plaque on the left leg, crossing the knee joint with central "porcelain"-like appearance and increased thickening of the skin

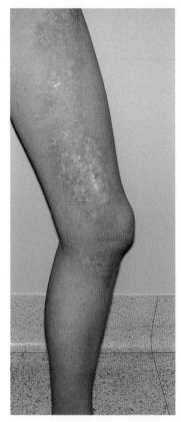

particularly of the upper aspect, but in addition there was a slightly violaceous hue. The range of motion of all joints of the left lower extremity was normal.

The laboratory evaluation revealed a normal complete blood count, differential and erythrocyte sedimentation rate (ESR), and tests for antinuclear antibody and rheumatoid factor were negative. The biopsy of the affected area showed markedly thickened and hyalinized collagen bundles with a scattered infiltrate of lymphocytes within the areas of thickened collagen, compatible with morphea. An ultrasound showed loss of normal echogenicity of the dermis and no differentiation of the two layers of the dermis. The hypodermis appeared normal. An MRI showed a focal linear area of stranding of subcutaneous fat involving the medial aspect of the left thigh, anterior to the sartorius muscle. There was no signal abnormality on T2 or inversion recovery sequences. There was no fasciitis, lipoatrophy, or muscle atrophy.

Given the extent of the morphea, the progression over the preceding few months, and the involvement of the knee joint, it was felt that systemic therapy was indicated. Treatment was started with methotrexate (MTX) 15 mg once weekly and intravenous pulse methylprednisolone (30 mg/kg/day) administered for three consecutive days, 4 weeks apart on three occasions.

Three months later, the patient did not feel that there had been much improvement; however, compared to the first visit's photographs, one could discern that

Fig. 5.2 Post-treatment appearance of the linear limb
morphea with marked hyperpigmentation and softening
of all the previously affected areas

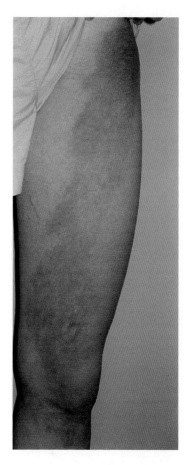

the lesions were less shiny and waxy in appearance and consistency. The borders of
the lesion on her lower extremity appeared less violaceous but the thickening of the
lesion persisted. Muscle bulk and leg length were normal. The dose of MTX was
increased to 20 mg weekly. Three months later, she reported expansion of the lesion
around the left knee and development of new lesions. MTX was changed from the
oral to the subcutaneous route and increased to 25 mg weekly.

Calcipotriene/betamethasone ointment was applied to her abdominal lesions.
Three months later she had hyperpigmentation of the lesions of her abdomen and
lower extremity and the violaceous hue had disappeared. No new lesions were
noted. While she continued to improve, she had two remaining areas of thickening
on her inner thigh. She was prescribed the immunomodulator imiquimod to be used
five times per week on these lesions. Over the next 4 months there was progressive
softening despite the fact that she was not compliant with the imiquimod treatment.
She continued on 25 mg of MTX subcutaneously every week.

After 3 years of treatment, the dose of MTX was tapered by 5 mg every 3 months.
Her morphea remained in remission (Fig. 5.2).

Discussion

Localized scleroderma (LSc), also known as morphea, is an uncommon disorder affecting children as well as adults. Studies from the Mayo Clinic reported an annual age- and sex-adjusted incidence rate of 2.7 per 100,000 population with the prevalence of approximately two per 1,000.[1] This is likely an underestimate, as mild cases may not receive medical attention. In the comprehensive Morphea Clinic at The Hospital for Sick Children, we have seen over 300 patients in a 20-year period. At the same time, we have seen approximately 400 cases of systemic lupus erythematosus (SLE) and 200 cases of juvenile dermatomyositis (JDM).

Localized scleroderma is much more common in the pediatric population than systemic sclerosis (SSc). While "hard skin" is the major feature of both LSc and SSc, the evolution of localized to systemic disease is extremely rare, and patients and families should be reassured that this almost never happens. The mean age of juvenile localized scleroderma is between 7 and 8 years of age. There is often a delay in diagnosis of at least 1 year. Females generally outnumber males by about 2 to 1. No differences are noted in age or gender by the type of onset or the site of the lesion.

The etiology of LSc is not known. Dysregulation of the immune system has been reported in many studies and includes activation of both T and B lymphocytes, with elevation of many serum cytokines and chemokines. Multiple autoantibodies have been found in patients with LSc, but they do not seem to correlate with the subtype of the disease, course, or prognosis. Several authors have suggested that trauma may be an inciting agent. *Borrelia burgdorferi* has been implicated in some cases in Europe and Japan but not in North America. In addition, several cases have been reported following radiation for breast cancer in adults.

Several schemes have been used to classify patients with LSc. The Pediatric Rheumatology European Society (PReS) has recently proposed a new classification for LSc (Table 5.1).[2] Of the various subtypes, linear lesions of the extremity are the most common followed by plaque lesions, facial lesions, and pansclerotic morphea.

Circumscribed or plaque morphea generally begins with oval patches on the trunk (Fig. 5.3). These are firm and indurated in the center with a shiny, waxy appearance, and may be superficial only or deep, involving fascia and even muscle. The border may be erythematous or violaceous.

Generalized morphea involves four or more individual plaques, larger than 3 cm, occurring in at least two separate anatomic sites (head-neck, right or left upper or lower limbs, anterior or posterior trunk).

Linear lesions may occur on an extremity or on the face/head, and are the most common subtype in most pediatric series. Extremity lesions are usually unilateral and typically present as a thickened band that may cross the flexor or extensor surface of joints. (Figs. 5.4 and 5.5) With time these lesions may impair joint movement due to tightening of the tissues around the joint. Joint contracture, loss of muscle bulk, and limb shortening are potential complications.

Table 5.1 Preliminary proposed classification of juvenile localized scleroderma (Consensus conference, Padua (Italy), 2004)

Main group	Subtype	Description
1. Circumscribed morphea	(a) Superficial	Oval or round circumscribed areas of induration limited to epidermis and dermis, often with altered pigmentation and violaceous, erythematous halo (lilac ring). They can be single or multiple
	(b) Deep	Oval or round circumscribed deep induration of the skin involving subcutaneous tissue extending to fascia and may involve underlying muscle. The lesions can be single or multiple
		Sometimes the primary site of involvement is in the subcutaneous tissue without involvement of the skin
2. Linear scleroderma	(a) Trunk/limbs	Linear induration involving dermis, subcutaneous tissue and, sometimes, muscle and underlying bone and affecting the limbs and/or the trunk
	(b) Head	En coup de sabre (ECDS). Linear induration that affects the face and/or the scalp and sometimes involves muscle and underlying bone
		Parry–Romberg or Progressive Hemifacial Atrophy. Loss of tissue on one side of the face that may involve dermis, subcutaneous tissue, muscle, and bone. The skin is mobile
3. Generalized morphea		Induration of the skin starting as individual plaques (4 or more and larger than 3 cm) that become confluent and involve at least 2 out of seven anatomic sites (head-neck, right upper extremity, left upper extremity, right lower extremity, left lower extremity, anterior trunk, posterior trunk)
4. Pansclerotic morphea		Circumferential involvement of limb(s) affecting the skin, subcutaneous tissue, muscle, and bone. The lesion may also involve other areas of the body without internal organs involvement
5. Mixed morphea		Combination of two or more of the previous subtypes. The order of the concomitant subtypes, specified in brackets, will follow their predominant representation in the individual patient (i.e., Mixed [linear-circumscribed])

Associated conditions: Lichen Sclerosus et Atrophicus (LSA) and Atrophoderma of Pasini and Pierini (APP) can be associated to the previous subtypes but are not included in the above classification

Reprinted from Laxer and Zulian.[2] with permission from Lippincott Williams & Wilkins

Fig. 5.3 Plaque morphea on the abdomen: central white discoloration corresponding to areas of "bound down" skin and violaceous borders

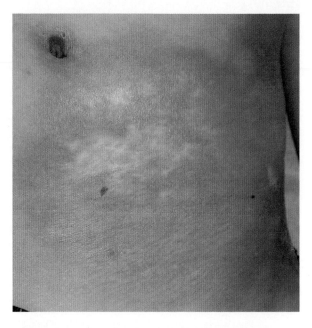

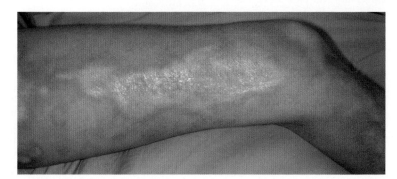

Fig. 5.4 Linear limb morphea: active lesion with central thickening, discoloration, and violaceous border

When lesions occur on the face and head they may take one of two forms: en coup de sabre lesions (ECDS) or Parry–Romberg Syndrome (also known as Progressive Hemifacial Atrophy). These appear to be two ends of a spectrum and often coexist in the same patient. ECDS lesions typically occur on the forehead (Fig. 5.6) and may extend into the scalp and cross the eye to the nose. When they involve the scalp they cause scarring alopecia. They are usually just off to the center of the midline and there may be a second accompanying lesion nearby giving the appearance of an inverted "V". The ECDS lesions are generally not as thick as other morphea lesions and may present only with a depression resulting from tissue loss. This may extend all the way to the skull and be felt as a bony ridge. Lesions can cross the

Fig. 5.5 Linear morphea of the hand: thickened band resulting in significant atrophy of the finger, dyspigmentation, and contracture

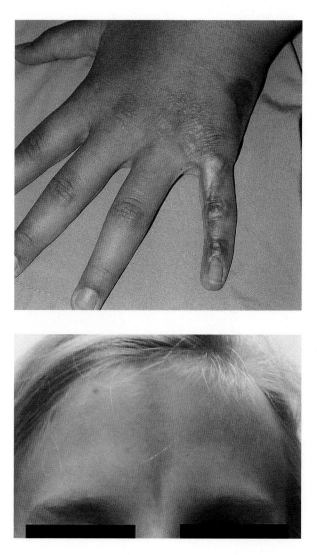

Fig. 5.6 En coup de sabre (ECDS) morphea: linear plaque on the middle of the forehead extending to the nose; marked depression, skin hyperpigmentation

eye and result in loss of hair on the eyebrow and eyelashes. Rarely, uveitis is found in these patients.

Occasionally, these lesions are associated with seizures, although the seizure focus may not correspond to the overlying skin lesions. CT and MRI scans of the brain may show changes in both affected and unaffected patients; as a result, we have not been doing them routinely but only in patients with central nervous system signs and/or symptoms. Abnormalities include small areas of calcification, T2 hyperintense lesions primarily in the subcortical white matter, and areas of brain atrophy.[3]

Parry–Romberg Syndrome presents with marked subcutaneous and deeper tissue (muscle, bone) atrophy, with no epidermal skin changes (Fig. 5.7). It involves the tissues below the forehead, but may occur concomitantly with ECDS lesions.

Fig. 5.7 Parry–Romberg syndrome: marked atrophy of the left side of the face with distortion of the facial contours, minimal superficial skin changes, and hyperpigmentation

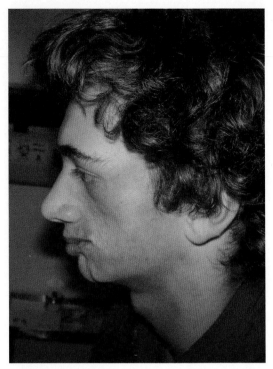

Associated features include ipsilateral atrophy of the tongue and hard palate. Even if the disease becomes inactive, significant asymmetry develops over time as the growth of the affected side is less than the normal side. This asymmetry leads to perceived "disease progression" and can pose clinical and therapeutic dilemmas.

Pansclerotic morphea is the least common but most severe subtype; typically there is extensive generalized full thickness involvement to bone, sparing only the digits. It is the most resistant to treatment. Squamous cell carcinoma has been reported, particularly in lesions that ulcerate.

Mixed lesions occur in up to 25% of patients and usually consist of plaques and linear lesions.[4] It is uncommon for patients with facial morphea to have lesions on the body as well.

Lesions may be warm to touch and may cause mild pruritus. Occasionally, patients present with marked tissue atrophy. If it is not treated early, growth discrepancies will occur with limb shortening and loss of fat and muscle mass.

Extracutaneous signs and symptoms (Table 5.2) occur in about 20–40% of patients.[5,6] Arthritis is the most common, and does not necessarily occur in the region of the LSc skin involvement. Neurologic involvement, including seizures and headache, is the next most frequent (seen almost exclusively in patients with facial lesions), followed by gastrointestinal abnormalities.

Congenital morphea is a rare condition which is often not diagnosed until several years of age. Facial lesions appear to be the most common and may be mistaken as capillary hemangiomas.[7]

Table 5.2 Major extracutaneous signs and symptoms in localized scleroderma

Arthritis/arthralgia
Neurologic
  Seizure
  Headaches
Other autoimmune conditions
Vascular
  Raynaud's phenomenon
  Vasculitis
  Deep vein thrombosis
Ocular
  Uveitis
  Lid atrophy
  Loss of eyebrows/eyelashes
Gastroesophageal reflux
Respiratory
  Cough
  Dyspnea

There is an increased incidence of rheumatic and/or autoimmune diseases in family members of patients with localized scleroderma. In one study, the prevalence of a positive family history was higher in patients with generalized morphea than with other subtypes.[4] In decreasing order of frequency, affected family members had rheumatoid arthritis, systemic sclerosis, and systemic lupus erythematosus of the rheumatic diseases. Psoriasis, vitiligo, and lichen sclerosis et atrophicus were also seen in family members.

There are no definitive tests that can make a diagnosis of LSc. There may be mild signs of systemic inflammation documented by an increase in the ESR, CRP, and serum immunoglobulin levels. Deeper lesions that extend to muscle occasionally present with elevations in the serum levels of muscle enzymes.

Skin biopsies should be performed if the diagnosis is in doubt. However, experienced clinicians can often make the diagnosis without a biopsy, based on the characteristic skin lesions and site of involvement. The characteristic histological features of localized scleroderma vary somewhat depending on the stage of the lesion. Early lesions are characterized by an intense cellular infiltrate consisting of lymphocytes, plasma cells, eosinophils, macrophages, and mast cells with an increase in collagen deposition. In later phase, the collagen thickens further and there is loss of rete pegs and hair follicles.

One of the many challenges has been how to determine disease activity and progression (Table 5.3). Signs of activity have generally been accepted to be warmth of the lesion and surrounding erythema or violaceous discoloration. An increase in size of the existing lesions and development of new lesions clearly suggests that the disease is active. However, lesions change very slowly over time making it difficult to assess changes from visit to visit and even short-term response to treatment. Some laboratory tests may reflect a degree of systemic inflammation and some, but not all, authors feel that an elevated ESR, eosinophil count, serum immunoglobulin

Table 5.3 Characteristic cutaneous features in different phases of localized scleroderma

Active	Chronic
• Smooth, shiny, waxy appearance	• Hyperpigmentation
• Surrounding erythema/violaceous discoloration	• Hypopigmentation
• Warmth	• Cutaneous/subcutaneous atrophy
• Thickening/induration	• No expansion (except for change related to growth)
• Expanding over time (not growth related)	• No new lesions
• Appearance of new lesions over time	

levels, and creatine phosphokinase (CPK) indicate ongoing disease activity. Nevertheless, many patients have completely normal lab results despite clinical signs of disease activity and progression over time.

As a result, both composite clinical and investigative measures have been developed to determine disease activity. The Localized Scleroderma Severity Index (LoSSI) measures surface area, skin thickness, erythema, and new lesion/extension, and has been found to be reliable and valid for assessing disease severity, showing high sensitivity to detect change over time, as did a Physician Global Assessment of disease activity.[8]

Infrared thermography measures the temperature of skin lesions, and while there is a high sensitivity, the specificity is low, likely due to atrophy in some of the lesions such that the blood flow may actually be closer to the surface. Laser Doppler flow and imaging studies may be more accurate than thermography.[9] Zulian and colleagues have developed a computerized skin score in which the ratio of the size of the lesion to the size of the limb is compared to the contralateral normal side.[10] Unfortunately, these are not routinely available in most centers. Clinical photographs may be helpful, but require technical expertise with identical lighting and surface markers to be able to compare the progress of the lesion over time.

Recently, high-frequency ultrasound using 8–15 MHz probes has been studied, suggesting that altered levels of echogenicity and vascularity may be associated with disease activity. Attempts to standardize techniques and interpretation and determine the validity and reliability are underway.[11]

The treatment of localized scleroderma depends on the extent of the disease and stage in the process, that is, whether or not the disease is still active. In addition, patients and parents must weigh the potential risks of treatment to the potential benefits that might be gained from halting the disease process. It is important to remember that the atrophy caused by the disease will rarely resolve, and that an area affected by atrophy may not grow to the same extent as the unaffected side. Similarly, skin dyspigmentation, particularly hyperpigmentation, will persist over time.

Supportive treatment measures are important. If joints are involved, appropriate physical and occupational therapy measures should be instituted to preserve range of motion and muscle strength. Patients with facial morphea may require specific counseling related to self-esteem. Cover-up make-up may be helpful in "camouflaging" some facial lesions. Timely consultation with a craniofacial surgeon should be considered for patients with facial lesions. Ophthalmology consultation is necessary to exclude asymptomatic anterior uveitis in patients with facial LSc, at least at the time of diagnosis and then annually.

While a number of both topical and systemic treatments have been reported to be effective, the lack of randomized controlled trials (RCTs) makes it difficult to make definitive treatment recommendations. In fact, the only two RCTs that have been published failed to demonstrate benefit (gamma interferon and systemic vitamin D3). Nevertheless, there is general consensus, based upon years of experience, that certain treatments are effective. Fortunately, many efforts are currently underway to better define treatment protocols and outcomes.

Topical treatments can be considered for plaque morphea that is active. Agents reported to be effective in uncontrolled studies include potent corticosteroids, calcipotriene, and the combination of the two. Recently, both topical tacrolimus[12] and the immune response modifier imiquimod have been demonstrated to soften indurated lesions.[13]

Indications for systemic treatment usually include the development of new lesions and progressive lesions that may cause functional or cosmetic complications. Thus, facial lesions and linear lesions that cross joints usually require systemic treatment. A survey conducted by the Childhood Arthritis and Rheumatology Research Alliance (CARRA) reported that most pediatric rheumatologists in North America treat localized scleroderma with a combination of MTX and corticosteroids.[14] Ultraviolet (UV) light therapy has also been reported to be effective and is used more often in Europe with adults. Although most studies have used UV-A treatment, UV-B has also shown benefit. These have been studied with and without psoralen and may be an alternative for patients who are not willing to take systemic treatment or who have side effects.[15] Long-term implications from light therapy in the pediatric population are unknown.

Several protocols have been reported that included MTX and corticosteroids.[16-19] Steroids may be given intravenously or orally, but generally are used only for the first few months to provide bridging treatment until the MTX may begin to take effect. Several different regimes of MTX have been reported as well with dosages ranging from 0.3 mg/kg per week up to 1 mg/kg per week (10–15 mg/m^2), usually up to a maximum of about 25 mg per week. Corticosteroids have been administered on a daily basis starting at 1–2 mg/kg, tapering over 3–6 months, or intravenously at 30 mg/kg per dose (maximum 1 g), ranging from daily, for three consecutive days, every 4 weeks for 3 months to one dose per week for several weeks. While the studies have been retrospective, over 90% of patients demonstrated a clinical response, for example, slowing the progress of the lesions and skin softening. Improvement is usually noticed by about 3 months and persists while patients remain on MTX. However, there is significant relapse rate after stopping, which may be as high as 30% (Pope et al., manuscript submitted). This suggests that treatment should be continued for at least 1 year after full clinical remission defined as softening of previously indurated lesions, absence of an erythematous/violaceous border, no progression of existing lesions, and no new lesion development.

Mycophenolate mofetil has been reported to be effective in a small group of patients who failed treatment with MTX.[20] This may also be the treatment of choice for patients with severe pansclerotic morphea, who have a very poor outcome. Autologous stem cell or allogeneic transplantation may be the only effective treatment for this group of patients.

D-penicillamine had been frequently used in the past although it is not currently in favor. Recently, case reports documenting success have appeared with a number of systemic medications including cyclosporine A,[21] bosentan,[22] infliximab,[23] and imatinib.[24] These might all be necessary in patients with disease unresponsive to methotrexate and MMF, and perhaps early in the treatment course for patients with pansclerotic morphea, where antithymocyte globulin[25] and stem cell transplantation may also need to be considered.

Occasionally, the effects of the LSc are so severe that surgical correction may be indicated. A variety of techniques for facial cosmetic and reconstructive surgery have been attempted. Short-term results suggest a good outcome and patients are generally satisfied.[26]

The quality of life of patients with LSc has been addressed only briefly. Patients have reported generally good self-esteem, and the overall health-related quality of life (HRQoL) seemed to be similar to a control group of healthy unaffected children. However, relatively few patients with facial morphea were included in these studies, and it is possible that this is the most affected subgroup in terms of HRQoL.[27,28]

References

1. Peterson LS, Nelson AM, Su WPD, Mason T, O'Fallon WM, Gabriel SE. The epidemiology of morphea (localized scleroderma) in Olmsted County 1960–1993. *J Rheumatol*. 1997;24: 73-80.
2. Laxer RM, Zulian F. Localized scleroderma. *Curr Opin Rheumatol*. 2006;18:606-613.
3. Kister I, Inglese M, Laxer RM, Herbert J. Neurologic manifestations of localized scleroderma: a case report and literature review. *Neurology*. 2008;71:1538-1545.
4. Zulian F, Athreya BH, Laxer R, et al. Juvenile localized scleroderma: clinical and epidemiological features in 750 children. An international study. *Rheumatology*. 2006;45:614-620.
5. Zulian F, Vallongo C, Woo P, et al. Localized scleroderma in childhood is not just a skin disease. *Arthritis Rheum*. 2005;52:2873-2881.
6. Christen-Zaech S, Hakim MD, Afsar S, Paller AS. Pediatric morphea (localized scleroderma): review of 136 patients. *J Am Acad Dermatol*. 2008;59:385-396.
7. Zulian F, Vallongo C, Feitosa De Oliverira SK, et al. Congenital localized scleroderma. *J Pediatr*. 2006;149:248-251.
8. Arkachaisri T, Vilaiyuk S, Li Z, et al. The localized scleroderma skin severity index and physician global assessment of disease activity: a work in progress toward development of localized scleroderma outcome measures. *J Rheumatol*. 2009;36:819-829.
9. Weibel L, Howell KJ, Visentin MT, et al. Laser doppler flowmetry for assessing localized scleroderma in children. *Arthritis Rheum*. 2007;56:3489-3495.
10. Zulian F, Meneghesso D, Grisan E, et al. A new computerized method for the assessment of skin lesions in localized scleroderma. *Rheumatology*. 2007;46:856-860.
11. Li SC, Liebling MS, Ramji FG, et al. Sonographic evaluation of pediatric localized scleroderma: preliminary disease assessment measures. *Pediatr Rheumatol online J*. 2010;8:14.

12. Vilela FA, Carneiro S, Ramos-e-Silva M. Treatment of morphea or localized scleroderma: review of the literature. *J Drugs Dermatol*. 2010;9:1213-1219.
13. Laxer RM, Babyn P, Doria A, Pope E. The efficacy of Imiquimod 5% cream in children and adolescents with plaque morphea. *Arthritis Rheum*. 2009;60(Suppl 10):1544.
14. Li SC, Feldman BM, Higgins GC, Haines KA, Punaro MG, O'Neil KM. Treatment of pediatric localized scleroderma: results of a survey of North American pediatric rheumatologists. *J Rheumatol*. 2010;37:175-181.
15. Kreuter A, Hyun J, Stucker M, Sommer A, Altmeyer P, Gambichler T. A randomized controlled study of low-dose UVA1, medium-dose UVA1, and narrowband UVB phototherapy in the treatment of localized scleroderma. *J Am Acad Dermatol*. 2006;54:440-447.
16. Uziel Y, Feldman BM, Krafchik BR, Yeung RSM, Laxer RM. Methotrexate and corticosteroid therapy for pediatric localized scleroderma. *J Pediatr*. 2000;136:91-95.
17. Fitch PG, Rettig P, Burnham JM, et al. Treatment of pediatric localized scleroderma with methotrexate. *J Rheumatol*. 2006;33:609-614.
18. Cox D, O'Regan G, Collins S, Byrne A, Irvine A, Watson R. Juvenile localized scleroderma: a retrospective review of response to systemic treatment. *Ir J Med Sci*. 2008;177:343-346.
19. Weibel L, Sampaio MC, Visentin MT, Howell KJ, Woo P, Harper JI. Evaluation of methotrexate and corticosteroids for the treatment of localized scleroderma (morphea) in children. *Br J Dermatol*. 2006;155:1013-1020.
20. Martini G, Ramanan AV, Falcini F, Girschick H, Goldsmith DP, Zulian F. Successful treatment of severe or methotrexate-resistant juvenile localized scleroderma with mycophenolate mofetil. *Rheumatology (Oxford)*. 2009;48:1410-1413.
21. Crespo MP, Betlloch I, Diaz JM, Costa AL, Nortes IB. Rapid response to cyclosporine and maintenance with methotrexate in linear scleroderma in a young girl. *Pediatr Dermatol*. 2009;26:118-120.
22. Roldan R, Morote G, Castro Mdel C, Miranda MD, Moreno JC, Collantes E. Efficacy of bosentan in treatment of unresponsive cutaneous ulceration in disabling pansclerotic morphea in children. *J Rheumatol*. 2006;33:2538-2540.
23. Diab M, Coloe JR, Magro C, Bechtel MA. Treatment of recalcitrant generalized morphea with infliximab. *Arch Dermatol*. 2010;146:601-604.
24. Moinzadeh P, Krieg T. Imatinib treatment of generalized localized scleroderma (morphea). *J Am Acad Dermatol*. 2010;63:e102-e104.
25. Song P, Gocke C, Wigley FM, Boin F. Resolution of pansclerotic morphea after treatment with antithymocyte globulin. *Nat Rev Rheumatol*. 2009;5:513-516.
26. Palmero ML, Uziel Y, Laxer RM, Forrest CR, Pope E. En coup de sabre scleroderma and Parry-Romberg syndrome in adolescents: surgical options and patient-related outcomes. *J Rheumatol*. 2010;37:2174-2179.
27. Uziel Y, Laxer RM, Krafchik BR, Yeung RS, Feldman BM. Children with morphea have normal self-perception. *J Pediatr*. 2000;137:727-730.
28. Orzechowski NM, Davis DM, Mason TG 3rd, Crowson CS, Reed AM. Health-related quality of life in children and adolescents with juvenile localized scleroderma. *Rheumatology (Oxford)*. 2009;48:670-672.

Chapter 6
An 8-Year-Old Girl with Tight Skin, Digital Ulcers, and Dysphagia

Ivan Foeldvari

Keywords Juvenile-onset systemic sclerosis (jSSc) • Outcome • Prognosis • Treatment

Case Study

Bluish discoloration of the fingers and later of the hands of a young girl was first noted at the age of 5 years. Over time the parents observed a change in texture and tightening of the skin of the fingers, hands, and later of the underarms. At the age of 6 years, a diagnosis of juvenile-onset systemic sclerosis (jSSc) was made at a pediatric rheumatology unit. The patient was noted at that time to be ANA positive (1:640) and to have anti-Scl-70 antibodies. Subsequently, she began to develop problems with swallowing. While growing normally in height, her weight was only at the third percentile. In the winter months she would develop open skin lesions on her fingertips.

She was first seen in consultation at our center at the age of 8 years. By then, she had already been treated with a combination of methotrexate, 10 mg/m² body surface area po weekly, with supplemental folic acid and azathioprine, 1.85 mg/kg body weight daily. Her main clinical issue at the time of the visit was dysphagia with poor weight gain.

There was no relevant family history of connective tissue diseases.

I. Foeldvari
Hamburger Zentrum Fuër Kinder- und Jugendrheumatologie,
Schön Klinik Eilbek, Dehnhaide 120, Hamburg 22081, Germany

R.M. Silver and C.P. Denton (eds.), *Case Studies in Systemic Sclerosis*,
DOI: 10.1007/978-0-85729-641-2_6, © Springer-Verlag London Limited 2011

Fig. 6.1 Hand of child with systemic sclerosis demonstrating shallow digital pitted scars on the second and third fingertips

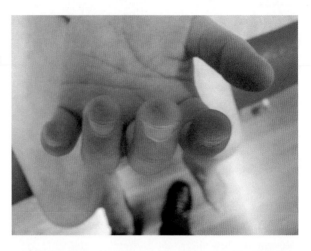

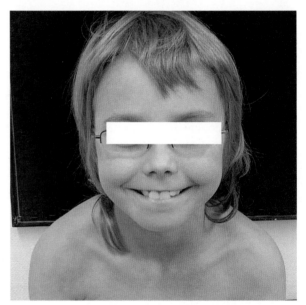

Fig. 6.2 Taut skin on the face of a child with systemic sclerosis

Physical Exam

General appearance was that of an 8 year-old girl in stable condition. Temperature: 36.8°C; pulse 80 bpm; blood pressure 113/62 mmHg. Body weight 20 kg (second percentile) and height 123.5 cm (tenth percentile). Skin: sclerodactyly; shallow digital pitting scars on bilateral second and third finger pads (Fig. 6.1), some with healing ulcerations; hide-bound skin on the distal forearms and over both hands; normal skin texture of both proximal arms and legs, chest and abdomen; under the right heel a white scar was present; she had palmar and plantar erythema; the modified Rodnan skin score was 15/51. HEENT: perioral skin tightening with reduced oral aperture of 4 cm (Fig. 6.2). Chest: no adventitial breath sounds. Cardiac: regular rate and rhythm with normal S1 and S2 heart sounds. Abdomen: no tenderness or distention. Extremities: no edema. Neurologic exam: normal. Musculoskeletal exam: mild flexion contractures of the fingers with inability to fully flatten the hands or to make a complete fist; finger–palm distance 0.5 cm; no joint tenderness or swelling. Firm, non-tender subcutaneous nodules were present over both elbows. Nailfold capillary microscopy revealed a few dilated capillary loops and capillary hemorrhages on the second to fourth digits of both hands; there was no capillary dropout but some megacapillaries were observed.

Laboratory Findings

CBC, chemistry panel and urinalysis: normal. ANA by IIF: positive with titer 1:640; anti-Scl-70 antibodies positive; other ENA antibodies and anti-dsDNA antibodies: negative. Anticardiolipin antibodies: negative. ECG: normal. Echocardiogram: normal except for trivial mitral insufficiency. PFTs: normal except decreased DLco (37% predicted). HRCT scan of chest: normal. Abdominal ultrasound: normal. Esophageal manometry: hypoperistalsis of the lower portion of the esophagus.

Course

A diagnosis of jSSc was confirmed and she was initially classified as having the limited subtype according to the LeRoy and Medsger classification,[1] recognizing that this classification system has not been validated in the pediatric population. The patient had no active digital ulcers at the time of the first visit. Her treatment was intensified with the methotrexate being increased to 15 mg/m^2 body surface area po weekly. Azathioprine was discontinued since it is not one of the suggested therapies according the EUSTAR/EULAR therapeutic recommendations for adult-onset SSc.[2] Because of her history of digital ulcers, low-dose aspirin 2 mg/kg daily was prescribed. The reduced DLco was thought to be erroneous, and this was supported by her ability to participate fully in physical exercises at school and by the normal HRCT chest scan. Because she was having problems with swallowing, esophageal scintigraphy was obtained and revealed no abnormalities. PFTs and echocardiography as well as serum chemistry, CBC, and urinalysis were recommended at 6 month intervals, according to the assessment protocol of the prospective juvenile-onset SSc inception cohort project (www.juvenile-scleroderma.com). Physiotherapy with regular stretching exercises and paraffin wax bath for the fingers was recommended for treatment of the early contractures. Regarding her growth disturbance, the main aim was to attempt to medically control her disease but with a plan that if her growth should not improve, then an evaluation by a pediatric endocrinologist regarding possible growth hormone treatment would be considered.

Over the next several months she developed calcinosis over both elbows and tips of the toes, as well as Gottron papules over the MCP and PIP joints of both hands. Raynaud's phenomenon increased in frequency without development of new fingertip ulcerations. Muscle strength was normal, and she had no elevation of muscle enzymes.

Discussion

This patient fulfills the criteria for the diagnosis of jSSc. She has skin induration and sclerosis as the major criterion and, in addition, she fulfills two minor criteria: (1) presence of ANA and anti-Scl 70 antibody, and (2) vascular changes with history of Raynaud's phenomenon and fingertip ulcerations[3] (Table 6.1). Interestingly, she initially was categorized as having limited cutaneous involvement (lSSc) according to the LeRoy and Medsger classification,[1] which is not the typical presentation of jSSc. In the cross-sectional survey of Martini et al.,[4] in which data from 153 patients with jSSc were collected, 90% were classified in the diffuse cutaneous subtype (dSSc). Diffuse cutaneous subtype predominance has been confirmed in other case series.[5,6] The patient subsequently developed overlap features of dermatomyositis, for example, Gottron papules, which may be a good prognostic sign according to a study of jSSc patients in the cohort from the Royal Free Hospital in London.[7] This patient has systemic sclerosis and not localized scleroderma, with bilateral and symmetric skin involvement and sclerodactyly. Furthermore, the anti-Scl-70 antibodies are quite specific for SSc, and such antibodies are not found in patients with localized scleroderma.[8] In localized scleroderma, there may be rare extracutaneous findings, for example, "white uveitis" and intracranial calcifications (see Chap. 5), but these differ from the extracutaneous features seen in children with systemic sclerosis (jSSc). It is important to differentiate jSSc from juvenile-onset localized scleroderma, the latter being

Table 6.1 The provisional classification criteria for juvenile systemic sclerosis

Major criterion	Minor criteria
• Induration[a]/Sclerosis[a]	• Vascular changes[a]
	• Pulmonary involvement[a]
	• Gastrointestinal involvement[a]
	• Renal involvement[a]
	• Cardiovascular involvement[a]
	• Musculoskeletal involvement[a]
	• Neurologic involvement[a]
	• Serology[a]

Modified from Zulian et al.[3] with permission from John Wiley & Sons Inc.
[a]Typical for systemic sclerosis – defined in the publication (Zulian et al. 2007)

much more common in the pediatric population (4.7–20 cases per 100,000 and 10 times more frequent than jSSc). Localized scleroderma is classified according to a newly proposed but not yet validated classification system.[8,9] It has, in most cases, a more benign course with the exception of pansclerotic morphea.[8] Extracutaneous involvement occurs in only about 10% of cases, mostly uveitis, arthritis, or neurologic involvement.[10] Localized forms of scleroderma rarely cross over to systemic sclerosis.

This patient had no significant internal organ involvement at the time of her most recent evaluation, which is another good prognostic factor.[7] Limited cutaneous subtype patients (lSSc) seem to have a better long-term prognosis. In three large data sets of jSSc patients followed to adulthood, it has been observed that the proportion of dSSc decreases over time while the proportion of lSSc patients increases over time.[7,11,12] This phenomenon reflects a survival benefit for the lSSc juvenile-onset subtype.

For this sort of patient with skin involvement only methotrexate is the first choice of therapy according to EULAR treatment recommendations for adult-onset SSc. Pediatric rheumatologists also prefer to use methotrexate. Although there have been no studies to determine the effective dose of methotrexate in patients with jSSc, experts often prescribe a dose of 15 mg/m^2 body surface area titrating up to 1 mg/kg body weight with a maximum of 50 mg weekly[13,14] as first-line immunosuppressive therapy. Such doses are generally well tolerated by children with other pediatric rheumatologic diseases, usually in combination with 1 mg folic acid daily.

The patient complained about problems swallowing. She had abnormal esophageal motility by manometric testing, but esophageal dysfunction was not documented by esophageal scintigraphy,[15,16] a technique that appears to be very sensitive in adult SSc patients. Esophageal scintigraphy has not, however, been validated in children with SSc. Other standard clinical and investigational tools may be difficult to interpret or have yet to be validated in the pediatric patient population.

The reduced DLco seemed discordant with her history of full physical function and otherwise normal PFT parameters. The normal HRCT chest scan and echocardiogram Doppler study also seemed to suggest that the DLco might be a false positive test result. The assessment of DLco in younger children can be quite difficult and, therefore, decreased values should always be viewed in clinical context before making treatment decisions based only on an isolated decrease in DLco. A recent study found good correlation between PFT and HRCT chest scan findings.[17] It should be remembered that DLco may reflect pulmonary vascular disease and normal HRCT chest findings should raise suspicion of possible pulmonary hypertension with prompt assessment including Doppler echocardiogram.

No outcome measures or clinical assessment tools, including those used in adult SSc patients, have yet been validated in jSSc patients. The modified Rodnan skin score (mRSS) may be elevated even in healthy children[18] due to their subcutaneous fat content.[19] Nailfold capillaroscopic findings cannot necessarily be interpreted as in adults; in a cross-sectional study of 110 healthy children aged 6–15 years, there was a significant trend for arterial and venous dimension to rise with age; this trend was not present for apical and loop diameters. Nailfold capillaroscopic results did not differ between males and females. When using capillary dimension as an outcome measure, age adjustment is required.[20] In another study of 17 healthy children, it was shown that both capillary density and capillary width were age-related. Younger children have fewer (for all children: 6.9 (0.9) capillaries/mm) and wider (for all children: 3.1 [2.2–9.4] mm) capillaries than older children. Some healthy children had tortuous, bizarre-shaped capillaries (tortuosity index median: 29% (5–49)).[21]

The 6-minute walk test (6MWT), a standard outcome measure and assessment tool for patients with pulmonary hypertension, has also not been validated in children. Two groups have looked at normal values in healthy children, but the normal values differ by age group so they cannot be applied yet to children with jSSc.[22,23] In both studies, the length of the walked distance correlated with the height of the patients, presumably with the length of the stride.

Other studies have begun to look at potential biomarkers of disease activity in jSSc patients. In one pilot study, serum concentrations of KL-6, a high-molecular-weight, mucin-like glycoprotein strongly expressed on type II pneumocytes, correlated in six jSSc patients with the presence of interstitial lung disease (defined by HRCT chest scan). Serum KL-6 expression was significantly higher in patients with interstitial lung disease than in patients without interstitial lung disease and/or in healthy controls.[24] B-type natriuretic peptide (BNP) seems to be a promising noninvasive marker of pulmonary hypertension, and BNP levels have been shown to correlate with pulmonary hypertension in children.[25-27]

Certain special considerations in the follow-up of children with jSSc, for example, weight and growth development and sexual maturation according to the Tanner stage, must be followed. If malnutrition were to occur from gastrointestinal tract involvement, then weight gain and growth delay might present problems. Currently, prospective data regarding this issue are lacking. Such parameters were not evaluated in prior retrospective cohorts of jSSc patients. Another important issue is the psychosocial development of the child, which might be influenced by alterations in facial and bodily appearance, especially during the phase of puberty. Again, at this time we have no data regarding this issue. These are among several parameters that will be assessed in the prospective jSSc inception cohort project (www.juvenile-scleriderma.com) currently in progress.

Special Issues in the Care for Children with Juvenile Systemic Sclerosis

Unfortunately, we have no evidence-based data on the treatment of children with jSSc. The approach to treatment and rehabilitation of these pediatric patients differs from that of adult SSc patients. Their care involves both the patient and the parents/caregivers.[6] The patient cannot give consent to treatment and rehabilitation plans, but only an assent; yet an understanding of the treatment by the patient is essential. The support of the concept by the parents and caregivers is essential too. Sometimes the patients and parents/caregivers have different fears and hopes regarding the side effects of the treatments and complications of the disease.

Treatment of Juvenile Systemic Sclerosis

We have no prospective or even good retrospective studies regarding efficacy of any treatment in jSSc except for one study on the treatment of severe digital ischemia.[28] There are some pilot data regarding the efficacy of methotrexate in children with jSSc.[13,14,29] Otherwise, we must rely on data from studies of adult SSc patients regarding treatment, as well as the current therapeutic guidelines from EULAR/ EUSTAR regarding the treatment of adults with SSc.[2] It must be taken into consideration that these guidelines are based on peer-reviewed and published data but inevitably do not encompass recent and emerging data, for example, pilot studies showing efficacy of rituximab[30] or tocilizumab[31] in the treatment of adult-onset SSc patients. There are obvious hazards in basing management of jSSc on adult-onset disease and even more when the limitations of the adult evidence base are considered. It bears mentioning that all these treatments are off-label for jSSc. Currently, there are no pediatric guidelines specifically for jSSc. Concepts from the treatment of adult SSc patients are applied, or concepts of treatment of pediatric patients with other rheumatic diseases are adopted.

Prognosis

Regarding the prognosis of jSSc, we can tell the parents that the disease has a more benign course than in adults. In two pediatric cohorts, the 5-year survival was between 90% and 95%. Most deaths in our cohort occurred in the first 2 years of the disease in association with multisystem involvement.[32] The eight patients who died had higher rates of pulmonary (75%), cardiovascular (100%), central nervous system (38%), and renal (50%) involvement. The male:female ratio was 1:1 and the median age at disease onset was 10.5 years. Interestingly, the fatal cases in the cohort of Martini et al. had a male:female ratio of 1:2.2 and a mean age of 10.4 years at disease onset.[33] Mean duration of disease until death was 4.6 years, but four died within the first 12 months of disease onset. The patients who died had a significantly shorter time interval to diagnosis of 8.8 months, compared to 23 months in the survivors. Those patients with a fatal outcome also had higher rates of pulmonary, gastrointestinal, and cardiac involvement. All were of the dSSc subset. Our patient had limited cutaneous involvement and, aside from the fingertip ulcers and Raynaud's phenomenon, she had no other proven organ involvement, which would seem to be a good prognostic factor. In the cohort of adult-aged patients from a major UK tertiary referral center for adult SSc patients, those jSSc patients with overlap features and with limited cutaneous involvement had a better survival.[7]

References

1. LeRoy EC, Krieg T, et al. Scleroderma (systemic sclerosis): classification, subsets and pathogenesis. *J Rheumatol*. 1988;15:202-205.
2. Kowal-Bielecka O, Landewe R, et al. EULAR recommendations for the treatment of systemic sclerosis: a report from the EULAR Scleroderma Trials and Research group (EUSTAR). *Ann Rheum Dis*. 2009;68(5):620-628.
3. Zulian F, Woo P, et al. The Pediatric Rheumatology European Society/American College of Rheumatology/European league against rheumatism provisional classification criteria for juvenile systemic sclerosis. *Arthritis Rheum*. 2007;57(2):203-212.
4. Martini G, Foeldvari I, et al. Systemic sclerosis in childhood: clinical and immunologic features of 153 patients in an international database. *Arthritis Rheum*. 2006;54(12):3971-3978.
5. Russo RA, Katsicas MM. Clinical characteristics of children with juvenile systemic sclerosis: follow-up of 23 patients in a single tertiary center. *Pediatr Rheumatol Online J*. 2007;5:6.
6. Aoyama K, Nagai Y, et al. Juvenile systemic sclerosis: report of three cases and review of Japanese published work. *J Dermatol*. 2007;34(9):658-661.
7. Foeldvari I, Nihtyanova SI, et al. Characteristics of patients with juvenile onset systemic sclerosis in an adult single-center cohort. *J Rheumatol*. 2010;37:2422-2426.
8. Zulian F, Athreya BA, et al. Juvenile localized scleroderma: clinical and epidemiological features in 750 children. An international study. *Rheumatology (Oxford)*. 2006;45:614-620.
9. Laxer RM, Zulian F. Localized scleroderma. *Curr Opin Rheumatol*. 2006;18(6):606-613.
10. Zulian F, Vallongo C, et al. Localized scleroderma in childhood is not just a skin disease. *Arthritis Rheum*. 2005;52(9):2873-2881.
11. Scalapino K, Arkachaisri T, et al. Childhood onset systemic sclerosis: classification, clinical and serologic features, and survival in comparison with adult onset disease. *J Rheumatol*. 2006;33(5):1004-1013.
12. Foeldvari I, Tyndall A, et al. Juvenile and young adult onset systemic sclerosis share the same outcome and organ involvement: data from the EUSTAR database on an adult cohort of systemic sclerosis patients. *Arthritis Rheum*. 2007;56(Suppl): S53/A51.
13. Foeldvari I, Lehmann TJA. Is methotrexate a new perspective in the treatment of juvenile progressive systemic scleroderma? *Arthritis Rheum*. 1993;36(Suppl):S218.
14. Lehman TJA. Systemic and localized scleroderma in children. *Curr Opin Rheumatol*. 1996;8:576-579.
15. Kaye SA, Siraj QH, et al. Detection of early asymptomatic esophageal dysfunction in systemic sclerosis using a new scintigraphic grading method. *J Rheumatol*. 1996;23:297-301.
16. Nakajima K, Kawano M, et al. The diagnostic value of oesophageal transit scintigraphy for evaluating the severity of oesophageal complications in systemic sclerosis. *Nucl Med Commun*. 2004;25(4):375-381.
17. Panigada S, Ravelli A, et al. HRCT and pulmonary function tests in monitoring of lung involvement in juvenile systemic sclerosis. *Pediatr Pulmonol*. 2009;44(12):1226-1234.
18. Foeldvari I, Wierk A. Healthy children have a significantly increased skin score assessed with the modified Rodnan skin scor. *Arthritis Rheum*. 2004;50(Suppl): S419, A1045.
19. de Rigal J, Escoffier E, et al. Assessment of aging of the human skin by in vivo ultrasound imaging. *J Invest Dermatol*. 1989;93:621-625.
20. Herrick ML, Moore T, et al. The influence of age on nailfold capillary dimension in childhood. *J Rheumatol*. 2000;27:797-800.
21. Dolezalova P, Young SP, et al. Nailfold capillary microscopy in healthy children and in childhood rheumatic diseases: a prospective single blind observational study. *Ann Rheum Dis*. 2003;62:444-449.
22. Li AM, Yin J, et al. Standard reference for the six-minute-walk test in healthy children aged 7 to 16 years. *Am J Respir Crit Care Med*. 2007;176(2):174-180.
23. Lammers AE, Hislop AA, et al. The 6-minute walk test: normal values for children of 4–11 years of age. *Arch Dis Child*. 2008;93(6):464-468.

24. Vesely R, Vargova V, et al. Serum level of KL-6 as a marker of interstitial lung disease in patients with juvenile systemic scleroderma. *J Rheumatol.* 2004;31:795-800.
25. Lammers AE, Hislop A, et al. Prognostic value of B-type natriuretic peptide in children with pulmonary hypertension. *Int J Cardiol.* 2009;135:21-26.
26. Van Albada ME, Loot FG, et al. Biological serum markers in the management of pediatric pulmonary arterial hypertension. *Pediatr Res.* 2008;63(3):321-327.
27. Bernus A, Wagner BD, et al. Brain natriuretic peptide levels in managing pediatric patients with pulmonary arterial hypertension. *Chest.* 2009;135(3):745-751.
28. Zulian F, Corona F, et al. Safety and efficacy of iloprost for the treatment of ischaemic digits in paediatric connective tissue diseases. *Rheumatology (Oxford).* 2004;43(2):229-233.
29. Lehman TJA. Methotrexate for the treatment of early diffuse scleroderma: comment on the article by Pope et al. *Arthritis Rheum.* 2002;46:845.
30. Smith V, Van Praet JT, et al. Rituximab in diffuse cutaneous systemic sclerosis: an open-label clinical and histopathological study. *Ann Rheum Dis.* 2010;69(1):193-197.
31. Shima Y, Kuwahara Y, et al. The skin of patients with systemic sclerosis softened during the treatment with anti-IL-6 receptor antibody tocilizumab. *Rheumatology (Oxford).* 2010;49(12): 2408-2412.
32. Foeldvari I, Zhavania M, et al. Favourable outcome in 135 children with juvenile systemic sclerosis: results of a multi-national survey. *Rheumatology (Oxford).* 2000;39(5):556-559.
33. Martini G, Vittadello F, et al. Factors affecting survival in juvenile systemic sclerosis. *Rheumatology (Oxford).* 2009;48:119-122.

Chapter 7
A 60-Year-Old Woman with Skin Thickening, Joint Contractures, and Peripheral Blood Eosinophilia

Marcy B. Bolster

Keywords Eosinophilic fasciitis • Diffuse fasciitis with eosinophilia • Eosinophilia • Fibrosis

Case Study

A 60-year-old woman presented with an 8-month history of skin changes of all extremities. She first noted swelling and discomfort of her forearms. The skin felt hardened to the touch and she recognized that she was unable to reach a full octave when playing her piano. She denied joint pain or specific joint swelling but noted that her forearms appeared "swollen" with involvement extending from the elbows to the wrists. Two months later she developed similar skin changes of her lower extremities extending from her knees to her ankles. She also reported that she had more difficulty rushing the net in her tennis league matches due to lower extremity discomfort. She denied symptoms of Raynaud's phenomenon, gastroesophageal reflux, diarrhea, oral ulcers, photosensitivity, shortness of breath, chest pain, or history of kidney disease. She had never undergone an MRI scan.

Her medical history was notable for osteopenia treated with calcium and vitamin D. She took no other medications and denied the use of tryptophan or other nutritional supplements. In the past year she had had a normal mammogram, pelvic exam, and had had a normal colonoscopy 4 years ago. She was a retired schoolteacher and continued to teach piano lessons. She was active in a local tennis league and denied any recent change in her exercise capacity. Family history was noncontributory.

M.B. Bolster
Division of Rheumatology and Immunology,
Medical University of South Carolina,
96 Jonathan Lucas Street, Suite 912, Charleston, SC 29425, USA

R.M. Silver and C.P. Denton (eds.), *Case Studies in Systemic Sclerosis*,
DOI: 10.1007/978-0-85729-641-2_7, © Springer-Verlag London Limited 2011

Fig. 7.1 "Peau d'orange" (*arrow*) of the forearm of a patient with eosinophilic fasciitis, characterized by induration and a lumpiness of the skin

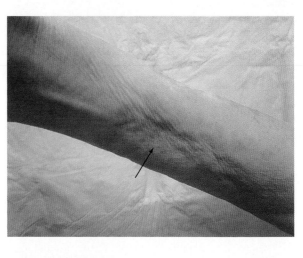

Fig. 7.2 A groove sign is evident on the forearm of a patient with eosinophilic fasciitis (*arrow*) and represents a tethering of the vein due to the inflammation and thickening of the fascia

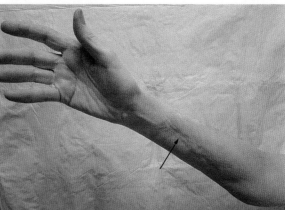

Physical Examination

Temperature 37°C, blood pressure 132/75 mmHg, pulse 85 bpm, respiratory rate 18/min. Skin examination revealed woody induration with warmth and mild erythema of the forearms. There was no sclerodactyly, digital pits, or telangiectasias. Woody induration also extended from the knees to the dorsum of both feet. Skin on the face, trunk, upper arms, and thighs was normal. In addition to the woody induration, the skin had a *peau d'orange* appearance over the forearms (Fig. 7.1) and distal lower extremities, characterized by a lumpy dimpled appearance. A "groove sign" (Fig. 7.2) was present on both forearms and over the distal right lower extremity. HEENT, lung, heart, and abdominal examination was unremarkable. Musculoskeletal exam revealed no evidence of joint swelling or tenderness, although flexion contractures were noted at the proximal interphalangeal (PIP) joints giving a "prayer sign"

Fig. 7.3 (**a**) A prayer sign is demonstrated in a patient with eosinophilic fasciitis when trying to oppose her palms and fingers. There is a space producing the "prayer sign" due to the fascia thickening resulting in proximal interphalangeal and metacarpophalangeal joint flexion contractures. (**b**) Following treatment with prednisone there has been marked improvement in the "prayer sign"

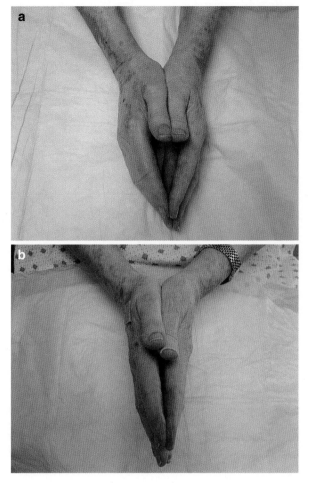

of the hands (Fig. 7.3). There was reduced range of motion of the ankle and subtalar joints without signs of synovitis. No tendon friction rubs were detected. Muscle strength was normal. Nailfold capillary microscopy was normal, specifically showing no dilated capillary loops or capillary dropout.

Laboratory and Pathology Findings

The CBC revealed a WBC count of 8,400 cells/mm^3, hemoglobin 13.6 g/dL, hematocrit 40%, platelets 350,000/mm^3. The WBC differential showed 60% granulocytes, 12% lymphocytes, and 28% eosinophils. Complete metabolic panel and urinalysis was normal. Antinuclear antibody (ANA) and rheumatoid factor (RF) tests were negative. Erythrocyte sedimentation rate (ESR) was elevated (65 mm/h). Full-thickness

Fig. 7.4 A photomicrograph demonstrating a hematoxylin and eosin stain. (**a**) En bloc skin to muscle biopsy revealing thickening of the fascia (20× magnification) and (**b**) a higher magnification (200×) of the same specimen revealing thickening of the fascia with an inflammatory cell infiltrate composed of lymphocytes and plasma cells, with scattered eosinophils

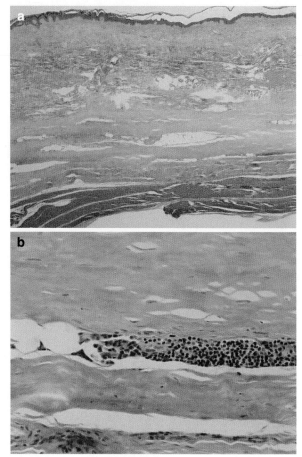

skin biopsy of the right forearm, obtained *en bloc* from skin to muscle, revealed thickening of the fascia with infiltration by inflammatory cells, including a predominance of lymphocytes and plasma cells with occasional eosinophils (Fig. 7.4).

Course

A diagnosis of eosinophilic fasciitis (EF or DFE, diffuse fasciitis with eosinophilia) was suspected on clinical grounds by the presence of woody induration of the skin of the extremities showing changes of *peau d'orange*, a groove sign, joint contractures, and a peripheral eosinophilia. Also supporting the diagnosis of EF was the absence of key symptoms and signs characteristic of SSc including Raynaud's phenomenon, gastroesophageal reflux, dyspnea, sclerodactyly, digital pitted scars, telangiectasias, tendon friction rubs, characteristic nailfold capillary changes, or positive ANA. EF was confirmed by full-thickness skin biopsy. The skin biopsy in this case study is typical of that seen in EF, notably with excess collagen deposition and inflammatory cell infiltration of the fascia. Lymphocyte and plasma cell infiltration are characteristic findings and there may additionally be a mild eosinophil infiltrate in the tissue. The eosinophilia of EF is typically, however, a peripheral blood eosinophilia.

The patient was treated initially with prednisone 50 mg daily (1 mg/kg/day) and hydroxychloroquine. Alendronate was added with supplemental calcium and vitamin D for bone health. She was referred for physical therapy and instructed in joint range of motion exercises. She will undergo ophthalmologic screening annually to screen for potential hydroxychloroquine toxicity. The planned glucocorticoid regimen includes initiating prednisone 50 mg daily for 1 month followed by a taper by 10 mg monthly until the patient is taking prednisone 20 mg daily. At this point, the taper will change to 5 mg decrements in prednisone dosing on a monthly basis.

Discussion

Eosinophilic fasciitis (EF, also known as diffuse fasciitis with eosinophilia or Shulman syndrome) was first described by Shulman in 1975.[1] It is a disease characterized by woody induration of the skin due to thickening and inflammation of the fascia and subcutaneous tissue, in association with a peripheral blood eosinophilia. EF is an uncommon disorder that must be differentiated from systemic sclerosis (scleroderma, SSc) and other fibrosing syndromes affecting the dermis and subcutis. There are typically three phases of the disease, beginning with an early edematous phase, progressing to the development of *peau d'orange*, and ultimately evolving to a woody induration and thickening of the skin. At the time of presentation the characteristic physical examination findings include a woody induration without sclerodactyly, the appearance of *peau d'orange*, and a groove sign. *Peau d'orange* (Fig. 7.1) and the groove sign (Fig. 7.2) are best observed with the extremity extended and elevated. Both findings represent the subcutaneous inflammation of EF. The groove sign occurs due to tethering of the vein by thickened fascia resulting in a flattening, and, in fact, an indentation over the course of the vein at the skin surface. Due to the thickening of the fascia, patients often develop joint flexion contractures[2] and may also experience compression neuropathies, most commonly carpal tunnel syndrome. Eosinophilic fasciitis has been observed to occur on rare occasions in patients with systemic sclerosis, and it is important to distinguish the classic physical findings of each disease in order to correctly approach patient management.

Hypothyroidism is another condition that commonly co-occurs with EF. Rarely, an inflammatory arthritis may be associated with EF. EF has also been associated with the occurrence of hematologic disorders,[3] and it may occur as a paraneoplastic process.[4,5] Absent in EF, however, is the visceral involvement typical of SSc, that is, lack of Raynaud's phenomenon, gastrointestinal dysmotility, and cardiopulmonary disease.

Fig. 7.5 A T2 weighted
axial MR image of the
proximal leg of a patient
with eosinophilic fasciitis
demonstrating diffuse fascial
edema

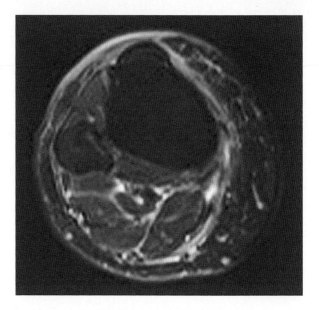

Laboratory findings in EF include a peripheral blood eosinophilia, elevated serum IgG, and elevated ESR.[1] The eosinophilia is usually detectable prior to the diagnosis and treatment of the patient, but the degree of eosinophilia may not always reflect the relative disease activity.[3]

The etiology of EF has not been clearly delineated. There has been a suspicion that EF may be triggered in some patients by heavy exertional activity, by certain medications including lipid-lowering agents, or that it could be related to Borrelia infection,[3,6,7] although no consistent precipitating factor has been confirmed.

EF should be differentiated from other fibrosing skin disorders including systemic sclerosis (*vide supra*), generalized morphea, nephrogenic systemic fibrosis, scleredema, and scleromyxedema, and these conditions are described elsewhere in this book. Generalized morphea may at times be difficult to differentiate from EF, though patients with generalized morphea typically have many plaques, which then may become confluent. The thickening and induration seen in morphea involve the dermis, thus these patients do not tend to have the woody induration seen in patients with the deeper histologic involvement characteristic of EF. Patients with generalized morphea may also have a peripheral blood eosinophilia and a weakly positive ANA. A full-thickness skin biopsy may be required to differentiate generalized morphea from EF.

The gold standard for confirming the diagnosis of EF is the full thickness, *en bloc*, biopsy of skin to muscle, which should ensure an adequate specimen that contains fascia. MRI is also being investigated as a reliable test in the diagnosis of EF and can demonstrate thickening and hyperintensity of the fascia on T1-weighted, T2-weighted, and STIR sequences as well as enhancement after intravenous contrast administration (Fig. 7.5).[2] MRI evidence of fascia thickening provides a noninvasive method for confirming a diagnosis as well as potentially documenting clinical improvement.[8-10] This may be an important option for patients who otherwise will undergo a deep, full-thickness biopsy followed by treatment of confirmed EF using high-dose glucocorticoids. The glucocorticoids may increase the risk of poor wound healing from the biopsy.

EF, unlike systemic sclerosis, is highly responsive to glucocorticoid therapy, particularly when initiated early at a more inflammatory stage of the disease.[2,11] The course of glucocorticoid therapy typically involves the initiation of high-dose glucocorticoids (1 mg/kg/day) followed by a taper over 9–12 months. On the contrary, high-dose glucocorticoid therapy is typically avoided in patients with systemic sclerosis due to the increased risk for developing normotensive renal crisis in patients with diffuse cutaneous disease.[12] In any patient initiating a course of glucocorticoids, consideration should be given for the patient's bone health. The American College of Rheumatology (ACR) has published new guidelines for the prevention of glucocorticoid-induced osteoporosis.[13] The patient in this case study was initiated on a bisphosphonate in addition to her calcium and vitamin D supplementation.

Hydroxychloroquine has been shown in open trials to be beneficial in the management of EF.[3] Due to its low toxicity and its potential efficacy, it is typically initiated at the onset of therapy as it can also serve as a steroid-sparing agent.

Some EF patients will experience refractory skin fibrosis. Risk factors for the development of refractory skin fibrosis include the presence of morphea-like skin lesions (more dermal involvement by the fibrosis), truncal skin involvement, and younger age of disease onset (<12 years old).[2,11] It also seems that earlier intervention with therapy at a time when the skin lesion may be at a more inflammatory stage may be advantageous in the avoidance of later persistent skin fibrosis.[11]

In patients who demonstrate difficulty with glucocorticoid tapering due to increased inflammation or thickening of skin disease, consideration can be given to the use of methotrexate or azathioprine as steroid-sparing agents. Other agents have been tried in the management of EF as anecdotal reports including cyclosporine A[14] and tumor necrosis factor (TNF) alpha inhibitors.[15] Mycophenolate mofetil has also been used and sometimes immunosuppressive agents are used in combination for refractory cases.[16]

In patients refractory to the combination of prednisone, hydroxychloroquine and methotrexate consideration can be given to the use of ultraviolet A-1 therapy. There are small trials that have provided support for the use of either psoralen-ultraviolet A (PUVA) photochemotherapy or Ultraviolet A1-retinoid therapy under the direction of a dermatologist.[17,18]

In summary, the diagnosis of EF should be considered in any patient presenting with a fibrosing skin disorder that involves the extremities but with acral sparing, and in the absence of Raynaud's phenomenon, gastroesophageal reflux, and dyspnea. Characteristic findings in patients with EF include woody induration, or a deeper induration (of the subcutis), *peau d'orange*, a "groove" sign, joint flexion contractures, compression neuropathies, and most patients will have a peripheral blood eosinophilia. The diagnosis is confirmed by full-thickness biopsy of skin to fascia and is characterized by fascia thickening (excessive collagen) and an inflammatory cell infiltrate mostly consisting of lymphocytes and plasma cells, with a more modest tissue infiltration by eosinophils. Potentially, MRI scans may provide diagnostic evidence of fascia thickening and inflammation. It is essential to correctly diagnose EF as this disorder, unlike other fibrosing skin disorders, is highly responsive to glucocorticoid therapy. Also important in the management of patients with EF is early and aggressive physical therapy in order to avoid reduced functional capacity related to joint flexion contractures. Glucocorticoids are the mainstay of therapy. Given its low toxicity profile and potential benefit in patients with EF, many will utilize the early addition of hydroxychloroquine. Other therapeutic considerations based on small case series in the literature include methotrexate, azathioprine, cyclosporine, mycophenolate mofetil, TNF alpha inhibitors, and phototherapy.

References

1. Shulman LE. Diffuse fasciitis with eosinophilia: a new syndrome? *Trans Assoc Am Physicians.* 1975;88:70-86.
2. Bischoff L, Derk CT. Eosinophilic fasciitis: demographics, disease pattern and response to treatment: report of 12 cases and review of the literature. *Int J Dermatol.* 2008;47(1):29-35.
3. Lakhanpal S et al. Eosinophilic fasciitis: clinical spectrum and therapeutic response in 52 cases. *Semin Arthritis Rheum.* 1988;17(4):221-231.
4. Chan LS, Hanson CA, Cooper KD. Concurrent eosinophilic fasciitis and cutaneous T-cell lymphoma. Eosinophilic fasciitis as a paraneoplastic syndrome of T-cell malignant neoplasms? *Arch Dermatol.* 1991;127(6):862-865.
5. Naschitz JE et al. Cancer-associated fasciitis panniculitis. *Cancer.* 1994;73(1):231-235.
6. Granter SR, Barnhill RL, Duray PH. Borrelial fasciitis: diffuse fasciitis and peripheral eosinophilia associated with Borrelia infection. *Am J Dermatopathol.* 1996;18(5):465-473.
7. Choquet-Kastylevsky G et al. Eosinophilic fasciitis and simvastatin. *Arch Intern Med.* 2001;161(11):1456-1457.
8. Moulton SJ et al. Eosinophilic fasciitis: spectrum of MRI findings. *AJR Am J Roentgenol.* 2005;184(3):975-978.
9. Angnew KL, Blunt D, Francis ND, Bunker CB. Magnetic resonance imaging in eosinophilic fasciitis. *Clin Exp Dermatol.* 2005;30:435-436.
10. Baumann F et al. MRI for diagnosis and monitoring of patients with eosinophilic fasciitis. *AJR Am J Roentgenol.* 2005;184(1):169-174.
11. Endo Y et al. Eosinophilic fasciitis: report of two cases and a systematic review of the literature dealing with clinical variables that predict outcome. *Clin Rheumatol.* 2007;26(9):1445-1451.
12. Steen VD, Medsger TA Jr. Case-control study of corticosteroids and other drugs that either precipitate or protect from the development of scleroderma renal crisis. *Arthritis Rheum.* 1998;41(9):1613-1619.
13. Grossman JM, Gordon R, Ranganath VK, Deal C, Caplan L, et al. American College of Rheumatology 2010 recommendations for the prevention and treatment of glucocorticoid-induced osteoporosis. *Arthritis Care Res.* 2010;62:1515-1526.
14. Bukiej A et al. Eosinophilic fasciitis successfully treated with cyclosporine. *Clin Rheumatol.* 2005;24(6):634-636.
15. Khanna D, Agrawal H, Clements PJ. Infliximab may be effective in the treatment of steroid-resistant eosinophilic fasciitis: report of three cases. *Rheumatology (Oxford).* 2010;49(6):1184-1188.

16. Loupasakis K, Derk CT. Eosinophilic fasciitis in a pediatric patient. *J Clin Rheumatol.* 2010;16(3):129-131.
17. Weber HO et al. Eosinophilic fasciitis and combined UVA1–retinoid–corticosteroid treatment: two case reports. *Acta Derm Venereol.* 2008;88(3):304-306.
18. Schiener R et al. Eosinophilic fasciitis treated with psoralen-ultraviolet A bath photochemotherapy. *Br J Dermatol.* 2000;142(4):804-807.

Chapter 8
A 35-Year-Old Man with Diffuse Scleroderma and Chemical Exposure

László Czirják and Cecília Varjú

Keywords Systemic sclerosis • Scleroderma • Solvent • Occupational • Exposure • Environmental

History

A 35-year-old man developed Raynaud's phenomenon at the age of 25. He also developed puffy fingers and swelling of the dorsum of both hands. He had worked as a car mechanic and polisher and was heavily exposed to chemicals both by inhalation and direct skin contact, including *n*-butyl acetate (an organic compound commonly used as a solvent in the production of lacquers and enamel paints), toluene, benzene, ethyl benzene, xylenes, acetone, and mineral spirits (also known as white spirit or Stoddard solvent). After 3 years of regular exposure to these particular solvents he developed severe Raynaud's phenomenon. His primary care physician referred him to the local county hospital, where he was noted to have sclerodactyly and facial scleroderma with decreased oral aperture, and where abnormal esophageal motility was detected by barium swallow. The forced vital capacity (FVC) was found to be normal (89% predicted). The ESR was normal, there was a slight elevation of C-reactive protein (16 mg/L), a positive ANA, and anti-topoisomerase (Scl-70) ELISA test was positive as well. The serum creatine kinase and lactate dehydrogenase levels were also slightly elevated. One month later the patient was sent to our department.

By the time of our first assessment, the patient had progressed to diffuse SSc with extensive skin involvement and severe Raynaud's phenomenon (Fig. 8.1), and he had also developed dyspnea on exertion (when going up about 20 steps). He did

L. Czirják (✉)
Department of Rheumatology and Immunology, University of Pécs,
Medical Center, Akác u. 1, Pécs H-7632, Hungary

R.M. Silver and C.P. Denton (eds.), *Case Studies in Systemic Sclerosis*,
DOI: 10.1007/978-0-85729-641-2_8, © Springer-Verlag London Limited 2011

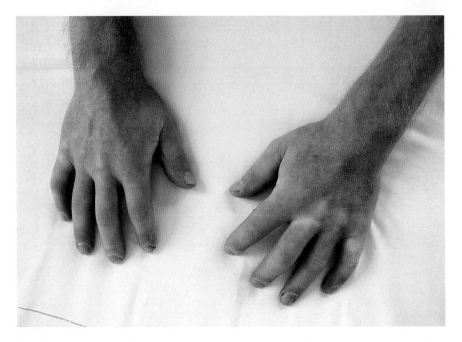

Fig. 8.1 Signs of severe Raynaud's phenomenon in a patient with solvent exposure and diffuse SSc

not complain of muscle pain, but he described proximal muscle weakness. The modified Rodnan skin score was 31/51, and typical scleroderma skin was present on the trunk as well as on the face and extremities. Joint contractures were present in both hands (Fig. 8.1). Radiographs of the hands and feet revealed no erosions, osteolysis, or subcutaneous calcification. PFT revealed an FVC of 86% predicted (normal), but the DLco (diffusing capacity of carbon monoxide) was markedly reduced at 39% predicted. A chest radiograph demonstrated bibasilar lung fibrosis, and HRCT of the chest showed a diffuse reticular pattern of the whole lung that was most predominant in the lower lobes.

With a diagnosis of early dSSc with interstitial lung involvement, we began treatment with monthly pulses of intravenous cyclophosphamide. He also was prescribed a proton pump inhibitor for his esophageal symptoms and a calcium channel blocker for the Raynaud's phenomenon. We advised the patient to give up his car painting activities and to avoid exposure to solvents; however, he declined to heed our precautions.

Despite pulse cyclophosphamide therapy his dyspnea worsened. In addition to interstitial lung disease, his clinical deterioration was felt to be due to the onset of arrhythmia and cardiac conduction abnormalities, including repetitive ventricular extrasystoles and supraventricular tachycardia detected by Holter monitoring. He did not have evidence of systolic or diastolic dysfunction. His cardiac arrhythmia was successfully treated by short-term administration of amiodarone and later by beta-blocker therapy.

Two years later, he began to experience retrosternal pain with occasional breathlessness that usually followed physical effort but sometimes occurred at rest. Invasive cardiac investigations showed no signs of coronary artery disease, and coronary vasospasm was not provoked during the catheterization procedure. Right heart catheterization (RHC) was also performed because of a borderline increase in estimated right ventricular systolic pressure by Doppler echocardiography, but pulmonary arterial hypertension was not confirmed by RHC hemodynamic measurements.

Pulse intravenous cyclophosphamide treatment was continued for 12 months (cumulative dose of 13 g), and then oral azathioprine was prescribed (2 mg/kg body weight). In the meantime, in spite of the immunosuppressive treatment, the FVC gradually declined from 86% to 60% predicted, while the chest HRCT scan revealed more extensive reticular features of fibrosis in the lower lobes and also in the right middle lobe. The latest HRCT scan performed 4 years after the initial scan showed a reticular pattern with honeycomb changes also predominantly in the lower lobes (Fig. 8.2 a, b).

In spite of advice to the contrary, the patient continued his work as a car polisher with regular exposure to solvents, and he did not avoid exposure to cold temperatures despite severe Raynaud's phenomenon with frequent occurrence of fingertip ulcers.

Over the next few years the patient remained stable with regard to pulmonary and cardiac function. FVC stabilized (approximately 55% predicted) and did not change during the next 3 years of follow-up. The modified Rodnan skin score peaked at 31/51 and then gradually regressed to 8/51, and currently skin tethering rather than

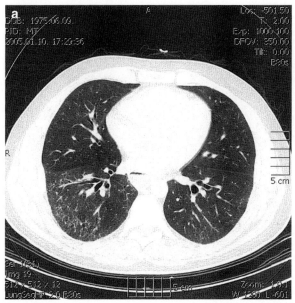

Fig. 8.2 High-resolution CT scan. (**a**) Reticulonodular pattern of the lungs typical for lung fibrosis and some ground glass opacification in a 35-year-old male with diffuse SSc and solvent exposure, first year following the onset of skin symptoms. (**b**) Four years later, the HRCT shows a reticular pattern with interval development of honeycomb changes

Fig. 8.2 (continued)

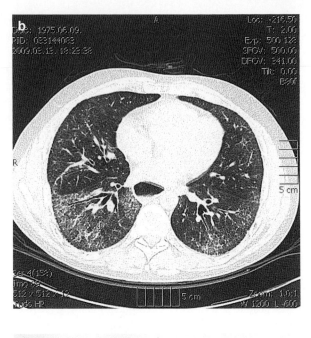

Fig. 8.3 Digital gangrene in a male patient who had occupational solvent exposure and developed diffuse SSc with severe Raynaud's phenomenon

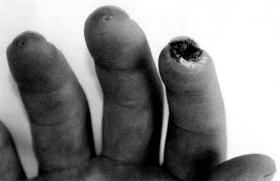

thickening predominates. Despite therapy, he developed multiple joint contractures in the metacarpophalangeal and proximal interphalangeal joints, and also a 5-degree flexion contracture in both knees. Raynaud's phenomenon has remained severe, with recurrent fingertip ulcers and an episode of digital gangrene (Fig. 8.3).

Discussion

Several occupational exposures including vinyl chloride, silica dust, epoxy resin, and organic solvents have been reported as potential provoking factors of SSc or scleroderma-like disorders (Table 8.1).[1-15] In our case study, the exposure to organic

Table 8.1 Pattern of skin involvement following an exposure to chemicals or drugs[1-24]

Provoking agent	Skin involvement	Idiopathic systemic scleroderma provoked by exposure	Systemic scleroderma-like skin involvement	Involvement of a well-defined skin area including pseudo-scleroderma	Morphea-like involvement
Cytostatic drugs					
Uracyl-tegafur	Limited cutaneous SSc type. No Raynaud's phenomenon	+			
Capecitabine (prodrug of 5-fluorouracyl), 5-fluorouracil, cytarabine, hydroxyurea, 6-mercaptopurine, cyclophosphamide, docetaxel, vinorelbine	Hand-foot syndrome with acral edema, swelling, desquamation, ulceration, and later development of scleroderma		+		
Taxane chemotherapy-induced scleroderma (docetaxel, paclitaxel)	Pitting edema of the extremities with a predilection of lower limbs; a subsequent development of sclerodermatous areas; fingers may be also involved	+	+		
Cytostatic agents other than taxanes: gemcitabine, melphalan, capecitabine	Predominantly morphea-like skin changes				+
Melphalan	Isolated limb perfusion with melphalan may induce scleroderma-like changes			+	
Doxorubicin + cyclophosphamide	Diffuse SSc with extensive skin involvement	+			

(continued)

Table 8.1 (continued)

Provoking agent	Skin involvement	Idiopathic systemic scleroderma provoked by exposure	Systemic scleroderma-like skin involvement	Involvement of a well-defined skin area including pseudo-scleroderma	Morphea-like involvement
Bleomycin, peplomycin	Acrosclerosis or morphea-like acral changes, pulmonary fibrosis, Raynaud's phenomenon	+			+
Appetite suppressants (phenmetrazine, diethylpropionhydrochloride, fenproporex)	Limited cutaneous SSc-like changes	+			
Other drugs					
D-penicillamine	Morphea-like changes in the trunk or generalized morphea or scleroderma of the extremities, shoulder girdle, hip			+	+
Valproic acid	Morphea-like digital skin changes or generalized morphea				+
Methysergide	Symmetric scleroderma in the legs and back			+	+
L-5-hydroxytryptophan and carbidopa	Arms legs. No sclerodactyly			+	
Ketobemidone	Woody induration, multiple irregular ulcers and scars surrounded by hyperpigmentation of the extremities			+	
Bromocriptine	Morphea-like changes				+
Local injection of vitamin K, corticosteroid, vitamin B12, pentazocin, progestin	Typical morphea at the site of injection				+

Contrast agents

Non-ionic, non-cyclic gadolinium containing contrast material (Nephrogenic systemic fibrosis)	Extremities predominantly; truncal involvement variable and less so than extremities; systemic involvement in some		+	+

Chemical agents

Solvents (trichloroethylene, perchlorethylene, benzene, or other organic compounds including amines, chlorinated solvents, formaldehyde derivatives)		+	+
Epoxy resin: bis(4-amino-3-methyl-cyclohexyl) methane	Erythema and edema evolving generalized dermal sclerosis. Alopecia. Muscle weakness and atrophy	+	

Other occupational exposures

Silica-induced scleroderma	Systemic scleroderma	+

"Historic" diseases

Vinyl chloride (Vinyl chloride disease)	Swollen fingers, skin induration, vasospasm, acro-osteolysis. Paresthesias, CNS symptoms, headache, memory loss, insomnia, thrombocytopenia, abnormal liver function	+

(continued)

Table 8.1 (continued)

Provoking agent	Skin involvement	Idiopathic systemic scleroderma provoked by exposure	Systemic scleroderma-like skin involvement	Involvement of a well-defined skin area including pseudo-scleroderma	Morphea-like involvement
L-Tryptophan dimer (Eosinophilia-myalgia syndrome)	Diffuse skin thickening, severe myalgia. Papules on trunk and face, sparing hands and feet. Blood eosinophilia			+	
Probable aniline derivatives of adulterated cooking oil (Toxic oil syndrome)	Acute phase: nonproductive cough, dyspnea, myalgia, arthralgia, headache, pruritus, rash. Eosinophilia. Intermediate phase: skin, subcutaneous edema, fibrosis. Contractures. Chronic phase: peripheral neuropathy, hepatomegaly, scleroderma-like skin changes, pulmonary hypertension			+	
Others					
Unknown agent following prosthetic knee joint implant	Scleroderma in the skin overlying the artificial joint			+	
Silicone breast implant (?)	SSc or UCTD	+			

solvents by inhalation and direct contact was considered to be a probable provoking factor for the development of SSc. Multiple reports from different parts of the world suggest that exposure to aliphatic or aromatic hydrocarbons, for example, trichloro-ethylene, perchloroethylene, toluene, benzene, xylene, as well as to white spirits, diesel fuels, aromatic mixes, or other organic compounds including amines, chlori-nated hydrocarbon solvents, and formaldehyde derivatives, may be scleroderma-provoking agents. A number of different case reports, case–control studies, and meta-analyses indicate that various solvents may be scleroderma-provoking agents,[1-18] and an increased relative risk in these reports suggests that exposure to organic solvents may be a risk factor for developing idiopathic systemic sclero-sis.[6,13,18] Among these particular solvents, trichloroethylene (TCE) seems to be a major possible provoking factor.

Patients with exposure to chemicals that seem to increase the relative risk for development of scleroderma have predominantly been male workers,[1,7,9,13-15] although female subjects may also be affected.[16] In our recent controlled study,[4] 16 out of 63 cases of SSc had had an exposure to chemicals. A borderline statistical significance was demonstrated compared to matched female controls ($p<0.05$). Patients with a history of chemical exposure often test positive for the anti-Scl-70 (topoisomerase) autoantibody.

Several other agents are able to provoke scleroderma or scleroderma-like dis-ease. Vinyl -chloride disease[9] was observed among workers exposed to this com-pound during its manufacturing process. Swollen fingers, skin induration, Raynaud's phenomenon, and acro-osteolysis were the most prevalent symptoms. The severity of bone loss and pattern of radiologic changes were often striking and different from the distal ischemia-associated tuft loss observed in cases of idiopathic systemic sclerosis. Upper abdominal complaints, thrombocytopenia, tiredness, and dizziness were often present. Paresthesias, CNS symptoms, headache, memory loss, insomnia and non-cirrhotic hepatic fibrosis were also noted in some patients. Vinyl chloride disease has largely ceased to exist now that exposure has been limited by changes made to the manufacturing process.

Exposure to silica-containing dust by inhalation also is associated with a higher risk of developing SSc.[9] Certain clinical features of occupational SSc may differ in some respects from idiopathic SSc; for example, the greater prevalence of pulmo-nary involvement in patients with silica dust exposure.[17,19] Concerning silica-induced SSc, the presence of muscle involvement, Raynaud's phenomenon, or esophageal dysphagia is less frequent[17] or similar in prevalence,[19] when compared with idio-pathic SSc. Antinuclear antibodies (ANA) and anti-topoisomerase (Scl-70) antibod-ies were found in similar frequency, in both occupationally induced and idiopathic scleroderma.[18]

Eosinophilia-myalgia syndrome (EMS) and toxic oil syndrome (TOS) are two other scleroderma-like syndromes provoked by chemical agents.[5] Nephrogenic sys-temic fibrosis (NSF) is another recently described environmental exposure reported to be associated with a scleroderma-like syndrome (see Chap. 9). Epoxy-resin inha-lation has been reported to occur in association with skin changes of generalized morphea.[16]

With regard to drugs, anticancer chemotherapeutic agents are being increasingly associated with vascular and cutaneous syndromes that resemble systemic sclerosis. This includes cytostatic agents such as taxanes, for example, docetaxel and paclitaxel, which may lead to scleroderma-like skin changes predominantly on the extremities and typically on the lower extremities. Other cytostatic agents, for example, gemcitabine, bleomycin, peplomycin, melphalan, capecitabine, and uracyl-tegafur, are also capable of provoking scleroderma-like, predominantly morphea, skin changes.[20-24] Appetite suppressants, valproic acid, methysergide, and other agents including bromocriptine, ethosuximide, and balicatib (cathepsin K inhibitor) have also been reported to provoke morphea-like skin changes. The opioid analgesic ketobemidone prescribed for chronic pain may cause woody induration and multiple irregular ulcers and scars surrounded by hyperpigmentation on the upper and lower extremities. Certain local injections (corticosteroid, vitamins K, and B12, pentazocine) also may provoke localized scleroderma-like skin changes.

In summary, our patient developed typical diffuse scleroderma with extensive skin involvement, interstitial lung disease, heart and esophageal involvement following chronic occupational exposure to organic solvents. Solvents should be considered a provoking factor for the development of idiopathic systemic sclerosis, although the exact mechanism whereby these various chemicals initiate the disease process is not well understood. The occupational case history should be carefully evaluated in all patients with either the systemic or localized form of scleroderma since a wide spectrum of chemicals and drugs have been implicated to provoke scleroderma or scleroderma-like disorders.

References

1. Garcia-Zamalloa AM, Ojeda E, Gonzalez-Beneitez C, Goni J, Garrido A. Systemic sclerosis and organic solvents: early diagnosis in industry. *Ann Rheum Dis*. 1994;53:618.
2. Nietert PJ, Sutherland SE, Silver RM, et al. Is occupational organic solvent exposure a risk factor for scleroderma? *Arthritis Rheum*. 1998;41:1111-1118.
3. Czirják L, Bokk Á, Csontos G, L rincz G, Szegedi G. Clinical findings in 61 patients with progressive systemic sclerosis. *Acta Derm Venereol*. 1989;69:533-536.
4. Czirják L, Kumánovics G. Exposure to solvents as a provoking factor for systemic sclerosis and Raynaud's phenomenon. *Clin Rheumatol*. 2002;21:114-118.
5. Bolster MB, Silver RM. Other fibrosing skin disorders. In: Clements PJ, Furst DE, eds. *Systemic Sclerosis*. Philadelphia: Lippincott Williams & Wilkins; 2004:121-9.
6. Aryal BK, Khuder SA, Schaub EA. Meta-analysis of systemic sclerosis and exposure to solvents. *Am J Ind Med*. 2001;40:271-274.
7. Bovenzi M, Barbone F, Pisa FE, et al. A case-control study of occupational exposures and systemic sclerosis. *Int Arch Occup Environ Health*. 2004;77:10-16.
8. Czirják L, Szegedi G. Benzene exposure and systemic sclerosis. *Ann Intern Med*. 1987;107:1181.
9. Nietert P, Silver R. Systemic sclerosis: environmental and occupational risk factors. *Cur Opin Rheumatol*. 2000;12:520-526.
10. Diot E, Lesire V, Guilmot JL, et al. Systemic sclerosis and occupational risk factors: a case-control study. *Occup Environ Med*. 2002;59:545-549.

11. Granel B, Zemour F, Lehucher-Michel MP, et al. Occupational exposure and systemic sclerosis. Literature review and result of a self-reported questionnaire. *Rev Méd Interne*. 2008;29:891-900.
12. Kütting B, Uter W, Drexler H. Is occupational exposure to solvents associated with an increased risk for developing systemic scleroderma? *J Occup Med Toxicol*. 2006;1:15.
13. Kettaneh A, Al Moufti O, Tiev KP, et al. Occupational exposure to solvents and gender-related risk of systemic sclerosis: a metaanalysis of case-control studies. *J Rheumatol*. 2007;34:97-103.
14. Czirják L, Dankó K, Schlammadinger J, Surányi P, Tamási L, Szegedi G. Progressive systemic sclerosis occurring in patients exposed to chemicals. *Int J Dermatol*. 1987;26:374-378.
15. Silman AJ, Jones S. What is the contribution of occupational environmental factors to the occurrence of scleroderma in men? *Ann Rheum Dis*. 1992;51:1322-1324.
16. Yamakage A, Ishikawa H. Generalized morphea-like scleroderma occurring in people exposed to organic solvents. *Dermatologica*. 1982;165:186-193.
17. Cowie RL. Silica-dust-exposed mine workers with scleroderma (systemic sclerosis). *Chest*. 1987;92:260-262.
18. Mora GF. Systemic sclerosis: environmental factors. *J Rheumatol*. 2009;36:2383-2396.
19. Rustin MH, Bull HA, Ziegler V, et al. Silica-associated systemic sclerosis is clinically, serologically and immunologically indistinguishable from idiopathic systemic sclerosis. *Br J Dermatol*. 1990;123:725-734.
20. Itoh M, Yanaba K, Kobayashi T, Nakagawa H. Taxane-induced scleroderma. *Br J Dermatol*. 2007;156:363-367.
21. Cleveland MG, Ajaikumar BS, Reganti R. Cutaneous fibrosis induced by docetaxel: a case report. *Cancer*. 2000;88:1078-1081.
22. Läuchli S, Trüeb RM, Fehr M, Hafner J. Scleroderma-like drug reaction to paclitaxel (Taxol). *Br J Dermatol*. 2002;147:619-621.
23. De Angelis R, Bugatti L, Cerioni A, Del Medico P, Filosa G. Diffuse scleroderma occurring after the use of paclitaxel for ovarian cancer. *Clin Rheumatol*. 2003;22:49-52.
24. Asano Y, Ihn H, Shikada J, Kadono T, Kikuchi K, Tamaki K. A case of peplomycin-induced scleroderma. *Br J Dermatol*. 2004;150:1213-1214.

Chapter 9
A 65-Year-Old Woman with Hardened Skin, Joint Contractures, and Yellow Scleral Plaques

Jonathan Kay

Keywords Nephrogenic systemic fibrosis • Chronic kidney disease • Contrast media • Gadolinium • Gadolinium DTPA • Gadodiamide • Imatinib

A 65-year-old woman who was receiving hemodialysis for stage 5 chronic kidney disease (GFR <15 mL/min/1.73 m^2), resulting from type 2 non-insulin-dependent diabetes mellitus and hypertension, presented with a 4-year history of progressive hardening of the skin on her arms and legs and flexion contractures of her fingers, elbows, and knees. Three months before she first noticed hardening of the skin on her lower legs, she had undergone MR angiography of her head and neck with Magnevist® (gadopentetate dimeglumine) contrast to evaluate new focal neurologic deficits. One year after the onset of the skin changes on her legs, she again underwent MR angiography with Magnevist® contrast, this time to evaluate the arteries in her pelvis and lower extremities. Over the subsequent 4 years, the skin on both legs and, subsequently, on both arms became firm to touch and unable to be pinched. She observed the skin on her arms and legs to be darker in color than unaffected skin.

As her skin changes progressed, she lost the ability to fully extend either knee and had difficulty walking independently. She used a walker to assist in ambulation and a wheelchair when she had to move any distance. She also developed fixed flexion contractures of the fingers of both hands and was unable to place either hand flat on a table top. She experienced increasing difficulty buttoning and had to use both hands to lift a cup to her mouth. She became unable to fully extend either elbow. Her skin changes were extremely painful, necessitating the regular use of propoxyphene-acetaminophen, 100–325 mg two tablets taken by mouth three times daily.

J. Kay
Rheumatology Division, Department of Medicine, UMass Memorial Medical Center,
University of Massachusetts Medical School, 119 Belmont Street,
Worcester, MA 01605, USA

R.M. Silver and C.P. Denton (eds.), *Case Studies in Systemic Sclerosis*,
DOI: 10.1007/978-0-85729-641-2_9, © Springer-Verlag London Limited 2011

The patient had no history of Raynaud's phenomenon and noted no skin changes on her face. When serological studies revealed a positive ANA, she was referred to a rheumatologist for further evaluation.

Physical Examination

Temperature 36.7°C; pulse 64 bpm; respirations 14 per minute; blood pressure 110/62 mmHg. Skin: cobblestoning of the skin on her lower back, buttocks, and both legs; hyperpigmentation, marked induration, and tethering of the skin on her arms and legs and in her perineum with firm fullness of the skin in each popliteal fossa, more pronounced on the right. HEENT: yellow scleral plaques nasal and temporal to the iris on her left eye, but not on her right eye; normal oral aperture. Chest: no adventitial breath sounds. Cardiac: regular rate with normal S1 and S2 heart sounds. Abdomen: nondistended and non-tender. Extremities: a nonfunctioning arteriovenous fistula was present on her left forearm and a functioning arteriovenous fistula was present on her left upper arm. Neurologic: decreased sensation to light touch on her legs in a stocking distribution to the mid-calf bilaterally; normal sensation in her upper extremities. Musculoskeletal: 60° flexion contracture of her right elbow and 30° flexion contracture of her left elbow; 30° flexion contractures of both knees; fixed flexion contractures of the fingers of both hands with the inability to flatten either hand; no joint tenderness or swelling. Nailfold capillary microscopy revealed normal capillary loops without capillary dropout.

Laboratory Findings

CBC: normal. Chemistry panel (predialysis): normal serum electrolytes, blood glucose 132 mg/dL, BUN 37 mg/dL, serum creatinine 4.54 mg/dL, serum calcium 9.8 mg/dL, and serum phosphorus 6.0 mg/dL. ANA by IIF positive (titer 1:160; homogeneous pattern); no antibodies to Scl-70; serum protein electrophoresis demonstrated a mild diffuse increase in gamma globulin but no monoclonal protein. Echocardiogram: Normal LV function; LV ejection fraction 60–65%; moderate-to-severe hypokinesis of the inferior base; indirect evidence of elevated left ventricular end diastolic pressures and of elevated left atrial pressures by way of abnormal mitral inflow pattern and abnormal pulmonary vein tracing; significant pulmonary hypertension with estimated RVSP 55 mmHg.

Course

A diagnosis of nephrogenic systemic fibrosis (NSF) was made based on the following clinical findings: hyperpigmentation, marked induration, and tethering of the skin on her arms and legs and in her perineum; fixed flexion contractures of her fingers, elbows, and knees; and yellow scleral plaques on her left eye. This diagnosis was supported by the timing of the onset of her condition, with the clinical features developing shortly after exposure to a gadolinium-containing contrast agent in the setting of stage 5 chronic kidney disease. Also supporting this diagnosis were the absence of Raynaud's phenomenon, lack of involvement of the skin on the face, and absence of paraproteinemia. Her low titer of circulating antinuclear antibodies was unassociated with the diagnosis of NSF.

Biopsy of skin from her forearm demonstrated "deep dermal and subcutaneous fibrosis with mildly increased fibroblasts, consistent with NSF in the appropriate clinical setting." Inductively coupled plasma mass spectroscopy demonstrated 54 ppm gadolinium in her skin biopsy specimen.

Treatment with oral imatinib mesylate 400 mg daily was initiated with rapid and marked reduction of her skin induration and tethering. Because imatinib mesylate is metabolized in the liver and its metabolites are more than 90% eliminated through the bile, the dose of imatinib mesylate does not need to be adjusted in the setting of renal dysfunction or dialysis treatment.[1] She also underwent physical therapy, including passive and active range of motion exercises, with subsequent improvement in her elbow and knee joint flexion contractures.

Discussion

Nephrogenic systemic fibrosis (NSF) was first observed in 1997, when several patients with stage 5 chronic kidney disease developed skin changes resembling scleromyxedema after renal transplantation at Sharp Memorial Hospital in San Diego, California.[2] Because it appeared to involve predominantly the skin, this disease was initially called "nephrogenic fibrosing dermopathy."[3] Typically, hyperpigmentation, induration, and tethering of skin begins on the distal lower extremities and progresses to involve both legs and arms.[4] The skin cannot be pinched and often has a cobblestone appearance that is caused by deep induration of the dermis of the upper arms and thighs. Follicular dimpling (*peau d'orange*) may be present in areas of affected skin on the extremities (Figs. 9.1 and 9.2). Hypopigmented, pink or flesh-colored macules or papules may coalesce into patches or thin plaques, most commonly on the arms. Truncal involvement is variable and usually to a much lesser degree than that of skin on the extremities. In contrast to scleromyxedema and scleroderma, the skin of the face is almost never involved. As affected skin around joints tightens, patients develop debilitating flexion contractures that significantly limit mobility, most characteristically involving the knees, fingers, and elbows (Fig. 9.3).

Following the identification of extracutaneous fibrosis involving lymph nodes, thyroid, esophagus, heart, lungs, liver, diaphragm, skeletal muscle, genitourinary tract, and dura mater, "nephrogenic fibrosing dermopathy" was renamed "nephrogenic systemic fibrosis."[5,6] Patients with NSF may develop interstitial pulmonary fibrosis. Also, as in this patient, thickening and fibrosis of the adventitial layer of the walls of small pulmonary arterioles can result in pulmonary hypertension.[7] When

Fig. 9.1 A patient with nephrogenic systemic fibrosis exhibiting fixed flexion contractures of her fingers, elbows, and knees. The skin on her forearms is hyperpigmented and that on her arms and legs is markedly indurated. Deep induration of the skin on her legs produces a cobblestone appearance, which is most pronounced medially, and follicular dimpling (*peau d'orange* changes)

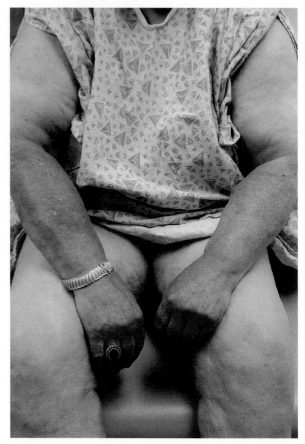

Fig. 9.2 Indurated skin on both legs of a patient with nephrogenic systemic fibrosis, with follicular dimpling (*peau d'orange* changes) and a cobblestone appearance that is most pronounced on the medial thighs. There also are flexion contractures of the knees

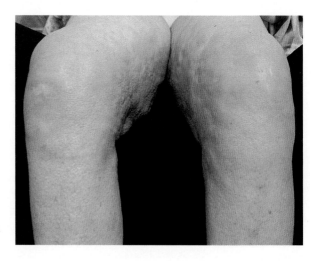

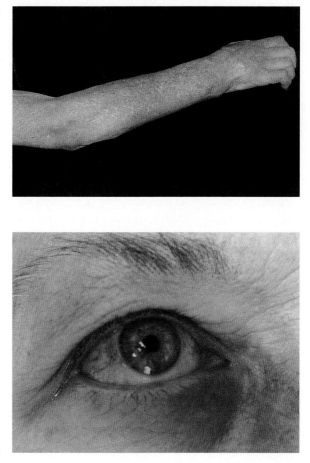

Fig. 9.3 Hyperpigmentation, induration, and tethering of skin on the arm of a patient with nephrogenic systemic fibrosis with fixed flexion contractures of the fingers and elbow

Fig. 9.4 Yellow scleral plaques, adjacent to the iris, with scleral capillary dilatation in a patient with nephrogenic systemic fibrosis

cutaneous changes of NSF are present in patients with stage 5 chronic kidney disease, the risk of dying within 2 years is increased by 2.5-fold compared to individuals receiving hemodialysis who do not have these skin changes.[8] This increased mortality most likely reflects involvement of vital organs, such as the heart and lungs.

Many patients with NSF have yellow plaques on their sclerae, adjacent to the iris, that often are accompanied by dilated conjunctival capillaries[9] (Fig. 9.4). These yellow scleral plaques resemble pingueculae, which develop in otherwise healthy individuals and are most prevalent with advanced age. Thus, in a younger individual with chronic kidney disease and characteristic skin changes, the presence of yellow scleral plaques provides additional support for the diagnosis of NSF.

Grobner first suggested a possible causative role for gadolinium-containing contrast agents in the pathogenesis of NSF after he observed five of nine patients in his hemodialysis unit who developed characteristic skin changes of NSF within days to weeks following MR angiography with Omniscan® (gadodiamide).[10] In a cohort of patients with stage 5 chronic kidney disease receiving hemodialysis in five outpatient centers, we demonstrated a very strong association between prior exposure to a gadolinium-containing contrast agent and the subsequent development of characteristic skin changes of NSF (Odds Ratio 14.7).[8] NSF has also occurred following the administration of other gadolinium-containing contrast agents, especially Magnevist® (gadopentetate dimeglumine) and OptiMARK® (gadoversetamide).[11] Within 3 months after the last Magnevist® administration, skin changes of NSF developed in 66% of 36 patients with stage 5 chronic kidney disease.[12] Among these patients, higher cumulative and higher total doses of gadolinium-containing contrast were associated with an increased risk of developing NSF. Thus, the association between gadolinium-containing contrast exposure and the onset of NSF among patients with chronic kidney disease appears to be both time- and dose-dependent.

NSF can be differentiated from most other fibrosing disorders based upon the characteristic appearance and anatomic distribution of its skin changes and the absence of clinical and laboratory findings typical of the other diseases. The absence of facial involvement and of Raynaud's phenomenon, as well as the normal nailfold capillary morphology in this patient, distinguishes NSF from scleroderma. Her circulating antinuclear antibodies are unrelated to her diagnosis of NSF, which is not an autoimmune disease. Other autoantibodies that occur in patients with diffuse or limited systemic sclerosis, such as anti-topoisomerase I and anticentromere antibodies, usually are absent in patients with NSF. Although the histological appearance of NSF may be indistinguishable from that of scleromyxedema, NSF does not usually involve the skin of the face or neck and is not associated with paraproteinemia. The skin on the upper back, which is typically indurated in patients with scleredema associated with diabetes mellitus (scleredema diabeticorum), also usually is not affected in NSF. Although the skin changes of chronic graft-versus-host disease resemble those of NSF, chronic graft-versus-host disease occurs in the setting of prior bone marrow transplantation and frequently involves the trunk. Morphea may present with localized, linear cutaneous fibrosis and hyperpigmentation, but lacks the typical symmetric distribution of NSF, as well as the systemic features of NSF. NSF may be mistaken for lipodermatosclerosis in patients who have skin changes involving only their legs; however, lipodermatosclerosis typically does not involve the skin on the arms or cause joint contractures. The clinical appearance of eosinophilic fasciitis on the extremities is similar to that of NSF, but peripheral eosinophilia is not a feature of NSF and these two conditions have different histologic appearances. Individuals with stage 5 chronic kidney disease and β_2-microglobulin amyloidosis may develop fixed flexion contractures of their fingers, but these are not accompanied by fibrosis of the overlying skin.

A deep punch biopsy of clinically affected skin helps to confirm the diagnosis of NSF. An increased number of spindle-shaped fibroblast-like cells in the dermis, demonstrating co-localization of staining for CD34 and procollagen I, is the most characteristic histopathological feature of NSF. These cells are thought to be derived from circulating fibrocytes that migrate to and differentiate in tissues containing gadolinium, where they secrete profibrotic growth factors and cytokines and contribute to extracellular matrix production.[13] The spindle cells intercalate around dermal collagen bundles, many of which are thickened, that typically are separated by adjacent clefts.[3] Preserved elastic fibers entwine these collagen bundles. Increased numbers of mono- and multinucleated cells, which stain with antibodies to both factor XIIIa and CD68, may also be present. These histological changes may extend into the subcutis layer. Dermal calcification, osteoclast-like giant cells, and osseous metaplasia may be observed.[14,15] When present, osseous tissue formed around elastic fibers (sclerotic bodies) is highly specific for NSF.[16] Few, if any, chronic inflammatory cells are present. Because not all biopsies of involved skin are diagnostic, especially early in the evolution of clinical findings, the failure to demonstrate characteristic histological features of NSF does not exclude the diagnosis; another biopsy performed several months later may corroborate the diagnosis. As in this patient's skin biopsy, gadolinium may be quantified by inductively coupled plasma mass spectroscopy.[17] However, this remains an investigational study that is not readily available in clinical practice.

Although several cases of NSF have been described with no history of antecedent exposure to a gadolinium-containing contrast agent, none of these case reports assessed skin biopsy specimens for tissue gadolinium content.[18-20] Thus, these patients may have received a gadolinium-containing contrast agent but did not recall or were not aware of such exposure. No case of NSF has yet been identified in which there has been neither a history of prior gadolinium-containing contrast exposure nor gadolinium demonstrated in tissue.

A number of treatments have been attempted but have failed to improve skin changes of NSF. These include potent topical corticosteroids, selective H2-receptor antagonists such as cimetidine and ranitidine, cyclosporine, prednisone, immunosuppressive agents, photopheresis, and plasmapheresis.[21,2223] Subjective skin softening has been described following extracorporeal photopheresis with ultraviolet-A light in 8 of 14 patients with NSF, 5 of whom exhibited improvement in ambulation.[24-26] Other treatments reported to improve skin changes and decrease pain in individual patients with NSF include pentoxyphylline,[10] sodium thiosulfate,[27] and rapamycin.[28]

As evidenced by the patient described above, imatinib mesylate treatment may lead to rapid improvement in skin induration and reduction in joint contractures in some patients with NSF.[23] These observations have been confirmed in an open-label trial in which imatinib mesylate was administered to 11 patients with NSF [www.ClinicalTrials.gov Identifier: NCT00677092].[29] Gadolinium deposited in the skin of patients with NSF might serve as a persistent stimulus for fibrosis that induces production of profibrotic cytokines. By selectively inhibiting signal transduction mediated by c-Abl, c-Kit, and the platelet-derived growth factor-BB receptor and by Smad-independent signaling through the TGFβ receptor, imatinib mesylate may decrease fibrosis in NSF.

Given that NSF was initially observed in patients who had recently received renal allografts, restoration of normal kidney function by renal transplantation does not appear to significantly improve tissue fibrosis in patients with NSF. It is not clear that performing hemodialysis after MRI with gadolinium-containing contrast, even immediately after the imaging procedure, will effectively reduce the risk of developing NSF in an individual whose kidney function is compromised. In patients with stage 5 CKD, only 78% of the gadolinium administered as Magnevist® is removed from the blood after a single 4 h hemodialysis session; 96% is removed after a second session and 99% is removed after a third session.[30] Because the rapidity with which free gadolinium dissociates from its chelate and becomes bound to tissue is unknown, even the small amount of gadolinium that remains after a hemodialysis treatment may be sufficient to deposit in tissue and induce fibrosis.

The only effective strategy to prevent the development of NSF is to avoid exposing individuals with impaired renal function to gadolinium-containing contrast agents. The United States Food & Drug Administration has placed a black box warning on all marketed gadolinium-containing contrast agents, informing about the risk of NSF and instructing that these agents not be administered to individuals with "chronic, severe kidney disease (GFR <30 mL/min/1.73 m²), or acute kidney injury." However, because NSF has occurred in individuals with stage 3 CKD (GFR 30–59 mL/min/1.73 m²),[31] administration of gadolinium-containing contrast agents probably should be avoided in patients with GFR <60 mL/min/1.73 m², unless the diagnostic information is critical and cannot be obtained by MRI without using gadolinium-containing contrast or by other imaging modalities.

In summary, one should consider the diagnosis of NSF in any patient with underlying chronic kidney disease who exhibits hyperpigmentation, marked induration, and tethering of skin on their extremities. Fixed flexion contractures of the fingers, elbows, or knees, and yellow scleral plaques may also be present. A temporal relationship between prior exposure to a gadolinium-containing contrast agent and the onset of clinical features of NSF supports the diagnosis. Skin biopsy demonstrating increased numbers of CD34+/procollagen I+ spindle-shaped fibroblast-like cells in the dermis and thickened collagen bundles separated by adjacent clefts confirms the diagnosis of NSF in a patient with characteristic clinical features. Systemic involvement contributes to significant morbidity and mortality. However, treatment with tyrosine kinase inhibitors may reverse existing fibrosis and prevent progression of disease in some NSF patients.

References

1. Gibbons J, Egorin MJ, Ramanathan RK, et al. Phase I and pharmacokinetic study of imatinib mesylate in patients with advanced malignancies and varying degrees of renal dysfunction: a study by the National Cancer Institute Organ Dysfunction Working Group. *J Clin Oncol.* 2008;26:570-576.
2. Fibrosing skin condition among patients with renal disease – United States and Europe, 1997–2002. *MMWR Morb Mortal Wkly Rep.* 2002;51:25-26.
3. Cowper SE, Su LD, Bhawan J, Robin HS, LeBoit PE. Nephrogenic fibrosing dermopathy. *Am J Dermatopathol.* 2001;23:383-393.
4. Cowper SE, Robin HS, Steinberg SM, Su LD, Gupta S, LeBoit PE. Scleromyxoedema-like cutaneous diseases in renal-dialysis patients. *Lancet.* 2000;356:1000-1001.
5. Koreishi AF, Nazarian RM, Saenz AJ, et al. Nephrogenic systemic fibrosis: a pathologic study of autopsy cases. *Arch Pathol Lab Med.* 2009;133:1943-1948.

6. Kay J, Bazari H, Avery LL, Koreishi AF. Case records of the Massachusetts general hospital. Case 6–2008. A 46-year-old woman with renal failure and stiffness of the joints and skin. *N Engl J Med.* 2008;358:827-838.

7. Jimenez SA, Artlett CM, Sandorfi N, et al. Dialysis-associated systemic fibrosis (nephrogenic fibrosing dermopathy): study of inflammatory cells and transforming growth factor beta1 expression in affected skin. *Arthritis Rheum.* 2004;50:2660-2666.

8. Todd DJ, Kagan A, Chibnik LB, Kay J. Cutaneous changes of nephrogenic systemic fibrosis: predictor of early mortality and association with gadolinium exposure. *Arthritis Rheum.* 2007;56:3433-3441.

9. Streams BN, Liu V, Liegeois N, Moschella SM. Clinical and pathologic features of nephrogenic fibrosing dermopathy: a report of two cases. *J Am Acad Dermatol.* 2003;48:42-47.

10. Grobner T. Gadolinium–a specific trigger for the development of nephrogenic fibrosing dermopathy and nephrogenic systemic fibrosis? *Nephrol Dial Transplant.* 2006;21: 1104-1108.

11. Broome DR. Nephrogenic systemic fibrosis associated with gadolinium based contrast agents: a summary of the medical literature reporting. *Eur J Radiol.* 2008;66:230-234.

12. Abujudeh HH, Kaewlai R, Kagan A, et al. Nephrogenic systemic fibrosis after gadopentetate dimeglumine exposure: case series of 36 patients. *Radiology.* 2009;253:81-89.

13. Cowper SE, Bucala R. Nephrogenic fibrosing dermopathy: suspect identified, motive unclear. *Am J Dermatopathol.* 2003;25:358.

14. Ruiz-Genao DP, Pascual-Lopez MP, Fraga S, Aragues M, Garcia-Diez A. Osseous metaplasia in the setting of nephrogenic fibrosing dermopathy. *J Cutan Pathol.* 2005;32:172-175.

15. Hershko K, Hull C, Ettefagh L, et al. A variant of nephrogenic fibrosing dermopathy with osteoclast-like giant cells: a syndrome of dysregulated matrix remodeling? *J Cutan Pathol.* 2004;31:262-265.

16. Bhawan J, Swick BL, Koff AB, Stone MS. Sclerotic bodies in nephrogenic systemic fibrosis: a new histopathologic finding. *J Cutan Pathol.* 2009;36:548-552.

17. High WA, Ayers RA, Cowper SE. Gadolinium is quantifiable within the tissue of patients with nephrogenic systemic fibrosis. *J Am Acad Dermatol.* 2007;56:710-712.

18. Wahba IM, Simpson EL, White K. Gadolinium is not the only trigger for nephrogenic systemic fibrosis: insights from two cases and review of the recent literature. *Am J Transplant.* 2007;7:2425-2432.

19. Weiss AS, Lucia MS, Teitelbaum I. A case of nephrogenic fibrosing dermopathy/nephrogenic systemic fibrosis. *Nat Clin Pract Nephrol.* 2007;3:111-115.

20. Anavekar NS, Chong AH, Norris R, Dowling J, Goodman D. Nephrogenic systemic fibrosis in a gadolinium-naive renal transplant recipient. *Australas J Dermatol.* 2008;49:44-47.

21. Baron PW, Cantos K, Hillebrand DJ, et al. Nephrogenic fibrosing dermopathy after liver transplantation successfully treated with plasmapheresis. *Am J Dermatopathol.* 2003;25: 204-209.

22. Swartz RD, Crofford LJ, Phan SH, Ike RW, Su LD. Nephrogenic fibrosing dermopathy: a novel cutaneous fibrosing disorder in patients with renal failure. *Am J Med.* 2003;114:563-572.

23. Kay J, High WA. Imatinib mesylate treatment of nephrogenic systemic fibrosis. *Arthritis Rheum.* 2008;58:2543-2548.

24. Gilliet M, Cozzio A, Burg G, Nestle FO. Successful treatment of three cases of nephrogenic fibrosing dermopathy with extracorporeal photopheresis. *Br J Dermatol.* 2005;152:531-536.

25. Richmond H, Zwerner J, Kim Y, Fiorentino D. Nephrogenic systemic fibrosis: relationship to gadolinium and response to photopheresis. *Arch Dermatol.* 2007;143:1025-1030.

26. Mathur K, Morris S, Deighan C, Green R, Douglas KW. Extracorporeal photopheresis improves nephrogenic fibrosing dermopathy/nephrogenic systemic fibrosis: three case reports and review of literature. *J Clin Apher.* 2008;23:144-150.

27. Yerram P, Saab G, Karuparthi PR, Hayden MR, Khanna R. Nephrogenic systemic fibrosis: a mysterious disease in patients with renal failure–role of gadolinium-based contrast media in causation and the beneficial effect of intravenous sodium thiosulfate. *Clin J Am Soc Nephrol.* 2007;2:258-263.

28. Swaminathan S, Arbiser JL, Hiatt KM, et al. Rapid improvement of nephrogenic systemic fibrosis with rapamycin therapy: possible role of phospho-70-ribosomal-s6 kinase. *J Am Acad Dermatol.* 2010;62:343-345.
29. Kay J, Sullivan ME, Patel TV. Efficacy and safety of oral imatinib mesylate in patients with nephrogenic systemic fibrosis [abstract]. *Arthritis Rheum.* 2009;60:458.
30. Okada S, Katagiri K, Kumazaki T, Yokoyama H. Safety of gadolinium contrast agent in hemodialysis patients. *Acta Radiol.* 2001;42:339-341.
31. Sadowski EA, Bennett LK, Chan MR, et al. Nephrogenic systemic fibrosis: risk factors and incidence estimation. *Radiology.* 2007;243:148-157.

Chapter 10
Painful Digital Ulcers in a Scleroderma Patient with Raynaud's Phenomenon

Fredrick M. Wigley and Peter K. Wung

Keywords Raynaud's phenomenon • Digital ischemia • Digital ulcer • Vasodilator • Scleroderma

Case Study

At age 28, a Caucasian woman noted for the first time that she was unusually sensitive to cold temperatures. She complained that while in the frozen food department of her favorite grocery store her fingers would become ice cold and pale in color. The pallor of the skin extended from the fingertips to the proximal fingers and was associated with numbness, a sensation of pins and needles, and pain on her distal fingers (Fig. 10.1a). When attempting to warm her hands the fingers first looked blue-black (Fig. 10.1b) and then in about 15 min after rewarming the fingers felt flushed and they looked blushed and red. She noted that not only direct cold exposure to the hands would trigger these color changes but also similar events occurred when she felt anxious or had a sense of her whole body being cold. After several weeks, she noted that her fingers were swollen such that her rings did not fit. Soon thereafter, even exposure to her office air conditioning, cold breezes, inactivity, and simple social interactions triggered more events. The discomfort on her fingertips made it difficult for her to use her computer. The number of times the fingers were cold and discolored averaged 6–10 times daily and seemed worse on her index and middle fingers and less so on the thumb. She then noted similar discomfort in her toes. Suddenly, a severe event happened on her right index finger with extreme pain

F.M. Wigley (✉)
Department of Medicine, Division of Rheumatology, Johns Hopkins
University School of Medicine, 5200 Eastern Avenue, Suite 4100,
Mason F. Lord Building, Center Tower, Baltimore, MD 21224, USA

R.M. Silver and C.P. Denton (eds.), *Case Studies in Systemic Sclerosis*,
DOI: 10.1007/978-0-85729-641-2_10, © Springer-Verlag London Limited 2011

Fig. 10.1 (**a**) Photo of the pallor (*white attack*) phase of Raynaud's phenomenon during which there is a reduction of total blood flow to the skin of the involved digits. (**b**) Photo of the cyanotic (*blue attack*) phase of Raynaud's phenomenon during which there is reduced blood flow in the thermoregulatory skin blood vessels

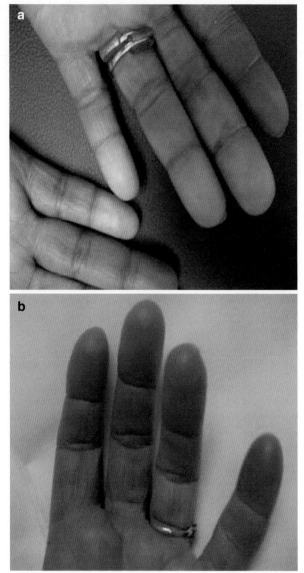

and discoloration that did not improve even after warming the fingers. The fingertip remained blue and then she developed a deep, painful ulcer on the palmer side of the fingertip. Her present and past medical history was otherwise negative. She was a nonsmoker, had no history or risk factors for vascular disease or no venous clotting events, and was not taking any medication. She had had two uneventful pregnancies. She denied trauma to the hands and had no exposure to toxins or illicit drugs. There was a negative family history for Raynaud's phenomenon or autoimmune diseases.

Physical Examination

Vital signs were normal with blood pressure equal in both arms. The general exam was otherwise normal except for signs of scleroderma with sclerodactyly and nail-fold capillary dilatation with a few telangiectasia on her lips and palmar surface of several fingers. The index finger was cold to touch, and pressure on the fingertip invoked pain. There was poor capillary refill after compression of the involved index fingertip, and a shallow ischemic ulcer was present (Fig. 10.2). The ulcer was about 3 mm deep with white-yellow discharge and surrounding erythema. Her pulses were strong and no vascular bruits were heard, but Allen's test demonstrated reduced flow through the ulnar artery compared to the radial artery at the wrist bilaterally.

Laboratory Findings

The complete blood count (CBC), general chemistries, and urinalysis were normal; the sedimentation rate was 40 mm/h and C-reactive protein was 2.5 mg/L. Serum protein electrophoresis and lipid profile were normal. Russell Viper Venom test and anticardiolipin antibodies were negative, but anti-beta2glycoprotein1 antibody of IgM isotype was present at high titer. ANA was positive at a titer of 1:1260 showing a centromere pattern. Anti-DNA, Ro, La, Smith, ribonuclear protein, topoisomerase, and RNA polymerase III antibodies were not present. Pulmonary function test (PFT) was normal with a forced vital capacity of 95% predicted and DLco of 98% predicted. Electrocardiogram and echocardiogram were also normal.

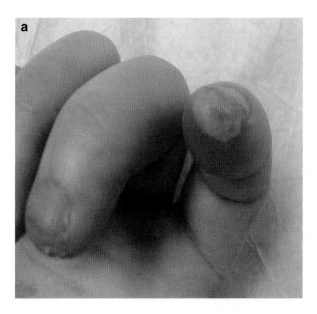

Fig. 10.2 (**a**) Early phase of a digital infarct in a patient with scleroderma. (**b**) Ischemic digital ulcer in a patient with scleroderma

Fig. 10.2 (continued)

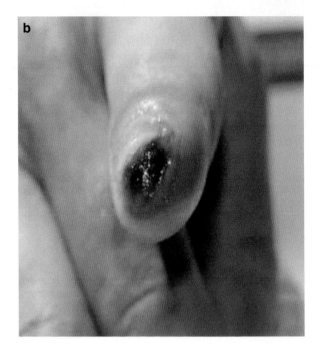

Course

A diagnosis of scleroderma was confirmed by the physical findings and laboratory testing that demonstrated limited skin disease and a positive anti-centromere antibody. Raynaud's phenomenon was the dominant problem and was associated with signs of peripheral vascular disease involving both the microcirculation and larger vessels with possible ulnar artery disease. Doppler studies and magnetic resonance imaging of the arteries (MRA) of the arm and hand demonstrated severe small artery disease of the palmar arch and digital vessels without significant correctable macrovascular disease. The patient was educated about cold avoidance and stress management as nondrug therapy for Raynaud's phenomenon. She was given a note to allow her have a space heater at work and given parking disability to allow her to park close to her office during the winter months. The active ulcer site was treated by cleaning with soap and water twice daily, followed by application of an antibacterial cream (muprocin 2%), and she was given oxycodone plus acetaminophen (5/500) to use as needed for pain. A topical preparation of lidocaine/prilocaine (2.5%/2.5%) was given to apply locally around the ulcer for pain control. She was started on a calcium channel blocker (amlodipine 5 mg), low-dose (81 mg) aspirin daily, and a statin (atrovastatin 10 mg). The initial ulcer healed in about 6 weeks, yet over the next several months new ulcers occurred on middle right finger and the left index finger. Amlopidine was titrated upward to maximal tolerated dose of 15 mg, but new ulcers continued to occur. Therefore, sildenafil 20 mg three times daily was added to the amlodipine, and atrovastatin was increased to 40 mg daily. She was well for several months but despite this therapy, she developed a painful left index finger with signs of critical ischemia and severe compromise to the distal finger. The digital tip began to ulcerate and the deeper tissue was threatened with signs of no blood flow. She was hospitalized and given intravenous epoprostenol sodium starting at 0.5 ng/kg/min and titrated to 2.0 ng/kg/min through a peripheral vein for 3 days. The finger rapidly improved and she was discharged on her usual medications. For the following year all the ulcers healed, no new ulcers occurred and she thought her Raynaud's phenomenon was overall much milder as documented by a reduction in Raynaud's Condition Score completed by the patient at her last visit.

Discussion

Raynaud's phenomenon (RP) is seen in over 95% of patients with SSc and is often the first symptom of the disease. It appears as triphasic color changes (pallor, cyanosis, and hyperemia) of the digits of the hands and feet and represents the clinical manifestation of disease of the thermoregulatory vessels and medium-sized and small arteries of the peripheral circulation. Normally, during local or whole body cooling, blood flow to the skin is reduced to prevent heat loss. This response to cold is mediated by reflex activation of the sympathetic nervous system and by a direct effect of cold on cutaneous blood vessels.[1]

Thermoregulation is further accomplished by numerous arteriovenous anastomoses (AVA), low-resistance conduits that allow shunting of blood from arterioles to venules at high flow rates. These thermoregulatory vessels allow a rapid shift of blood to the skin (a blush) when hot and into deeper tissue circulation and away from the surface when exposed to cold. Cyanosis is seen with reduced blood flow to the skin secondary to vasoconstriction of superficial thermoregulatory arteries in the skin. Pallor of the skin is seen because of a compromise to both capillary and total digital artery blood flow and, as such, white attacks are associated with tissue ischemia and are of greater clinical importance.

Scleroderma vascular disease is secondary to an obliterative vasculopathy causing not only vasospasm but also structural disease of the involved vessels.[2] Pathological studies show luminal narrowing of greater than 75% in digital arteries due to intimal fibrosis and luminal occlusion with thrombi.[3] Three major biological processes occur in RP associated with scleroderma: (1) cold-induced vasoconstriction of the peripheral blood vessels occurs via sympathetic stimulation as part of the normal biological response to prevent heat loss; (2) a nonvasculitic vasculopathy is associated with endothelial dysfunction and a fibrotic proliferation of the intimal layer of small arteries, ultimately leading to narrowing of the vessel's lumen; and (3) occlusion of the involved vessels (arteries, arterioles, and capillaries) occurs either secondary to advancing vasculopathy or thrombosis. These three pathways result in critical ischemia, loss of digital tissue, and fibrosis. Management of critical ischemia attempts to address these underlying mechanisms and prevent tissue loss.

Raynaud's phenomenon is seen clinically as attacks triggered by cold exposure or emotional stress. A typical attack will continue with physical signs of ischemia (pallor or cyanosis) until rewarming or removal of provoking stress. It takes about 15 min for recovery, but unlike patients with primary RP who have mild episodes that rarely interfere with daily activities, patients with SSc experience intense and frequent, often painful attacks. The presence of pain is an indication of critical ischemia that precedes tissue injury. A sign of critical ischemia is persistence of sharp demarcation of pallor of the distal finger associated with pain. In addition, the examiner can apply pressure to the fingerpad of the patient's involved digit. If there is a lack of any rebound blood flow on compression and release of pressure, then there is a no-flow state of critical ischemia that heralds tissue infarction. Digital ulcers are representative of vascular involvement in scleroderma and occur in about 30–50% of patients with scleroderma.[4] A variety of ulcers are often present on the hands of patients with scleroderma. Such ulcers are found at the tips of the fingers and on the dorsal surface of the proximal interphalangeal (PIP) and metacarpophalangeal (MCP) joints.[5] The digital tip lesions are typically a consequence of ischemia and can be associated with pain, digital pits, and loss of digital pulp. In contrast, the ulcers located on the dorsum of the PIP and MCP joints are thought to be related to trauma imposed upon the atrophic skin of contracted joints. A positive Allen's test in the wrists is suggestive of medium-sized vessel involvement and should be performed on routine examination of all patients with severe Raynaud's phenomenon and refractory digital ulcers.

Noninvasive assessment of the peripheral circulation will supplement the physical examination and may provide clues as to the cause and size of the vessels involved. Doppler ultrasound is a useful tool and a relatively cost-effective way to evaluate patients with digital ischemia. Magnetic resonance angiography (MRA) is a newer imaging modality that can demonstrate vascular wall changes. MRA shows dramatic arterial changes in patients with SSc compared to other forms of RP.[6] Occasionally, digital subtraction arteriography may be used to exclude features of vasculitis and define the distal circulation more precisely.

Therapeutics

The primary goal in the management of RP is the prevention of digital ischemia through the use of nonpharmacological and pharmacological measures (Fig. 10.3). In the setting of acute digital ischemia, rapid intervention using both treatment modalities is required.

Nonpharmacological Therapies

The primary and most important nonpharmacologic therapy for prevention is the avoidance of cold ambient temperatures, particularly transitioning from a warm or hot environment to a cold one. Additionally, strategies to keep the body and

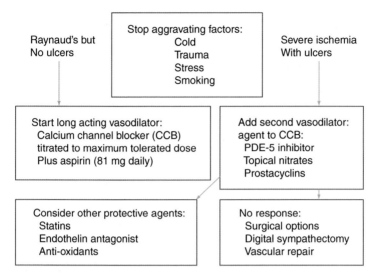

Fig. 10.3 Scheme for managing scleroderma digital ischemia

extremities warm (e.g., dressing warmly or wearing insulating gloves) should be employed. Patients who have an acute ischemic event are best treated by having them rest in a warm environment (home or hospital) while insulating them from any cold temperature (e.g., warm blankets). Other potential therapies include minimizing emotional distress thus reducing sympathetic tone and eliminating any vasoconstricting agents (e.g., use of tobacco or sympathomimetic drugs). Although behavioral therapies (biofeedback autogenic training and classical conditioning) are reported to be helpful, their benefit is controversial and they play no role in the management of acute ischemia related to scleroderma.[7]

Pharmacological Therapies

Calcium channel blockers are considered to be the first-line therapeutic agents in the treatment of RP.[8] This class of medication works primarily by inducing arterial vasodilatation through relaxation of smooth muscle cells; however, they provide additional benefits by reducing oxidative stress and inhibiting platelet activation. The majority of published studies evaluating the efficacy of calcium channel blockers in RP have employed dihydropyridines (e.g., nifedipine, amlodipine, nisoldipine, isradipine, and felodipine). The current recommendation is to use an extended release formulation of nifedipine or amlodipine for treatment of nonurgent RP. The dose should be titrated to clinical efficacy, and common side effects (hypotension, headache, pedal edema) should be monitored.

Nitroglycerin is a potent vasodilator and has been used for many years in the management of RP. Although different formulations exhibit some degree of efficacy, they are all associated with a substantial degree of side effects including headache, dizziness, or local skin irritation. When used, a small amount of 2% nitroglycerin cream may be helpful on a finger with critical ischemia, while taking care to avoid direct contact with any open ulcer. New preparations of topical nitroglycerin gel (e.g., MQX-503) are being studied and show promise.[9]

The three drugs available in the class of a cyclic guanine monophosphate phosphodiesterase type 5 inhibitor include sildenafil, tadalafil, and vardenafil. Sildenafil is thought to be potentially effective in the treatment of RP by sustaining the vasodilatory effect of nitric oxide.[10] In contrast, a recent randomized, placebo-controlled trial using tadalafil suggested no benefit over placebo.[11] Thus, the exact role of these agents has yet to be fully defined.

Prostaglandins are efficacious in the treatment of RP because they are strong vasodilators, inhibit platelet aggregation, and could enhance vascular function through other mechanistic pathways. Intravenous iloprost (a prostacyclin analogue) is efficacious in the treatment of RP.[12] In Europe, iloprost is now available and used via various protocols for severe RP and digital ulcers. In the USA, other prostacyclin analogues, for example, epoprostenol and treprostinil, are available but not yet approved by the FDA for use in RP. Evidence suggests that intermittent use of prostacyclin analogues, either by intravenous or subcutaneous delivery, can treat digital ischemic events. However, oral iloprost, beraprost, and cicaprost showed no significant benefit over placebo. A trial testing a new formulation of oral treprostinil is underway for the treatment of digital ulcers in patients with scleroderma.

Angiotensin-converting enzyme inhibitors and angiotensin receptor blockers can potentially modulate RP. However, a study of quinapril showed no benefit for the occurrence of digital ulcers or the frequency or severity of RP episodes.[13] A study did find that the angiotensin receptor blocker, losartan, was comparable to nifedipine in reducing the severity and frequency of RP attacks.[14]

Bosentan, an endothelin-1 receptor antagonist, was shown in two published clinical trials of SSc patients with digital ulcers to be effective in reducing new digital ulcers formation but did not appear to improve healing of existing ulcers compared to placebo[15,16] While bosentan is now approved in Europe for treatment of SSc with digital ulcers, larger studies will be needed to determine efficacy and long-term outcomes; but these short-term findings are encouraging.

Statins (HMG-CoA reductase inhibitors) can modify endothelial dysfunction, reduce thrombogenicity, reduce certain inflammatory functions, and potentially increase the number of endothelial progenitor cells, thereby improving vascular remodeling after injury. A recently published randomized placebo-controlled study in scleroderma patients showed that atorvastatin significantly reduced the number of digital ulcers and severity of RP.[17]

Other agents that may be helpful include serotonin receptor uptake inhibitors, other phosphodiesterase inhibitors (pentoxifylline; cilostazol); and sympatholytic agents (prazosin, an α1-adrenergic-receptor blocker). Antiplatelet agents (aspirin or clopidogrel) may reduce thrombosis and further vascular injury.

Chronic anticoagulation is not recommended unless there is a concomitant hypercoagulable disorder.

Surgical Interventions

Sympathectomy is a viable option for patients with RP who are unresponsive to medical therapy and should be considered if a critical ischemic event does not quickly respond to medical management. Localized digital sympathectomy with lysis of fibrosis around the vessel is effective for acute ischemia[18] and has mostly replaced central sympathectomy. Improvement of RP after digital sympathectomy can be transient or prolonged. If macrovascular disease is present, the patient should be referred to vascular surgery to consider any surgically correctable lesion.[19] Recently, some patients have reported benefit from local botulinum toxin injection around digital arteries. This may improve pain and potentially reduce vasospasm and may be a chemical sympathectomy. However, more studies are needed to define the role if botulinum toxin injections for RP.

Severe Raynaud's Phenomenon with Digital Ulcers

In patients with digital ulcers and severe RP, we again stress supportive therapy, initiation of low-dose aspirin, and titration of a long-acting calcium channel blocker to the highest dose tolerated. If the patient is still experiencing recurrent ulcers or moderate to severe RP once the calcium channel blocker is at the highest dose tolerated, we then add a second agent. Usually, our second agent is a topical nitrate or a phosphodiesterase inhibitor such as sildenafil; however, both should not be used together as there is a risk of severe hypotension. Intermittent infusion of a prostacyclin analogue (e.g., iloprost or epoprostenol) is considered appropriate in conjunction with the calcium channel blocker. Studies suggest that continued benefit may be seen for about 10 weeks following a 5-day (6 h each day) infusion of iloprost. Alternatively, bosentan, a endothelin-1 antagonist can be used to prevent new digital ulcers. If a combination of medications is not effective for a nonhealing ulcer or chronic digital ischemia, then we pursue digital sympathectomy.

Treatment of Critical Digital Ischemia

Patients who present with signs and symptoms of critical digital ischemia require immediate attention in order to prevent ulceration or digital loss. In addition to initiating nonpharmacologic therapies, starting or maximizing a vasodilator such as a rapid acting calcium channel blocker is strongly recommended. Antiplatelet therapy (daily aspirin or clopidogrel) and unfractionated or low molecular weight heparin should be initiated for 1–3 days if signs of larger vessel occlusion are present. Chemical sympathectomy performed by injection of lidocaine or bupivacaine locally at the base of a digit may rapidly reduce pain and reverse vasospasm. Local nitroglycerin gel applied to the affected digit may also provide some benefit. Although botulinum toxin injections are reported to improve digital ulcer healing and RP,[20] the experience with this treatment is too limited and thus not recommended during an acute crisis. A prostaglandin or prostaglandin analogue can be initiated if the above measures are not helpful. Epoprostenol, iloprost, and treprostinil (prostacyclin analogues) can be administered through a peripheral line continuously for 3–5 days in a closely monitored setting.

References

1. Charkoudian N. Mechanisms and modifiers of reflex induced cutaneous vasodilation and vasoconstriction in humans. *J Appl Physiol*. 2010;109(4):1221-1228.
2. Wigley FM. Vascular disease in scleroderma. *Clin Rev Allergy Immunol*. 2009;36:150-175.
3. Rodnan GP, Myerowitz RL, Justh GO. Morphologic changes in the digital arteries of patients with progressive systemic sclerosis (scleroderma) and Raynaud phenomenon. *Medicine Baltimore*. 1980;59:393-408.
4. Steen V, Denton CP, Pope JE, et al. Digital ulcers: overt vascular disease in systemic sclerosis. *Rheumatology Oxford*. 2009;48(suppl 3):iii19-iii24.
5. Hummers LK, Wigley FM. Management of Raynaud's phenomenon and digital ischemic lesions in scleroderma. *Rheum Dis Clin North Am*. 2003;29:293-313.
6. Allanore Y, Seror R, Chevrot A, et al. Hand vascular involvement assessed by magnetic resonance angiography in systemic sclerosis. *Arthritis Rheum*. 2007;56:2747-2754.
7. Malenfant D, Catton M, Pope JE. The efficacy of complementary and alternative medicine in the treatment of Raynaud's phenomenon: a literature review and meta-analysis. *Rheumatology Oxford*. 2009;48:791-795.
8. Thompson AE, Shea B, Welch V, et al. Calcium-channel blockers for Raynaud's phenomenon in systemic sclerosis. *Arthritis Rheum*. 2001;44:1841-1847.
9. Chung L, Shapiro L, Fiorentino D, et al. MQX-503, a novel formulation of nitroglycerin, improves the severity of Raynaud's phenomenon: a randomized, controlled trial. *Arthritis Rheum*. 2009;60:870-877.
10. Fries R, Shariat K, von Wilmowsky H, et al. Sildenafil in the treatment of Raynaud's phenomenon resistant to vasodilatory therapy. *Circulation*. 2005;112:2980-2985.
11. Schiopu E, Hsu VM, Impens AJ, et al. Randomized placebo-controlled crossover trial of tadalafil in Raynaud's phenomenon secondary to systemic sclerosis. *J Rheumatol*. 2009;36:2264-2268.
12. Wigley FM, Wise RA, Seibold JR, et al. Intravenous iloprost infusion in patients with Raynaud phenomenon secondary to systemic sclerosis. A multicenter, placebo-controlled, double-blind study. *Ann Intern Med*. 1994;120:199-206.
13. Gliddon AE, Doré CJ, Black CM, et al. Prevention of vascular damage in scleroderma and autoimmune Raynaud's phenomenon: a multicenter, randomized, double-blind, placebo-controlled trial of the angiotensin-converting enzyme inhibitor quinapril. *Arthritis Rheum*. 2007;56:3837-3846.
14. Dziadzio M, Denton CP, Smith R, et al. Losartan therapy for Raynaud's phenomenon and scleroderma: clinical and biochemical findings in a fifteen-week, randomized, parallel-group, controlled trial. *Arthritis Rheum*. 1999;42:2646-2655.

15. Korn JH, Mayes M, Matucci-Cerinic M, et al. Digital ulcers in systemic sclerosis: prevention by treatment with bosentan, an oral endothelin receptor antagonist. *Arthritis Rheum.* 2004;50:3985-3993.
16. Matucci-Cerinic M, Denton CP, Furst DE, et al. Bosentan treatment of digital ulcers related to systemic sclerosis: results from the RAPIDS-2 randomized, double-blind, placebo-controlled trial. *Ann Rheum Dis.* 2011;70(1):32-38.
17. Abou-Raya A, Abou-Raya S, Helmii M. Statins: potentially useful in therapy of systemic sclerosis-related Raynaud's phenomenon and digital ulcers. *J Rheumatol.* 2008;35:1801-1808.
18. Bogoch ER, Gross DK. Surgery of the hand in patients with systemic sclerosis: outcomes and considerations. *J Rheumatol.* 2005;32:642-648.
19. Taylor MH, McFadden JA, Bolster MD, Silver RM. Ulnar artery involvement in systemic sclerosis (scleroderma). *J Rheumatol.* 2002;29:102-106.
20. Van Beek AL, Lim PK, Gear AJ, et al. Management of vasospastic disorders with Botulinum toxin A. *Plast Reconstr Surg.* 2007;119:217-226.

Chapter 11
Rapidly Progressive Skin Disease in a Patient with Diffuse Systemic Sclerosis

Elena Schiopu and James R. Seibold

Keywords Systemic sclerosis • Skin fibrosis • Surrogate markers • Occupational therapy

Case Study

A 28-year-old male physician presented with a 4-month history of biphasic color changes of Raynaud's phenomenon (RP) of the fingers, new onset of mild dysphagia, and morning stiffness involving his hands and wrists. At initial assessment, physical exam revealed normal vital signs, mild pitting edema of the fingers, spotty digital cyanosis, nailfold capillary dilatation with minimal drop out, normal mouth aperture of 65 mm, reduction in the wrist flexion/extension by 15°, and incomplete ability to make a fist but no frank synovial thickening. Clinical assessment of skin thickening (modified Rodnan skin score, MRSS) revealed subtle changes over the fingers and possibly the face (total MRSS of 3/51).

Laboratory Findings

Complete blood count (CBC), chemistry panel, hepatitis serology, and urinalysis were normal. Antinuclear antibody (ANA) by immunofluorescense was positive (1:1280, homogeneous pattern) and anti-topoisomerase I (anti-Scl-70) antibody was positive. RF was negative.

J.R. Seibold (✉)
Division of Rheumatology, University of Connecticut Health Center,
Scleroderma Research Consultants, LLC,
97 Deer Run, Avon, CT 06001, USA

R.M. Silver and C.P. Denton (eds.), *Case Studies in Systemic Sclerosis*,
DOI: 10.1007/978-0-85729-641-2_11, © Springer-Verlag London Limited 2011

Fig. 11.1 Bilateral hand involvement in dSSc with skin tightness and flexion contractures involving proximal interphalangeal (PIP), metacarpophalangeal (MCP), and wrist joints

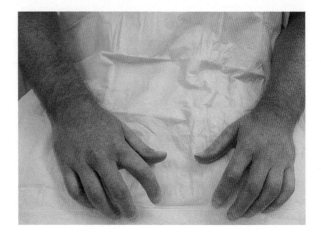

Course

An initial diagnosis of undifferentiated connective tissue disease (UCTD) (suspected early systemic sclerosis) was made and the patient was advised to obtain baseline cardiopulmonary studies, to use lifestyle modification for RP and booked for follow-up in the clinic at 3 months. The patient had his first pulmonary function test (PFT) shortly after his initial visit which showed: forced vital capacity (FVC) of 106% of predicted, total lung capacity (TLC) of 100% of predicted, and diffusion capacity (DLco) of 113% of predicted. He was then lost to follow-up until he returned to clinic 9 months later, having noticed significant tightness of his skin during the previous month. He reported rapid progression of skin thickening including worsening over his face and fingers and new areas of involvement including his arms and legs. Other symptoms included worsening heartburn, new onset of erectile dysfunction, generalized muscle weakness and pain, and significant generalized fatigue. The physical examination revealed worsening MRSS (now 14/51) and confirmed new involvement of the skin on the forearms, upper arms and legs; digital pitting scars; tendon friction rubs over the wrists; worsening flexion contractures of his metacarpophalangeal (MCP), proximal interphalangeal (PIP), and wrist joints (see Fig. 11.1). There were new findings of bibasilar end-expiratory crackles by auscultation of the chest.

At this point, his diagnosis was changed to that of diffuse cutaneous systemic sclerosis (dSSc). His cardiopulmonary workup included repeated PFTs, which confirmed significant deterioration compared with previous assessment (see Table 11.1), a Doppler echocardiogram which revealed normal left and right ventricular function and a small pericardial effusion, and a high-resolution CT scan of the chest which showed intra- and inter-septal thickening, mild bronchiectasis and ground glass opacities consistent with nonspecific interstitial pneumonia (NSIP). The patient was initiated on mycophenolate mofetil (MMF, total dose of 2 g/day), a proton pump inhibitor for his pyrosis, and was referred to Occupational Therapy for evaluation and treatment

Table 11.1 Weight, modified Rodnan skin score (MRSS) and pulmonary function test (PFT) parameters changes at consecutive clinic visits

Clinic visits	Weight (lb)	MRSS	% predicted FVC	% predicted TLC	% predicted DLco
Month 0 (initial visit)	228.1	3	106	100	113
Month 9	232.1	14	87	83	73
Month 12	213.6	33	74	73	58
Month 14	200.3	38	69	70	54
Month 16	180.2	35	57	61	56

MRSS modified Rodnan skin score, *FVC* forced vital capacity, *TLC* total lung capacity, *DLco* diffusion capacity

of his hand involvement. He was encouraged to maintain an active lifestyle with accent on aerobic exercise, a balanced diet (frequent, small meals, with focus on high protein, high energy foods), and he was instructed to check his blood pressure weekly. However, when assessed 3 months later, the patient's skin tightness had progressed dramatically (see Table 11.1), he had significant weight loss, with new shortness of breath, and his percent predicted FVC had decreased by 14%. We increased the dose of MMF to 3 g/day and reviewed other treatment options. The patient did not wish to consider monthly intravenous cyclophosphamide. The patient's pulmonary and skin involvement continued to worsen (see Table 11.1) and a decision was made by the patient, after reviewing the available protocols and options, to undergo high-dose immunosuppression therapy and autologous hematopoietic cell transplantation as part of a US-based randomized controlled trial.

Discussion

The etymology of the word "scleroderma" derives from two Greek words: "skleros" (hard) and "derma" (skin). The skin thickening is a central clinical event in SSc and it is used as a diagnostic and classification tool, as well as a measure of disease severity and response to therapy.

In the case described, we assessed the skin thickness objectively using the MRSS. Trained clinicians palpate the skin from 17 body areas and assign each area a score from 0 to 3 (0 = normal, 1 = mild, 2 = moderate, 3 = severe); the MRSS is obtained by adding all the scores. The inter- and intra-observer variability is low and sufficiently reproducible, so the MRSS can be used as a measure of disease outcome, especially when a single evaluator is involved.[1]

The extent of skin involvement has been the primary basis of the SSc traditional classification as limited (lSSc) and diffuse (dSSc). The more recent clinical and immunological observations point toward a spectrum of SSc family of diseases in which the degree of skin sclerosis serves as a surrogate for visceral involvement.

Although the pathogenesis of SSc is still unknown, abnormal fibroblast activation followed by excessive deposition of collagen in the dermis and the subcutaneous tissue is the hallmark of skin thickening in dSSc. Rodnan compared the weight of skin biopsy cores obtained from 147 SSc patients to the weight of skin biopsy cores obtained from the same anatomical area from 58 controls and found a close correlation between the clinical estimation of the skin thickness and the total dermal collagen content (which was higher especially during the indurative phase of dSSc).[2] Another trial found strong correlations between MRSS and both the wet and dry weights of forearm skin biopsies obtained at entry from 141 SSc patients enrolled in a prospective, double blind study of ketanserin versus placebo in SSc.[3] In this study, the dry weight as a percentage of wet weight was the same (30.7%) in lSSc and dSSc, despite the wet weight being higher in the dSSc biopsies, supporting the usefulness of MRSS to differentiate between SSc subtypes. Both of these studies only evaluated correlations between skin scores and the amount of collagen measured by weighing the skin biopsies. A more recent clinicopathological study of dSSc found close correlations between the MRSS and the histological extent of skin fibrosis as well as the TGF-β signaling in SSc fibroblasts (as measured by increased Smad3 phosphorylation levels).[4] In conclusion, the MRSS is well validated and it reflects the underlying pathology of SSc.

Durometers are handheld devices that have been used to objectively measure skin thickening and hardening in SSc. Durometer-measured skin thickness correlates well with MRSS, thus lending content and construct validity to MRSS as well as ultrasound-measured skin thickness, and it is sensitive to change.[5] Merkel et al. further demonstrated that durometer measurements are reliable, valid, and demonstrate better sensitivity to change compared with MRSS.[6]

The most striking clinical change in the case described here is the rapid and profound skin involvement. The initial question as part of the decision-making process should be: What is the significance of the rapid skin thickening in a patient with SSc? Does it *a priori* signal greater visceral damage? Is it always associated with higher morbidity and lower survival?

The Pittsburgh Scleroderma Databank has been instrumental in answering some of these questions. Nine hundred and fifty-three patients with dSSc were followed prospectively for 23 years and severe organ involvement by specific criteria was recorded.[7] More than 70% of severe skin (defined as MRSS>40/51) and kidney involvement occurred during the first 3 years of the disease, and 45–55% of the severe lung, heart, and GI tract involvement happened during the first 3 years as well. The percentage of patients developing severe organ involvement beyond 3 years was significantly lower. Survival was extremely poor in patients with severe organ involvement, although the patients with severe skin involvement had the best outcome (54% at 9 years), and the subgroup of patients with severe skin involvement without additional organ damage had a 72% survival at 9 years. This study confirms that severe organ involvement occurs early in dSSc, therefore careful monitoring of renal function along with cardiopulmonary testing in the initial stages of the disease is important, and that a high skin score alone does not predict a poor outcome.

A paper derived from the high-dose versus low-dose D-penicillamine trial assessed the clinical implications of skin thickness in a cohort of 134 patients with dSSc.[8] A baseline MRSS $\geq 20/51$ and presence of lung involvement were the only two risk factors for early mortality. More so, the MRSS $\geq 20/51$ at baseline and large joint contractures are the best predictors for scleroderma renal crisis and heart involvement. The 2-year follow-up data on 68 patients who completed the study showed that improvement in skin score in patients with dSSc was associated with better hand function, contractures, and overall functional ability.

The skin thickening in dSSc is known to have an unpredictable course but it is generally accepted that the skin involvement worsens during the early inflammatory stages of the disease, followed by a plateau phase with little changes, and then by spontaneous improvement in the fibrotic stage. Little is known about the relationship between skin softening and prognosis of the disease. If higher skin scores in dSSc are associated with worse mortality, is skin softening protective against new organ damage? The Pittsburgh Scleroderma Databank data from 278 dSSc patients showed that 63% of the subjects who had more than 25% improvement in their MRSS at 2 years also had significantly better survival at 5 and 10 years.[9] An interesting observation is that there was no significant difference in the occurrence of severe organ involvement during the 2 years of follow-up to explain the worse survival among the "non-improvers." Seibold et al. reported that softening of the skin was significantly paralleled by improved patient function and hand extension during the 6-month double-blind, placebo-controlled trial of human recombinant relaxin.[10] These studies suggest that skin softening is associated with better survival and function, regardless of the degree of progression of the internal organ involvement.

Another study created a latent linear trajectory model of the skin involvement, recognizing three different patterns in patients with dSSc: high baseline MRSS with no subsequent improvement; high baseline score with improvement; low baseline score with later improvement.[11] Although this study had the limitations of a retrospective design, the results were similar to those from the Pittsburgh Scleroderma Databank[9]: no difference in occurrence of severe internal organ involvement was noted between improvers and non-improvers but significantly higher mortality among non-improvers ($p=0.005$). A simple conclusion that could be drawn from these observations is that worse skin involvement is an independent predictor of a higher mortality in dSSc, possibly via the decreased overall patient level of functioning.

Our patient experienced a rapid evolution of his skin thickening: his MRSS increased by 22 within an interval of only 5 months. How important is the pace of the skin thickening in predicting outcomes in dSSc?

Domsic et al. utilized the Pittsburgh Scleroderma Clinic prospective data to introduce the concept of skin thickness progression rate (STPR) as the ratio between the MRSS at the first visit and the duration of skin thickening (in years).[12] For example, based on our patient's MRSS of 14/51 for a month after he first noticed swelling of his fingers, his STPR was 14/0.083 years, or 168 per year, which would be within the range of rapid STRP (defined as STPR > 45 per year). In this study, the rapid STPR group had the highest number of deaths at 1, 2, and 5 years of follow-up

(17%, 24%, and 35%, respectively). A significantly higher proportion of patients in the rapid STPR group developed scleroderma renal crisis (SRC), cardiac and gastrointestinal involvement at years 1 and 2 after the initial visit. When multivariate regression analysis was performed to evaluate for predictors of severe internal organ involvement, rapid STPR was found to be an independent predictor of SRC at 1 year, but no other predictive value was found even with sensitivity analysis. This study stresses again the heterogeneity of dSSc as a syndrome and the need for a combined index of baseline measures to predict the severity of the disease.

Confirming the same conclusion, recently published data from the German Systemic Sclerosis Network (DSSN) showed no significant correlation between the MRSS and potentially life-threatening complications in a heterogeneous cohort of patients with SSc, which included both the diffuse and the limited subtypes.[13]

Our patient had a positive anti-topoisomerase I antibody which, especially when associated with rapid STPR, is associated with reduced survival.[14]

The most important clinical decision when faced with such a patient is the choice of therapy. There are presently no proven disease modifying therapies for SSc and choice of treatment is often determined by organ-based diseases such as lung fibrosis. The natural progression to skin softening over time in dSSc makes interpretation of placebo-controlled clinical trials very difficult. Our patient developed skin and lung involvement concomitantly, so we tried to choose an intervention that would address both organs while stabilizing the progression of the disease. Cyclophosphamide has been evaluated in both the intravenous and the oral forms, especially in the setting of SSc lung disease. The Scleroderma Lung Study (oral)[15] showed statistically significant improvement in the FVC at 18 months but no difference at 2 years (which may have been related to the fact that treatment lasted only 1 year); beneficial effects on the skin were noted as well. The Fibrosing Alveolitis in Scleroderma Trial (FAST[intravenous]))[16] showed a trend of FVC improvement at 1 year (except for a post hoc subanalysis with additional adjustment for weight) and did not evaluate change in MRSS. Mycophenolate mofetil is thought to be safer than cyclophosphamide and seemed to reduce skin score and progression to severe lung disease when compared to other immunosuppressive drugs in a large retrospective cohort of patients with dSSc.[17] Methotrexate, currently used in SSc musculoskeletal involvement (arthritis and myositis), has a modest effect on skin involvement.[18] Postlethwaite et al. showed no significant differences in skin score in a large placebo-controlled trial of oral bovine type I collagen in patients with dSSc.[19] High-dose immunosuppressive therapy (HDIT) and hematopoietic stem cell transplantation (HSCT) is used as an attempt to "re-set" the immune system and modify the course of SSc. A long-term follow-up study conducted in the USA using total body irradiation as part of the HSCT conditioning regimen showed improvement in the skin score at 12 months.[20] Long-term European data showed significant skin score reduction and the 5- and 7-year survival was 96.2 and 84.8%, respectively.[21] Other biological and antifibrotic therapies have been studied with variable effects on the skin involvement.[22]

In summary, a traditional focus on the importance of skin involvement in SSc might not hold true in the current era that defines SSc as a spectrum of diseases.

Although still associated with high mortality, a high MRSS at baseline predicts the occurrence of SRC, but no other internal organ damage – an observation that contradicts the old idea that skin could serve as a surrogate for visceral involvement. The same is true in the subset of patients that experience rapid skin involvement. The degree of disability due to more severe skin involvement is significant and tends to improve when the skin score improves. Certain therapies seem to have a beneficial effect on the skin involvement but their side effects might not justify their use for skin thickening alone, but rather if the lung parenchyma is involved as well. The question of whether the MRSS should be used as an outcome measure in dSSc or merely as a surrogate for disease activity is only partially answered by the currently available data.

References

1. Clements P, Lachenbruch P, Siebold J, et al. Inter and intraobserver variability of total skin thickness score (modified Rodnan TSS) in systemic sclerosis. *J Rheumatol.* 1995;22:1281-1285.
2. Rodnan G, Lipinski E, Luksick J. Skin thickness and collagen content in progressive systemic sclerosis and localized scleroderma. *Arthritis Rheum.* 1979;22:130-140.
3. Furst D, Clements P, Steen V, et al. The modified Rodnan skin score is an accurate reflection of skin biopsy thickness in systemic sclerosis. *J Rheumatol.* 1998;25:84-88.
4. Verrecchia F, Laboureau J, Verola O, et al. Skin involvement in scleroderma – where histological and clinical scores meet. *Rheumatology Oxford.* 2007;46:833-841.
5. Kissin E, Schiller A, Gelbard R, et al. Durometry for the assessment of skin disease in systemic sclerosis. *Arthritis Rheum.* 2006;55:603-609.
6. Merkel P, Silliman N, Denton C, et al. Validity, reliability, and feasibility of durometer measurements of scleroderma skin disease in a multicenter treatment trial. *Arthritis Rheum.* 2008;59:699-705.
7. Steen V, Medsger TJ. Severe organ involvement in systemic sclerosis with diffuse scleroderma. *Arthritis Rheum.* 2000;43:2437-2444.
8. Clements P, Hurwitz E, Wong W, et al. Skin thickness score as a predictor and correlate of outcome in systemic sclerosis: high-dose versus low-dose penicillamine trial. *Arthritis Rheum.* 2000;43:2445-2454.
9. Steen V, Medsger TJ. Improvement in skin thickening in systemic sclerosis associated with improved survival. *Arthritis Rheum.* 2001;44:2828-2835.
10. Seibold J, Korn J, Simms R, et al. Recombinant human relaxin in the treatment of scleroderma. A randomized, double-blind, placebo-controlled trial. *Ann Intern Med.* 2000;132:871-879.
11. Shand L, Lunt M, Nihtyanova S, et al. Relationship between change in skin score and disease outcome in diffuse cutaneous systemic sclerosis: application of a latent linear trajectory model. *Arthritis Rheum.* 2007;56:2422-2431.
12. Domsic R, Rodriguez-Reyna T, Lucas M, Fertig N, Medsger TJ. Skin thickness progression rate: a predictor of mortality and early internal organ involvement in diffuse scleroderma. *Ann Rheum Dis.* 2010;70:104-109.
13. Hanitsch L, Burmester G, Witt C, et al. Skin sclerosis is only of limited value to identify SSc patients with severe manifestations–an analysis of a distinct patient subgroup of the German Systemic Sclerosis Network (DNSS) Register. *Rheumatology Oxford.* 2009;48:70-73.
14. Perera A, Fertig N, Lucas M, et al. Clinical subsets, skin thickness progression rate, and serum antibody levels in systemic sclerosis patients with anti- topoisomerase I antibody. *Arthritis Rheum.* 2007;56:2740-2746.

114   E. Schiopu and J.R. Seibold

15. Tashkin D, Elashoff R, Clements P, et al. Cyclophosphamide versus placebo in scleroderma lung disease. *N Engl J Med*. 2006;354:2655-2666.
16. Hoyles R, Ellis R, Wellsbury J, et al. A multicenter, prospective, randomized, double-blind, placebo-controlled trial of corticosteroids and intravenous cyclophosphamide followed by oral azathioprine for the treatment of pulmonary fibrosis in scleroderma. *Arthritis Rheum*. 2006;54:3962-3970.
17. Nihtyanova S, Brough G, Black C, Denton C. Mycophenolate mofetil in diffuse cutaneous systemic sclerosis–a retrospective analysis. *Rheumatology Oxford*. 2007;46:442-445.
18. Pope J, Bellamy N, Seibold J, et al. A randomized, controlled trial of methotrexate versus placebo in early diffuse scleroderma. *Arthritis Rheum*. 2001;44:1351-1358.
19. Postlethwaite A, Wong W, Clements P, et al. A multicenter, randomized, double- blind, placebo-controlled trial of oral type I collagen treatment in patients with diffuse cutaneous systemic sclerosis: I. oral type I collagen does not improve skin in all patients, but may improve skin in late-phase disease. *Arthritis Rheum*. 2008;58:1810-1822.
20. Nash RA, Crofford LJ, Abidi M, et al. High-dose immunosuppressive therapy and autologous hematopoietic cell transplantation for severe systemic sclerosis: long-term follow- up of the US multicenter pilot study. *Blood*. 2007;110:1388-1396.
21. Vonk MC, Marjanovic Z, van den Hoogen FH, et al. Long-term follow-up results after autologous haematopoietic stem cell transplantation for severe systemic sclerosis. *Ann Rheum Dis*. 2008;67:98-104.
22. Quillinan N, Denton C. Disease-modifying treatment in systemic sclerosis: current status. *Curr Opin Rheumatol*. 2009;21:636-641.

Chapter 12
A 28-Year-Old Woman with Early Diffuse Scleroderma and Shortness of Breath

Otylia Kowal-Bielecka and Krzysztof Kowal

Keywords Diffuse SSc • Interstitial lung disease • Pulmonary hypertension • Pulmonary function tests • Echocardiography

Case Study

A 28-year-old woman presented with arthralgia, Raynaud's phenomenon, fatigue, and shortness of breath with exercise. She also reported difficulty closing her fists and bending her knees. Her disease began 10 months before with pain in the knees, puffiness and pain of both hands, and Raynaud's phenomenon. Weakness and dyspnea developed later. At the beginning, dyspnea was present only during vigorous physical exercise, but later she experienced dyspnea with mild physical exercise such as climbing one flight of stairs. Her general practitioner noted that the patient's skin was thickened and referred her to a rheumatologist. The preliminary diagnosis was SSc with dyspnea as a consequence of the disease.

The detailed medical history revealed that the patient had been suffering from systemic hypertension for 5 years, which was controlled with a beta-blocker. She had a long-life history of obesity. One year earlier dyslipidemia was diagnosed. She had never smoked.

Family history was negative for systemic rheumatic disease. She had no recent history of respiratory infection. There was no history of exposure to toxic substances at home or at work.

O. Kowal-Bielecka (✉)
Department of Rheumatology and Internal Medicine, Medical University of Bialystok,
Sklodowskiej-Curie 24a, Bialystok 15-276, Poland

R.M. Silver and C.P. Denton (eds.), *Case Studies in Systemic Sclerosis*,
DOI: 10.1007/978-0-85729-641-2_12, © Springer-Verlag London Limited 2011

Physical Examination

Temperature 36.6°C; pulse 88 bpm; respirations 14 per min; blood pressure 130/80 mmHg. Height 177 cm, weight 103 kg, BMI 32.9.

Skin of the face, hands, forearms, arms, legs, and anterior trunk was thickened and hyperpigmented. Digital pitting scars were present on the finger pads. Head and neck exam was remarkable only for microstomia. Chest examination revealed normal breath sounds and no adventitial sounds were heard. Heart examination was normal.

Musculoskeletal examination revealed contractures of the hand joints and restriction in movement of the knees and hand joints. Tendon friction rubs were palpable over both knees. Neurological examination was normal except for mild weakness of the muscles of the shoulder and pelvic girdles.

Laboratory Findings

Erythrocyte sedimentation rate (ESR): 44 mm/h; Complete blood count: WBC $5.7 \times 10^3/mm^3$, RBC $3.7 \times 10^6/mm^3$, hemoglobin concentration10.1 g/dL; platelets $206 \times 10^3/mm^3$; reticulocyte count and blood smear normal. Chemistry: normal except for elevated triglycerides and elevated CK (600 IU/L). Urinalysis, renal function test, including creatinine concentration and creatinine clearance, as well as coagulation tests were within normal limits. Antinuclear antibody was positive (1:1280) with a speckled pattern; anti-centromere antibodies (ACA) and anti-topoisomerase I antibodies (anti-Scl-70) were negative.

Cardiopulmonary Testing

Pulmonary function tests (PFTs) revealed normal spirometry forced vital capacity (FVC 3.97 L, 94.3% predicted; forced expiratory volume in one second FEV1 3.62 L, 98.3% predicted; FEV1/FVC 1.04). Diffusing capacity of the lungs for carbon monoxide, DLco was diminished (58% of predicted). Chest radiograph was normal. High resolution computed tomography (HRCT) of the lungs revealed small linear subpleural lines and "ground glass" opacities located mainly in the lower parts of the lungs, consistent with interstitial lung disease. Echocardiography with Doppler revealed normal cardiac valves and normal ejection fraction, diminished relaxation of the left ventricle, tricuspid regurgitation with an estimated pulmonary artery systolic pressure (PASP) of 41 mmHg. Resting ECG was normal.

Submaximal exercise testing was stopped at 5 METS (normal for age and sex: 10 METS) due to shortness of breath and fatigue without chest pain or any abnormalities on ECG, and without fall in oxygen hemoglobin saturation measured by pulse oximetry. Right heart catheterization (RHC) revealed a normal mean pulmonary artery pressure (22 mmHg) and normal capillary wedge pressure (13 mmHg). Left heart catheterization revealed no abnormalities of the coronary arteries.

Other Tests

Capillaroscopy of the nailbeds revealed avascular areas with megacapillaries and hemorrhages. Electromyography revealed features of primary muscle injury suggestive of myositis.

Course

A diagnosis of diffuse systemic sclerosis (dSSc) was made based on the presence of widespread skin thickening, tendon friction rub, digital pitting scars, high titer ANA, and characteristic changes on capillary microscopy.

In light of the rapid progression of her disease with involvement of internal organs including the respiratory system, together with the presence of predictors of poor prognosis, this patient was considered to be a candidate for intensive immunosuppressive therapy. She received one infusion of methylprednisolone (intravenously 1 g) followed by cyclophosphamide (intravenously, 0.6 g/m^2 of body surface area monthly) together with prednisone (orally, 15 mg daily, decreased after 1 month to 10 mg daily). Vasodilators were started as treatment for Raynaud's phenomenon and an ACE-inhibitor for diastolic dysfunction and hypertension. The patient was advised to adhere to a low fat, nutritious diet, check blood pressure on a daily basis, and have blood counts, creatinine concentration and urinalysis performed monthly. After 6 months of cyclophosphamide therapy, her dyspnea and functional capacity had improved, the hemoglobin concentration and CK levels had normalized, while her skin score and lung function remained stable. The patient's immunosuppressive medication was changed to azathioprine (orally 100 mg daily) after six monthly infusions of cyclophosphamide. Low-dose prednisone and vasodilators were continued. Further monitoring of blood pressure, lung, and kidney function and echocardiography was recommended.

Discussion

Diagnosis of Shortness of Breath in Early Diffuse SSc

Systemic sclerosis (scleroderma, SSc) is classified into two major clinical subsets: diffuse cutaneous SSc (dSSc) and limited cutaneous SSc (lSSc).[1] These two subsets differ with respect to extent of skin disease, pattern of internal organ involvement,

Fig. 12.1 Proximal skin involvement in early diffuse systemic sclerosis (visible thickened shiny skin with hyper- and hypopigmentation over the anterior chest)

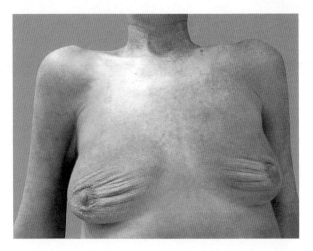

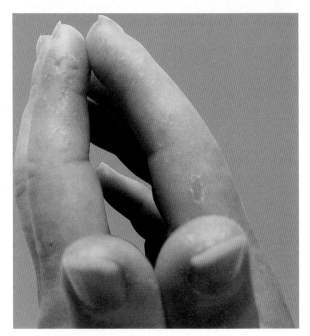

Fig. 12.2 Fingers of patient with early diffuse systemic sclerosis (visible edema and contractures of the fingers, pitting scars on the lateral surface of the fingers)

and prognosis.[1,2] Diffuse SSc is characterized by widespread skin thickening involving, in addition to face and distal extremities, areas proximal to elbows and/or knees, including arms, thighs, and/or trunk. Usually skin changes progress rather rapidly, reaching maximal thickness within several months.[2] Thickened skin is frequently discolored due to the presence of areas of hyper- and hypopigmentation (Fig. 12.1). Severe skin thickening may lead to joint contractures in the hands and other joints (Fig. 12.2).

Diffuse SSc is associated with high risk of early internal organ involvement. In a series of over 900 patients with dSSc severe skin, lung, heart, gastrointestinal, and/ or kidney disease most often occurred in the first 3 years of the disease.[3] SSc patients who developed severe organ complications had significantly worse survival compared with SSc patients without severe complications.[3] High or rising skin score, palpable tendon friction rubs, elevated ESR, heart or kidney involvement, and diminished lung function were all found to be independent predictors of mortality in early dSSc.[4]

Due to the particularly high risk of the development of severe internal organ involvement which determines further prognosis, the first 3 years may be considered to be the "early phase" of dSSc, during which time particular attention must be paid to potential internal organ involvement.[2,3] Early diagnosis is essential so that appropriate treatments can be instituted possibly prior to the occurrence of irreversible tissue damage. Such an approach is of key importance since available treatment strategies can sometimes be effective in preventing progression of individual SSc-related organ injuries, rather than reversing existing manifestations of chronic fibrosis.

Shortness of breath in a patient with early dSSc, such as presented in this case study, should therefore always raise concern for potential lung or heart involvement, including acute pulmonary edema associated with scleroderma renal crisis. As in this patient, exercise testing for detecting and assessing severity of lung or heart involvement may be difficult to interpret in dSSc patients, since severe skin, joint, and muscle involvement as well as the presence of general fatigue may limit the amount of physical effort a patient may exert, even in the absence of cardiopulmonary complications.[5]

Interstitial lung disease (ILD, pulmonary fibrosis) is the most frequent pulmonary complication in dSSc and the main cause of death in SSc.[6,7] The clinical course of SSc-ILD is rather variable. HRCT of the lungs reveals features of ILD in up to 90% of patients with early dSSc, while only about 40% of SSc patients exhibit a restrictive ventilatory defect.[8,9] The greatest loss of lung volume takes place within the first 3–5 years of the disease.[9] Since the course of ILD in a given SSc patient is often difficult to predict, serial PFTs are advised in early dSSc patients to identify those who might develop progressive ILD, and to follow their response to treatment. Demonstration of significant loss of lung volume over time is a more sensitive indicator of lung involvement than any single measurement alone. SSc-ILD is characterized by a restrictive PFT pattern defined as a decrease in FVC and total lung capacity (TLC) with the FEV1/FVC ratio approximating 1. DLco is diminished proportionally to lung volumes.

Diminished lung volumes/capacities are by no means specific for ILD and might be found in other diseases involving lung parenchyma such as pneumonia and tuberculosis, or they might reflect impaired chest wall mechanics due to severe truncal skin or muscle involvement. Low FVC and FEV1 are also seen in obstructive pulmonary diseases such as chronic obstructive pulmonary disease (COPD); however,

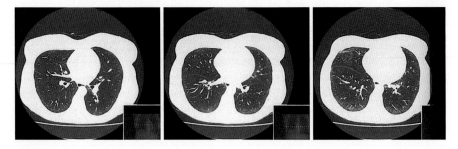

Fig. 12.3 Serial high resolution computed tomography scans of the lungs in early diffuse systemic sclerosis showing subpleural lines and ground glass opacities consistent with interstitial lung disease more pronounced in the lower parts of the lungs

the diagnosis of COPD can easily be established using spirometry and imaging studies. In obstructive lung disease the FEV1 is reduced more drastically than FVC leading to decreased FEV1/FVC ratio (<0.7).

In the authors' studies, features of airway obstruction were found in as many as 23.5% of patients with dSSc and in 8% of patients with lSSc[10] Recently, a new clinical syndrome consisting of ILD combined with emphysema has been described in patients with idiopathic pulmonary fibrosis and patients with connective tissue diseases including SSc.[11,12] This syndrome is frequently found in smokers and is characterized by severe dyspnea, diminished DLco, and relatively well-preserved lung volumes.[11]

Bronchoalveolar lavage (BAL) can provide important insight into the nature of pulmonary involvement through sampling of cells and fluids from the lower respiratory tract. In SSc-ILD patients, increased percentages of neutrophils, eosinophils, and/or lymphocytes are frequently found by cytological analysis of BAL fluid (BALF). An abnormal BALF cellular profile, in particular granulocytosis, is usually associated with more severe physiologic and radiologic changes.[13] At present, there is insufficient evidence to support widespread usage of BALF analysis in routine clinical practice. However, BAL is useful in differential diagnosis of other entities which might coexist with SSc-ILD, for example, infection, pulmonary hemorrhage, hypersensitivity pneumonitis, or malignancy.[13]

Radiological assessment is helpful for identification of the extent and type of lung involvement. On chest imaging, SSc-ILD manifests as reticular abnormalities or ground glass opacities, most prominent in the lung bases, but an ordinary radiograph lacks sensitivity in detecting early ILD.[8] HRCT of the lungs is much more sensitive, allows more appropriate evaluation of the extent of lung involvement and might be helpful in revealing coexisting pathology such as emphysema, discrete atelectasis, or fine bronchiectasis. HRCT manifestations of SSc-ILD include linear thickening of interlobar septa, bronchiectases, areas of diminished ventilation ("ground glass" opacities), or severe fibrosis with secondary destruction of lung parenchyma, so-called "honey combing" (Fig. 12.3). In the present case study, the HRCT scan established a diagnosis of early SSc-ILD, yet the severity of interstitial changes did not seem to satisfactorily explain the severe degree of dyspnea reported by the patient, thus raising the possibility of other potential causes for dyspnea.

Pulmonary hypertension is another possible cause of dyspnea in SSc patients (see Chap. 13). Pulmonary hypertension may develop as an isolated form (pulmonary arterial hypertension, PAH) or may be secondary to ILD or left heart involvement, for example, diastolic dysfunction.[6] PAH is detected in approximately 8–12% of SSc patients by RHC.[6] It has been thought to appear mainly in patients with long-standing limited SSc, but recent studies indicate that PAH is present in dSSc also, and in almost 50% of all patients with SSc-PAH, it developed within the first 5 years from onset of the initial non-Raynaud's phenomenon symptom.[14] Pulmonary hypertension due to left heart disease has been found in approximately 10% of SSc patients and its incidence is similar to that of PAH in the overall SSc population.[15,16] Pulmonary hypertension secondary to ILD has been identified by echocardiography (PASP>45 mmHg) in up to 21% of dSSc patients (29% of dSSc patients with pulmonary fibrosis),[17] although it should be noted that echocardiographic estimates of PASP may not always be accurate and are not sufficient to establish the diagnosis of PAH. According to recent studies, the 3-year survival is only 47–64% in SSc-related PAH, and only 28–39% when pulmonary hypertension occurs in association with SSc-ILD.[18,19]

Heart involvement might develop in SSc as a "primary" event (see Chap. 15), as a consequence of lung or kidney disease, or due to coexisting coronary artery disease.[20] Coronary angiography was performed in this case study patient because of several traditional risk factors for atherosclerosis and nondiagnostic results of submaximal exercise testing; large vessel coronary artery disease was excluded as a possible cause of diastolic dysfunction and dyspnea; however, small vessel disease from SSc, beyond the detection of coronary angiography, may certainly have existed and contributed to this patient's symptoms.

Severe anemia may be a cause of decreased exercise capacity and shortness of breath. Microangiopathic anemia is one of the laboratory features of scleroderma renal crisis.[21] However, anemia in dSSc may develop in different ways: it may be a reflection of chronic inflammation, iron deficiency, malabsorption, or gastrointestinal hemorrhage.

Myopathy occurring as a primary event or from atrophy of disuse, joint disease, or treatment with steroids can result in limited physical capacity and dyspnea. Myositis with proximal muscle weakness, elevated CK levels and/or abnormal electromyography, as in the present patient, is found in approximately 17% of SSc cases and is associated with significantly higher risk of myocardial involvement including congestive heart failure.[22] Severe weakness of respiratory muscles from myositis may lead to hypoventilation with subsequent respiratory failure. Involvement of pharyngeal muscles increases the risk of aspiration with development of pneumonia.

Finally, it should be kept in mind that multiple causes of dyspnea may coexist, especially in patients with systemic autoimmune diseases such as SSc in whom multiple organ systems are often affected. Thus, a multidisciplinary approach involving consultants from rheumatology, pulmonology, cardiology, radiology, and sometimes gastroenterology and hematology is often required to define the precise cause(s) for a dSSc patient's complaints of dyspnea and reduced exercise capacity.

Management

Early dSSc patients, due to rapid progression of skin disease and high risk of developing severe internal organ complications, usually require treatment.[2] No disease-modifying drug, however, has been shown to be efficacious in all SSc patients; therefore, the strategy for treating dSSc is based mainly on managing specific organ complications.[23,24] According to recent guidelines, immunosuppressive treatment is recommended for SSc patients with severe and/or progressing ILD, as well as for those in the early phase of the disease, since they are at higher risk for progression of lung disease.[25]

Thus far, only cyclophosphamide has been demonstrated to be an effective treatment for SSc-ILD.[26,27] In the Scleroderma Lung Study (SLS) involving 158 patients with symptomatic ILD and cytological or radiological features of alveolitis, cyclophosphamide (given orally, 1–2 mg/kg/day for 12 months) significantly improved lung function tests (FVC, TLC), dyspnea, and quality of life. The placebo-corrected mean improvement in FVC and TLC was 2.5% and 4.1%, respectively.[26] A similar magnitude of effect on FVC (placebo-corrected 4.2% improvement) was seen in the FAST trial in which cyclophosphamide was given intravenously at a dose of 600 mg/m^2 monthly for 6 months, together with prednisolone (20 mg on alternate days) and followed by oral azathioprine (2.5 mg/kg/day) for another 6 months. In the FAST study, the treatment effect was not statistically significant ($p=0.08$), possibly due to insufficient statistical power of the study.[27] Follow-up of the SLS patients revealed that improvement in lung function continued to increase through 6 months but dissipated by 1 year after discontinuation of cyclophosphamide.[28] Altogether, these observations suggest that longer immunosuppressive therapy, possibly with less toxic agents, will be required to maintain benefits achieved with cyclophosphamide treatment. Whether other immunosuppressive drugs are effective treatments for SSc-ILD remains to be established. Recent retrospective analyses and small uncontrolled studies suggest that mycophenolate mofetil might prevent progression of SSc-ILD.[29,30]

Unlike in other connective tissue disease, steroids should be used with caution in SSc patients since such treatment has been associated with scleroderma renal crisis.[24,25,31,32]

The patient described in this case had severe and progressive skin disease, ILD with declining exercise capacity and lung function, muscle involvement, and other features of active disease (e.g., tendon friction rubs, elevated ESR, anemia), which prompted immunosuppressive treatment. Cyclophosphamide was used due to its potential efficacy in SS-ILD and to achieve control of disease activity as soon as possible. Since the patient was at high risk of developing scleroderma renal crisis, only low to moderate doses of steroids, except for the initial bolus, were used in combination with cyclophosphamide, and blood pressure and kidney function were closely monitored. To minimize its toxicity, cyclophosphamide was given by an intravenous regimen and later switched to azathioprine as soon as subjective improvement, stabilization of lung function, and normalization of CK were achieved. For diastolic dysfunction, an ACE inhibitor was prescribed. In addition, traditional risk factors of atherosclerosis were managed.

In summary, patients with early dSSc are characterized by rapid progression of skin changes and high risk of developing of severe internal organ involvement, including lung, heart, and kidney disease. Therefore, dyspnea in a patient with early dSSc should always raise awareness of these complications and lead to appropriate diagnostic procedures. Even if the baseline tests fail to reveal definite abnormalities, regular monitoring of lung, heart, and kidney function is recommended especially during the early years of dSSc to identify particular organ involvement at the earliest possible stage. This is of key importance for introducing appropriate treatment aimed at preventing progression of the disease. A recent retrospective analysis of 520 SSc patients from a single center revealed that the 5-year survival of patients with dSSc had significantly increased, from 69% for dSSc patients whose disease was diagnosed between 1990 and 1993, to 84% for those in whom disease was diagnosed between 2000 and 2003.[33] Improvement of survival appears to be, at least in part, due to better detection of pulmonary complications as a result of systematic annual screening for this and other organ-based complications.[33]

Immunosuppressive drugs are at present a cornerstone of therapy for early dSSc patients, with particular agents chosen depending on the pace of progress of skin disease and particular organ involvement. Additional therapies targeting specific complications might be used in individual patients based on their particular profile of organ involvement.

References

1. LeRoy EC, Black C, Fleischmajer R, et al. Scleroderma (systemic sclerosis): classification, subsets and pathogenesis. *J Rheumatol.* 1988;15:202-205.
2. Medsger TA Jr. Classification, prognosis. In: Clements PJ, Furst DE, eds. *Systemic Sclerosis.* 2nd ed. Philadelphia: Lippincott Williams & Wilkins; 2004:17-28.
3. Steen VD, Medsger TA Jr. Severe organ involvement in systemic sclerosis with diffuse scleroderma. *Arthritis Rheum.* 2000;43:2437-2444.
4. Steen VD, Medsger TA Jr. The value of the Health Assessment Questionnaire and special patient-generated scales to demonstrate change in systemic sclerosis patients over time. *Arthritis Rheum.* 1997;40:1984-19991.
5. Garin MC, Highland KB, Silver RM, et al. Limitations to the 6-minute walk test in interstitial lung disease and pulmonary hypertension in scleroderma. *J Rheumatol.* 2009;36:330-336.
6. Hant FN, Herpel LB, Silver RM. Pulmonary manifestations of scleroderma and mixed connective tissue disease. *Clin Chest Med.* 2010;31:433-449.
7. Steen VD, Medsger TA. Changes in causes of death in systemic sclerosis 1972–2003. *Ann Rheum Dis.* 2007;66:940-944.
8. Warrick JH, Bhalla M, Schabel SI, Silver RM. High resolution computed tomography in early scleroderma lung disease. *J Rheumatol.* 1991;18:1520-1528.
9. Steen VD, Conte C, Owens GR, Medsger TA Jr. Severe restrictive lung disease in systemic sclerosis. *Arthritis Rheum.* 1994;37:1283-1289.
10. Kowal K, Kowal-Bielecka O, Sierakowski S, Bodzenta-Lukaszyk A. Lung involvement in systemic sclerosis (SSc) – analysis of spirometry results. *Int Rev Allergol Clin Immunol.* 2002;8:237-239.
11. Cottin V, Cordier JF. The syndrome of combined pulmonary fibrosis and emphysema. *Chest.* 2009;136:1-2.

12. Cottin V, Nunes H, Mouthon L, et al. Combined pulmonary fibrosis and emphysema syndrome in connective tissue disease. *Arthritis Rheum*. 2011;63:295-304.
13. Kowal-Bielecka O, Kowal K, Highland KB, Silver RM. Bronchoalveolar lavage fluid in scleroderma interstitial lung disease: technical aspects and clinical correlations: review of the literature. *Semin Arthritis Rheum*. 2010;40:73-88.
14. Hachulla E, Launay D, Mouthon L, et al. Is pulmonary arterial hypertension really a late complication of systemic sclerosis? *Chest*. 2009;136:1211-1219.
15. Hachulla E, Gressin V, Guillevin L, et al. Early detection of pulmonary arterial hypertension in systemic sclerosis: a French nationwide prospective multicenter study. *Arthritis Rheum*. 2005;52:3792-3800.
16. Hachulla E, de Groote P, Gressin V, et al. The three-year Incidence of pulmonary arterial hypertension associated with systemic sclerosis in a multicenter nationwide longitudinal study in France. *Arthritis Rheum*. 2009;60:1831-1839.
17. Trad S, Amoura Z, Beigelman C, et al. Pulmonary arterial hypertension is a major mortality factor in diffuse systemic sclerosis, independent of interstitial lung disease. *Arthritis Rheum*. 2006;54:184-191.
18. Condliffe R, Kiely DG, Peacock AJ, et al. Connective tissue disease-associated pulmonary arterial hypertension in the modern treatment era. *Am J Respir Crit Care Med*. 2009;179:151-157.
19. Mathai SC, Hummers LK, Champion HC, et al. Survival in pulmonary hypertension associated with the scleroderma spectrum of diseases: impact of interstitial lung disease. *Arthritis Rheum*. 2009;60:569-577.
20. Meune C, Vignaux O, Kahan A, Allanore Y. Heart involvement in systemic sclerosis: evolving concept and diagnostic methodologies. *Arch Cardiovasc Dis*. 2010;103:46-52.
21. Denton CP, Lapadula G, Mouthon L, Müller-Ladner U. Renal complications and scleroderma renal crisis. *Rheumatology Oxford*. 2009;48(suppl 3):iii32-iii35.
22. Follansbee WP, Zerbe TR, Medsger TA Jr. Cardiac and skeletal muscle disease in systemic sclerosis (scleroderma): a high risk association. *Am Heart J*. 1993;125:194-203.
23. Kowal-Bielecka O, Veale DJ. DMARDs in systemic sclerosis: do they exist? In: Distler O, ed. *Scleroderma-Modern Aspects of Pathogenesis, Diagnosis and Therapy*. 1st ed. Bremen, London, Boston: Uni-Med; 2009:89-95.
24. Kowal-Bielecka O, Landewé R, Avouac J, et al. EULAR recommendations for the treatment of systemic sclerosis: a report from the EULAR Scleroderma Trials and Research group (EUSTAR). *Ann Rheum Dis*. 2009;68:620-628.
25. Wells AU, Hirani N. On behalf of the British Thoracic Society. Interstitial Lung Disease Guideline Group, a subgroup of the British Thoracic Society Standards of Care Committee, in collaboration with the Thoracic Society of Australia and New Zealand and the Irish Thoracic Soc Interstitial lung disease guideline: the British Thoracic Society in collaboration with the Thoracic Society of Australia and New Zealand and the Irish Thoracic Society. *Thorax*. 2008;63:v1-v58.
26. Tashkin DP, Elashoff R, Clements PJ, Scleroderma Lung Study Research Group, et al. Cyclophosphamide versus placebo in scleroderma lung disease. *N Engl J Med*. 2006;354:2655-2666.
27. Hoyles RK, Ellis RW, Wellsbury J, et al. A multicenter, prospective, randomized, double-blind, placebo-controlled trial of corticosteroids and intravenous cyclophosphamide followed by oral azathioprine for the treatment of pulmonary fibrosis in scleroderma. *Arthritis Rheum*. 2006;54:3962-3970.
28. Tashkin DP, Elashoff R, Clements PJ, et al. Effects of 1-year treatment with cyclophosphamide on outcomes at 2 years in scleroderma lung disease. *Am J Respir Crit Care Med*. 2007;176:1026-1034.
29. Nihtyanova SI, Brough GM, Black CM, Denton CP. Mycophenolate mofetil in diffuse cutaneous systemic sclerosis–a retrospective analysis. *Rheumatology Oxford*. 2007;46:442-445.
30. Derk CT, Grace E, Shenin M, et al. A prospective open-label study of mycophenolate mofetil for the treatment of diffuse systemic sclerosis. *Rheumatology Oxford*. 2009;48:1595-1599.

31. Steen VD, Medsger TA Jr, Osial TA, et al. Factors predicting development of renal involvement in progressive systemic sclerosis. *Am J Med*. 1984;76:779-786.
32. Steen VD, Medsger TA Jr. Case-control study of corticosteroids and other drugs that either precipitate or protect from the development of scleroderma renal crisis. *Arthritis Rheum*. 1998;41:1613-1619.
33. Nihtyanova SI, Tang EC, Coghlan JG, Wells AU, Black CM, Denton CP. Improved survival in systemic sclerosis is associated with better ascertainment of internal organ disease: a retrospective cohort study. *QJM*. 2010;103:109-115.

Chapter 13
Late Limited Systemic Sclerosis Patient Who Develops Shortness of Breath on Exertion

Jérôme Le Pavec and Marc Humbert

Keywords Systemic sclerosis • Pulmonary arterial hypertension • Systemic sclerosis-related pulmonary arterial hypertension

Case Study

A 64-year-old female patient was admitted to the hospital due to progressive dyspnea on exertion. In the context of longstanding esophageal dysfunction and Raynaud's phenomenon, she had been noted to test positive for anticentromere antibodies and diagnosed with limited cutaneous systemic sclerosis (lSSc) 10 years earlier.

Physical Examination

Physical examination showed a blood pressure of 100/70 mmHg, a heart rate of 98 bpm, a loud second heart sound (S2), no peripheral edema, a normal jugular venous pressure, facial telangiectasia and sclerodactyly. Dyspnea was classified as New York Heart Association (NYHA) functional class III (Table 13.1). On a 6-minute walk test (6MWT), the patient walked only 200 m.

M. Humbert (✉)
Department of Respiratory Medicine, Antoine Béclère, Assistance Publique,
Hôpitaux de Paris, 157 rue de la Porte de Trivaux, Clamart 92140, France

R.M. Silver and C.P. Denton (eds.), *Case Studies in Systemic Sclerosis*,
DOI: 10.1007/978-0-85729-641-2_13, © Springer-Verlag London Limited 2011

Table 13.1 The New York Heart Association classification

Class	Patient symptoms
I	No limitation of physical activity. Ordinary physical activity does not cause undue fatigue, palpitation, or dyspnea (shortness of breath)
II	Slight limitation of physical activity. Comfortable at rest, but ordinary physical activity results in fatigue, palpitation, or dyspnea
III	Marked limitation of physical activity. Comfortable at rest, but less than ordinary activity causes fatigue, palpitation, or dyspnea
IV	Unable to carry out any physical activity without discomfort. Symptoms of cardiac insufficiency at rest. If any physical activity is undertaken, discomfort is increased

Reprinted with permission from The Heart Failure Society of America © 2009 HFSA, Inc.

Laboratory Findings

The abnormal laboratory findings at the time of her admission included 950 ng/mL of N-terminal pro b-type natriuretic peptide (N-TproBNP; normal <450 ng/mL). Chest radiograph and high-resolution computed tomography (HRCT) of the chest showed mild bibasilar parenchymal infiltrates and enlargement of the main pulmonary artery diameter (Fig. 13.1). Pulmonary function tests revealed normal forced vital capacity (FVC; 105% of predicted) and decreased diffusion capacity for carbon monoxide (DLco; 30% of predicted). An echocardiogram demonstrated normal left ventricular size and function, but a dilated right ventricle and atrium with tricuspid regurgitation. The estimated tricuspid regurgitation velocity (TRV) jet was 3.3 m/s. No evidence of shunt was detected. A nuclear perfusion lung scan showed homogenous distribution of tracer, with no segmental defects. Right heart catheterization (RHC) demonstrated severe pulmonary arterial hypertension (PAH) with mean pulmonary arterial pressure (mPAP) of 58 mmHg, mean pulmonary capillary wedge pressure (PCWP) of 12 mmHg, cardiac output (CO) of 4.0 L/min and pulmonary vascular resistance (PVR) of 920 dyn·s/cm^5. There was no acute vasodilator response with nitric oxide (NO) inhalation (10 ppm).

Course

In the absence of other associated conditions, the work-up confirmed SSc-associated PAH (SSc-PAH). The patient was treated with the orally administered nonselective endothelin-receptor antagonist bosentan. Long-term hemodynamic effects were evaluated by repeated RHC after 4 months. Mean pulmonary arterial pressure was 37 mmHg, PVR was 521 dyn·s/cm^5, and CO was 4.3 L/min.

Systemic arterial pressure was not affected. N-TproBNP level was decreased by 235 ng/mL. The results of pulmonary function tests remained unchanged. The 6-minute

Fig. 13.1 High-resolution computed tomography of the chest showing mild bibasilar parenchymal infiltrates and significant increase in the diameter of the main pulmonary artery

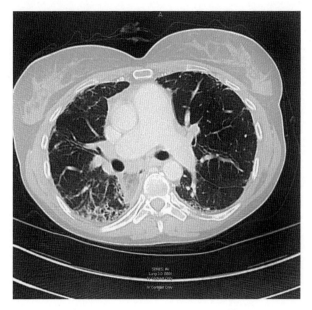

walk distance (6MWD) increased dramatically to 420 m at 4 months. The patient had symptomatic improvement and the NYHA functional class was class II.

Discussion

PAH, defined as a mPAP greater than 25 mmHg, PCWP less than 15 mmHg, and PVR greater than 240 dyn·s/cm[5], is a progressive disease of the pulmonary vasculature that leads to right heart failure and death.[1] In the current clinical classification of pulmonary hypertension (PH), connective tissue disease-associated PAH is an important subgroup of cases and accounts for up to half of the cases of PAH seen in most large centers (Table 13.2).[1]

In prospective studies using RHC for diagnosis, the prevalence of SSc-PAH is between 7.8% and 12%.[2,3] In the French PAH registry, connective tissue disease (75% of cases corresponding to SSc) accounted for 15.3% of all PAH cases.[4]

Recent advances in our understanding of the pathogenesis of PAH in general have led to development of specific therapies targeting the pulmonary vasculature. Although these therapies have shown, to varying degrees, improvements in symptoms, functional capacity, and quality of life, few have demonstrated a survival benefit. Further, patients with SSc-PAH have a divergent response to therapy and overall worse outcome than patients with idiopathic PAH. Although the reasons for these clinical differences remain unclear, there may be several explanations ranging from

Table 13.2 Updated clinical classification of pulmonary hypertension (Dana Point, 2008; Simplified version)

1. Pulmonary arterial hypertension (PAH)
    1.1. Idiopathic PAH
    1.2. Heritable
        1.2.1. BMPR2
        1.2.2. ALK1, endoglin (with or without hereditary hemorrhagic telangiectasia)
        1.2.3. Unknown
    1.3. Drug- and toxin-induced
    1.4. Associated with
        1.4.1. Connective tissue diseases
        1.4.2. HIV infection
        1.4.3. Portal hypertension
        1.4.4. Congenital heart diseases
        1.4.5. Schistosomiasis
        1.4.6. Chronic hemolytic anemia
    1.5. Persistent pulmonary hypertension of the newborn
    1.6. Pulmonary veno-occlusive disease (PVOD) and/or pulmonary capillary hemangiomatosis (PCH)
2. Pulmonary hypertension owing to left heart disease
3. Pulmonary hypertension owing to lung diseases and/or hypoxia
4. Chronic thromboembolic pulmonary hypertension (CTEPH)
5. Pulmonary hypertension with unclear multifactorial mechanisms including myeloproliferative disorders, splenectomy, sarcoidosis, pulmonary Langerhans cell histiocytosis...

Reprinted from Simonneau et al.[1] with permission from Elsevier

inadequacy of currently employed outcome measures for SSc-PAH to distinguish structural differences in the pulmonary vasculature and right heart involvement. Thus, there remains significant room for improvement in the assessment and treatment of SSc-PAH.

Assessment of SSc-PAH

Because the prevalence of PAH in SSc is high, this population is considered at high risk and therefore worthy of a specific diagnostic approach to detect the presence of disease at an earlier stage, when therapeutic intervention may potentially improve outcomes. While HRCT of the chest has become an important part of the routine detection of interstitial lung disease, it may also provide valuable informations for the positive diagnosis of PAH. Indeed, a diameter larger than 29 mm demonstrates 87% sensitivity and 89% specificity for PAH.[5] The ratio of the main pulmonary artery to aortic diameter greater than 1:1 correlates strongly with elevated mPAP, particularly in patients below 50 years of age and those who have severe PAH.[6]

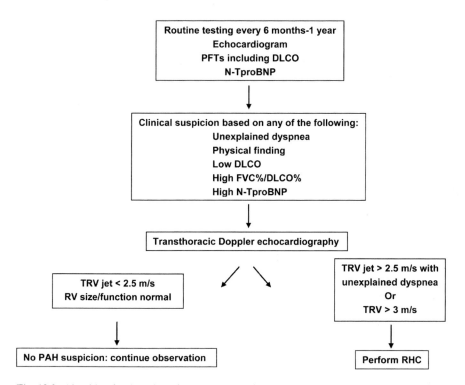

Fig. 13.2 Algorithm for detection of pulmonary arterial hypertension (PAH) in patients with systemic sclerosis (SSc). Proposed algorithm for performance of routine clinical tests in patients with SSc that may allow early detection of PAH or other causes of dyspnea (e.g., cardiac dysfunction). *PFTs* pulmonary functional tests, *DLco* single breath diffusing capacity of carbon monoxide, *FVC* forced vital capacity, *RV* right ventricle, *TRV* tricuspid regurgitation jet velocity, *RHC* right heart catheterization (Reprinted with permission of the American Thoracic Society.[7] Copyright © American Thoracic Society)

An algorithm for detection of PAH in patients with SSc may be helpful if based on a combination of symptoms and screening echocardiography. In a large study encompassing 21 referral centers in France, SSc patients with a TRV jet by transthoracic echocardiography greater than 3 m/s, or between 2.5 and 3 m/s, if accompanied by unexplained dyspnea, were systematically referred for RHC. This approach allowed detection of incident cases of SSc-PAH with less severe disease (as judged on hemodynamic data) compared with patients with known disease. Therefore, unexplained dyspnea should prompt a search for PAH in these patients, in particular in the setting of a low single-breath DLco or declining DLco over time, echocardiographic findings suggestive of the disease (elevated TRV jet or dilated RV or RA), or elevated levels of N-TproBNP[2] (Fig. 13.2). Of note, TRV jet is not measurable in up to 20% of SSc patients[2] and should prompt one to perform RHC in the presence of any indirect signs of PAH. However, whether early diagnosis and treatment of patients with SSc-PAH improves outcomes is still uncertain.[7]

In addition to the challenges in diagnosing SSc-PAH, currently available markers of disease severity and clinical tools to assess response to therapy, which may be reliable in idiopathic PAH, are either limited or lacking in SSc-PAH. Thus, compared with idiopathic PAH, SSc-PAH patients tend to have seemingly less severe alterations in hemodynamics and a poorer survival despite similar 6MWD between the two groups.[4,8,9] These findings question the ability of the 6MWT as well as traditional baseline hemodynamics (obtained by RHC) to accurately assess the severity of SSc-PAH.

Because of its simplicity, reproducibility, and validity in reflecting severity in idiopathic PAH patients, the 6MWT has been widely accepted, and is recommended and routinely used in the baseline assessment of PAH patients, for prognostication and monitoring response to therapy.[10] However, this test has never been properly and independently validated in SSc-PAH.[11] Furthermore, what constitutes a clinically relevant change in 6MWD and whether results should be expressed as absolute or percentage of predicted values remain to be determined. Further limitations to the utility of the 6MWT in PAH-SSc include the impact of musculoskeletal disease and subclinical interstitial lung disease upon distance achieved.[12] This makes it imperative to consider 6MWT in context, and changes in exercise capacity may be more meaningful than absolute distances in serial evaluation of SSc-PAH.

Cardiopulmonary hemodynamic abnormalities are required for the diagnosis of PAH and offer the best established indicators of the severity of the illness.[13] However, while these data have generally been validated in idiopathic PAH, they remain of unclear utility in SSc-PAH. Indeed, recent studies have highlighted the lack of correlation between baseline hemodynamic data and clinical evolution in SSc-PAH patients. In a retrospective analysis comparing baseline hemodynamic data in idiopathic PAH and SSc-PAH patients, patients with SSc-PAH had significantly lower mPAP and PVR by RHC, and equally depressed cardiac index compared to idiopathic PAH patients; however, follow-up indicated they were four times more likely to die compared to idiopathic PAH patients despite comparable therapy.[8] Taken together, these results suggest that in the setting of SSc, the ability of RHC to evaluate the severity of PAH may be limited.

The development of treatments for PAH has brought to the forefront the question of how to best assess and monitor the efficacy of long-term therapy. There is a clear need for better noninvasive and clinically relevant markers of disease severity and some are already being tested.[14]

Over the past few years, N-TproBNP has been studied in various PAH populations and found to be useful in predicting development of PAH and survival in patients with SSc.[15] N-TproBNP serum levels are significantly higher in SSc-PAH (compared to idiopathic PAH patients) despite less severe hemodynamic perturbations,[16] for reasons that remain unclear, but would suggest more profound cardiac dysfunction.

A strong correlation between hyponatremia, as a marker of neurohormonal activation, and right ventricular dysfunction and survival was demonstrated in a cohort of PAH patients.[17] SSc-PAH patients were more likely to be hyponatremic than idiopathic PAH patients despite similar hemodynamics, suggesting possible differences in neurohormonal activation between the two groups. These as well as other specific markers of disease and disease severity need to be identified.

Tricuspid annular systolic excursion (TAPSE), which measures the displacement of the tricuspid annulus from end-diastole to end-systole by echocardiography, correlates with right ventricular function and remodeling, and predicts survival in PAH.[18] Preliminary studies suggest that SSc-PAH patients exhibit lower TAPSE measurements and worse prognosis compared to other PAH patients.[19] Its value as an outcome measure needs further validation.

Cardiac MRI has become the gold standard for quantitative evaluation of right ventricle structural changes; it allows accurate and reproducible measurements of ventricular dimensions, wall thickness, and myocardial mass without relying on geometric assumptions.[20] It enables precise analysis of the different patterns of heart involvement in SSc by differentiating morphological, functional, perfusion, and delayed contrast enhancement abnormalities. Compared to other imaging modalities, cardiac MRI detected significantly compromised RV function in a higher number of asymptomatic SSc patients and may become an invaluable tool in detecting subclinical involvement in such patients.[21]

Current Medical Therapies for SSc-PAH

With improved understanding of the pathogenesis of PAH, novel therapies targeting select pathways have been developed, with a focus on the chronically impaired endothelial function affecting vascular tone and remodeling.[22]

Vasodilator therapy using high-dose calcium channel blockers is an effective long-term therapy for idiopathic PAH patients, but only for the minority of such patients who demonstrate acute vasodilation during hemodynamic testing,[23] and an even smaller number (<3%) of SSc-PAH patients.[4,24] Therefore, high-dose calcium channel blocker therapy is usually not indicated for patients with SSc-PAH, although most patients often receive these drugs at low dosage, typically for Raynaud's phenomenon.

Continuous intravenous epoprostenol, which improves exercise capacity and hemodynamics compared with conventional therapy in SSc-PAH even if no demonstrable effect on survival has ever been shown,[25] remains a valuable therapeutic option for patients with SSc-PAH with NYHA class IV, and in NYHA class III patients who demonstrate no improvement on oral therapy.[26]

Regarding endothelin receptor antagonists, a recent analysis of patients with connective tissue disease-associated PAH included in randomized clinical trials showed that bosentan demonstrated a trend toward improvement in 6MWD (however, far from the effects observed in idiopathic PAH patients[27]) and improved survival compared to historical cohorts.[28] There are three oral ERA licensed in Europe and two in the United States, and these include ETRA selective and nonselective antagonists. There is no clear evidence of superiority for any of these agents, although some cohort comparison and open-label clinical trial data have explored this.[29]

Randomized clinical trials of phosphodiesterase inhibitors such as sildenafil and tadalafil have included patients with PAH related to connective tissue diseases (e.g., SSc-PAH). In a post hoc subgroup analysis of 84 patients with PAH related to connective tissue disease, data from the Sildenafil Use in PAH (SUPER) study suggest a modest effect of sildenafil on exercise capacity, hemodynamic measures, and functional class after 12 weeks of treatment.[30] The specific effects of tadalafil on SSc-PAH or PAH related to other connective tissue diseases is unknown.[31]

It is now common practice in various pulmonary hypertension centers to add drugs when patients fail to improve on monotherapy. A small, nonrandomized study examined the effect of adding sildenafil in patients with idiopathic PAH or SSc-PAH who had failed initial monotherapy with bosentan.[32] While the combination improved 6MWD and functional class in idiopathic PAH patients, the outcome in SSc-PAH patients was less favorable. However, clinical deterioration may have been slowed in these patients. Importantly, there were significantly more side effects in SSc-PAH subjects compared to idiopathic PAH, including hepatotoxicity. Besides, there are many open questions regarding combination therapy, including the choice of combination agents, the optimal timing, when to switch and when to combine. In the setting of idiopathic PAH, experts recommend combination therapy of established PAH drugs by expert centers only, for patients not responding adequately to monotherapy.[33]

Patients with SSc have long been considered suboptimal candidates for lung or heart-lung transplantation. Presumed heightened risk in the postoperative period arising from SSc-related gastroesophageal reflux, renal impairment, or skin fibrosis likely contributes to this perception. However, the results of two recent studies suggest that lung transplantation, in carefully selected patients, may represent a viable therapeutic option for patients with end-stage lung dysfunction resulting from SSc.[34,35] Transplant experts recommend that advanced cases of SSc-PAH that are potential candidates for transplantation should be evaluated on an individual basis.

Future Directions for Medical Therapies

The recognition of aberrant proliferation of endothelial and smooth muscle cells in PAH has prompted the study of antineoplastic drugs, initially in experimental models and now in clinical trials. Two strategies are currently under investigation in randomized controlled trials: disruption of the platelet-derived growth factor (PDGF) pathway and the vascular endothelial growth factor (VEGF) pathway. Imatinib, which was originally developed to inhibit the Bcr-Abl kinase in the treatment of chronic myelogenous leukemia, is also a PDGF and c-kit tyrosine inhibitor that is currently under investigation for the treatment of PAH. A few case reports[36,37] have suggested its usefulness, including one in a patient with SSc-PAH and another in a patient with pulmonary veno-occlusive disease (PVOD).[38] It is also noteworthy that imatinib and other tyrosine kinase inhibitors are currently being studied for the treatment of SSc-related ILD and skin disease based on the notion that dysregulated proliferation and increased growth factors are prevalent in SSc and may be involved in the pathogenesis of SSc.

In summary, despite major advances in the understanding and management of PAH, SSc-PAH remains a condition with poor response to modern therapy. Currently available markers of disease severity and clinical tools to assess therapeutic response are either limited or lacking. There is an urgent need to identify specific pathogenic mechanisms and design novel physiologic, molecular, and imaging biomarkers that will allow a better understanding of the underlying pathogenesis and serve as reliable tools to design targeted therapy and adequately monitor response in this devastating syndrome.

References

1. Simonneau G, Robbins IM, Beghetti M, et al. Updated clinical classification of pulmonary hypertension. *J Am Coll Cardiol*. 2009;54(1 suppl):S43-S54.
2. Hachulla E, Gressin V, Guillevin L, et al. Early detection of pulmonary arterial hypertension in systemic sclerosis: a French nationwide prospective multicenter study. *Arthritis Rheum*. 2005;52(12):3792-3800.
3. Mukerjee D, St George D, Coleiro B, et al. Prevalence and outcome in systemic sclerosis associated pulmonary arterial hypertension: application of a registry approach. *Ann Rheum Dis*. 2003;62(11):1088-1093.
4. Humbert M, Sitbon O, Chaouat A, et al. Pulmonary arterial hypertension in France: results from a national registry. *Am J Respir Crit Care Med*. 2006;173(9):1023-1030.
5. Tan RT, Kuzo R, Goodman LR, Siegel R, Haasler GB, Presberg KW. Utility of CT scan evaluation for predicting pulmonary hypertension in patients with parenchymal lung disease. Medical College of Wisconsin Lung Transplant Group. *Chest*. 1998;113(5):1250-1256.
6. Ng CS, Wells AU, Padley SP. A CT sign of chronic pulmonary arterial hypertension: the ratio of main pulmonary artery to aortic diameter. *J Thorac Imaging*. 1999;14(4):270-278.
7. Le Pavec J, Humbert M, Mouthon L, Hassoun PM. Systemic sclerosis-associated pulmonary arterial hypertension. *Am J Respir Crit Care Med*. 2010;181(12):1285-1293. Official Journal of The American Thoracic Society.
8. Fisher MR, Mathai SC, Champion HC, et al. Clinical differences between idiopathic and scleroderma-related pulmonary hypertension. *Arthritis Rheum*. 2006;54(9):3043-3050.
9. Girgis RE, Mathai SC, Krishnan JA, Wigley FM, Hassoun PM. Long-term outcome of bosentan treatment in idiopathic pulmonary arterial hypertension and pulmonary arterial hypertension associated with the scleroderma spectrum of diseases. *J Heart Lung Transplant*. 2005;24(10):1626-1631.
10. Snow JL, Kawut SM. Surrogate end points in pulmonary arterial hypertension: assessing the response to therapy. *Clin Chest Med*. 2007;28(1):75-89. viii.
11. Pamidi S, Mehta S. Six-minute walk test in scleroderma-associated pulmonary arterial hypertension: are we counting what counts? *J Rheumatol*. 2009;36(2):216-218.
12. Garin MC, Highland KB, Silver RM, Strange C. Limitations to the 6-minute walk test in interstitial lung disease and pulmonary hypertension in scleroderma. *J Rheumatol*. 2009;36(2): 330-336.
13. D'Alonzo GE, Barst RJ, Ayres SM, et al. Survival in patients with primary pulmonary hypertension. Results from a national prospective study. *Ann Intern Med*. 1991;115:343-349.

14. Distler O, Behrens F, Pittrow D, et al. Defining appropriate outcome measures in pulmonary arterial hypertension related to systemic sclerosis: a Delphi consensus study with cluster analysis. *Arthritis Rheum.* 2008;59(6):867-875.
15. Williams MH, Handler CE, Akram R, et al. Role of N-terminal brain natriuretic peptide (N-TproBNP) in scleroderma-associated pulmonary arterial hypertension. *Eur Heart J.* 2006;27(12):1485-1494.
16. Mathai SC, Buesco M, Hummers L, et al. N-terminal pro-brain natriuretic peptide is a unique marker of poor survival in scleroderma-related pulmonary arterial hypertension. *Eur Respir J.* 2010;35(1):95-104.
17. Forfia PR, Mathai SC, Fisher MR, et al. Hyponatremia predicts right heart failure and poor survival in pulmonary arterial hypertension. *Am J Respir Crit Care Med.* 2008;177(12):1364-1369.
18. Forfia PR, Fisher MR, Mathai SC, et al. Tricuspid annular displacement predicts survival in pulmonary hypertension. *Am J Respir Crit Care Med.* 2006;174(9):1034-1041.
19. Brown L, Osman N, Sibley C, et al. Right ventricular structure and function in pulmonary arterial hypertension associated with systemic sclerosis. *Proc Am Thorac Soc.* 2008;A442.
20. Boxt LM. Radiology of the right ventricle. *Radiol Clin North Am.* 1999;37(2):379-400.
21. Bezante GP, Rollando D, Sessarego M, et al. Cardiac magnetic resonance imaging detects subclinical right ventricular impairment in systemic sclerosis. *J Rheumatol.* 2007;34(12):2431-2437.
22. Humbert M, Sitbon O, Simonneau G. Treatment of pulmonary arterial hypertension. *N Engl J Med.* 2004;351(14):1425-1436.
23. Sitbon O, Humbert M, Jais X, et al. Long-term response to calcium channel blockers in idiopathic pulmonary arterial hypertension. *Circulation.* 2005;111(23):3105-3111.
24. Montani D, Savale L, Natali D, et al. Long-term response to calcium-channel blockers in non-idiopathic pulmonary arterial hypertension. *Eur Heart J* 2010;31(15):1898-1907.
25. Badesch DB, Tapson VF, McGoon MD, et al. Continuous intravenous epoprostenol for pulmonary hypertension due to the scleroderma spectrum of disease. A randomized, controlled trial. *Ann Intern Med.* 2000;132(6):425-434.
26. Hassoun PM. Therapies for scleroderma-related pulmonary arterial hypertension. *Expert Rev Respir Med.* 2009;3(2):187-196.
27. Barst RJ, Rubin LJ, Long WA, et al. A comparison of continuous intravenous epoprostenol (prostacyclin) with conventional therapy for primary pulmonary hypertension. The Primary Pulmonary Hypertension Study Group. *N Engl J Med.* 1996;334(5):296-302.
28. Denton CP, Humbert M, Rubin L, Black CM. Bosentan treatment for pulmonary arterial hypertension related to connective tissue disease: a subgroup analysis of the pivotal clinical trials and their open-label extensions. *Ann Rheum Dis.* 2006;65(10):1336-1340.
29. Valerio CJ, Handler CE, Kabunga P, Smith CJ, Denton CP, Coghlan JG. Clinical experience with bosentan and sitaxentan in connective tissue disease-associated pulmonary arterial hypertension. *Rheumatology Oxford.* 2010;49(11):2147-2153.
30. Badesch DB, Hill NS, Burgess G, et al. Sildenafil for pulmonary arterial hypertension associated with connective tissue disease. *J Rheumatol.* 2007;34(12):2417-2422.
31. Galie N, Brundage BH, Ghofrani HA, et al. Tadalafil therapy for pulmonary arterial hypertension. *Circulation.* 2009;119(22):2894-2903.
32. Mathai SC, Girgis RE, Fisher MR, et al. Addition of sildenafil to bosentan monotherapy in pulmonary arterial hypertension. *Eur Respir J.* 2007;29(3):469-475.
33. Galie N, Hoeper MM, Humbert M, et al. Guidelines for the diagnosis and treatment of pulmonary hypertension. *Eur Respir J.* 2009;34(6):1219-1263.
34. Schachna L, Medsger TA Jr, Dauber JH, et al. Lung transplantation in scleroderma compared with idiopathic pulmonary fibrosis and idiopathic pulmonary arterial hypertension. *Arthritis Rheum.* 2006;54(12):3954-3961.

35. Shitrit D, Amital A, Peled N, et al. Lung transplantation in patients with scleroderma: case series, review of the literature, and criteria for transplantation. *Clin Transplant.* 2009;23: 178-183.
36. Ghofrani HA, Seeger W, Grimminger F. Imatinib for the treatment of pulmonary arterial hypertension. *N Engl J Med.* 2005;353(13):1412-1413.
37. Souza R, Sitbon O, Parent F, Simonneau G, Humbert M. Long term imatinib treatment in pulmonary arterial hypertension. *Thorax.* 2006;61(8):736.
38. Overbeek MJ, van Nieuw-Amerongen GP, Boonstra A, Smit EF, Vonk-Noordegraaf A. Possible role of imatinib in clinical pulmonary veno-occlusive disease. *Eur Respir J.* 2008;32(1):232-235.

Chapter 14
A Diffuse Scleroderma Patient Who Presents with Shortness of Breath and Enlarged Cardiac Silhouette

Yannick Allanore and Christophe Meune

Keywords Heart • Pericarditis • Chest pain • Dyspnea • Echocardiography

Case Study

A 61-year-old woman presented for a routine annual follow-up of her disease. She had been diagnosed 4 years before as having systemic sclerosis. Initial symptoms consisted of hand stiffness and swelling with carpal tunnel syndrome, Raynaud's phenomenon of recent onset, dysphagia and gastroesophageal reflux, and dyspnea. Skin involvement included sclerodactyly with forearm and arm lesions and also truncal skin thickness. Blood tests showed positive antinuclear antibodies with anti-topoisomerase I specificity. She was treated with methotrexate (20 mg weekly), nifedipine (60 mg daily) and omeprazole (40 mg daily). Four years after presentation she complained of worsening dyspnea and chest pain. Although the patient did not have dyspnea at rest, modest effort worsened dyspnea with evident shortness of breath that could be classified at functional class III.

Physical Examination

Temperature 36.8°C; pulse 90 bpm; respirations 18 per min; blood pressure 130/80 mmHg. Skin: puffy fingers with thickness of the skin in particular on upper arms and trunk with Rodnan skin score 28/51. HEENT: perioral skin furrowing with

Y. Allanore (✉)
Department of Rheumatology A and INSERM U1016, Université Paris Descartes,
Hôpital Cochin, 27 rue Faubourg Saint Jacques, Paris 75679, France

R.M. Silver and C.P. Denton (eds.), *Case Studies in Systemic Sclerosis*,
DOI: 10.1007/978-0-85729-641-2_14, © Springer-Verlag London Limited 2011

Fig. 14.1 X-ray: the cardiac silhouette appears enlarged and interstitial lung disease (reticulations) is present

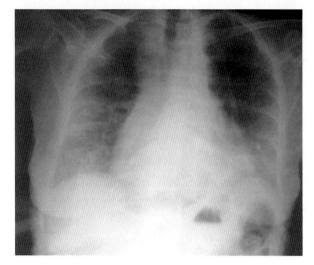

reduced oral aperture. Chest: diffuse crackles. Cardiac: regular rate and rhythm with normal S1 and S2 heart sounds. Abdomen: nondistended and nontender. Extremities: no edema. Musculoskeletal: mild flexion contractures of the fingers with inability to flatten hand; no joint tenderness or swelling.

Laboratory Findings

Complete blood count (CBC), chemistry panel, and urinalysis were normal, in particular creatinine concentration was 80 mmol/L (creatinine clearance 68 mL/min). Troponin concentration was 0.01 ng/mL (99th percentile for the method is at 0.07 ng/mL) and NT-proBNP concentration was 97 pg/mL (97th percentiles of normal values below 287 pg/mL for subjects aged 55–64 years). Chest radiograph: interstitial lung disease with enlarged cardiac silhouette (Fig. 14.1). CT scan: severe and diffuse interstitial lung disease (ILD) with both ground glass and reticular lesions (Fig. 14.2) and also pericardial effusion (Fig. 14.3). Pulmonary function test (PFTs): FVC 1.80 L (80% predicted); FEV1 1.53 L (83% predicted); DLco 6.11 (31% predicted), DLco/VA 2.26 (53% predicted). Echocardiogram: normal LV ejection fraction, normal RA and RV dimensions, estimate of RVSP 40 mmHg, a >10 mm circumferential pericardial effusion without signs of tamponade (Fig. 14.4).

Course

A diagnosis of diffuse cutaneous systemic sclerosis (dSSc) was already known; it was supported by the onset of Raynaud's phenomenon concomitant with the onset of skin disease, the proximal and truncal distribution of skin thickness, and the

Fig. 14.2 CT scan: interstitial lung disease with ground glass opacities, reticular markings, and bronchiectasis

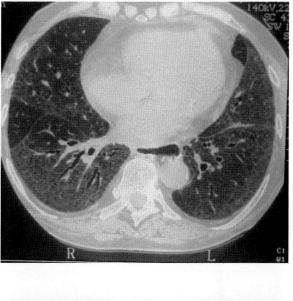

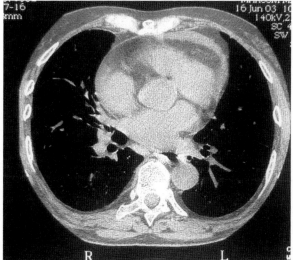

Fig. 14.3 CT scan: moderate-sized, circumferential pericardial effusion

presence of anti-topoisomerase I antibodies. In accordance, interstitial lung disease was present early in the course of disease. Subsequently, she complained of worsening shortness of breath together with intermittent chest pain. Chest pain was not evocative of acute myocardial infarction, and normal cardiac markers and ECG definitely ruled out ischemic heart disease. The chest pain was not suggestive of gastroesophageal reflux (heartburn, regurgitation, dysphagia), and she was being treated with PPI therapy. Therefore, chest pain in this case was possibly a symptom of the recently discovered pericarditis. Typical pericardial pain has the following characteristics: sharp or dull constant pain at the center of the chest, sometimes

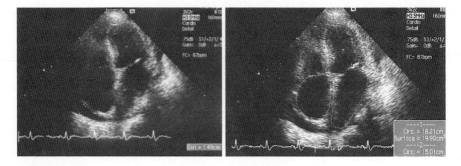

Fig. 14.4 Echocardiogram: circumferential pericardial effusion measuring >10 mm, predominant along the right heart chambers

referred to the left shoulder, and usually worsened by deep breathing, lying down, or swallowing.

Worsening dyspnea was the patient's other major complaint. There was no history or sign for respiratory infection or pulmonary embolism. Lung CT-scan showed ground glass and reticulation but lung volumes remained normal. Echocardiography revealed a pericardial effusion without apparent ventricular dysfunction, but the estimated systolic pulmonary artery pressure was near the upper accepted value of 40 mmHg. It should be noted that the presence of a large pericardial effusion limits the accurate measurement of several echocardiographic parameters: contractility, ejection fraction, left ventricular relaxation, pulmonary artery pressure (because of reduced preload and possible swinging heart). PFTs revealed low DLco and DLco/VA, in the setting of normal spirometry suggesting pulmonary vascular disease. The normal NTproBNP concentration was indicative of the lack of increased cardiac strain. We, therefore, considered pericarditis to be the most likely cause of both her chest pain and dyspnea. We treated the patient with colchicine 2 mg daily for 3 days followed by 1 mg daily for 10 days, in addition to her current medications. Nonsteroidal anti-inflammatory drugs could have been considered but because of the known history of esophagitis, we preferred colchicine. Unfortunately, there was no clinical or echocardiographic improvement 10 days later. Therefore, we initiated oral prednisone at 20 mg daily for 3 days, tapering to 10 mg daily after 2 weeks. Systemic pressure was unchanged and no rise in serum creatinine concentration was observed. Clinical improvement occurred quickly and after a few days chest pain disappeared and dyspnea returned to functional class II. Repeat echocardiography confirmed that the pericardial effusion had decreased in size. The patient returned home and was advised rest.

The patient called her doctor 3 months later because of worsening dyspnea. She came to the department and clinical examination was unchanged. However, cardiac markers revealed an increase NT-proBNP value of 750 pg/mL, and echocardiography showed a higher value for systolic pulmonary artery pressure that was now nearly 50 mmHg, with very small pericardial effusion. Right heart catheterization was performed and demonstrated pulmonary arterial hypertension.

Discussion

All cardiac layers, endocardium, myocardium, and pericardium, may be involved in SSc resulting in pericardial effusion, atrial and ventricular arrhythmias, conduction system defects, valvular impairment, myocardial ischemia, myocardial hypertrophy, and heart failure.[1,2] Renal and pulmonary involvement can also adversely affect cardiac status.

Pericarditis often causes chest pain and sometimes other symptoms. Autopsy studies have commonly revealed pericardial abnormalities including pericarditis with or without effusion, fibrous or fibrinous involvement, or pericardial adhesions.[3] In a series of 44 patients, pericarditis was present in 31 (77.7%), with dense fibrinous deposits characteristic of uremic pericarditis seen in only two cases, one of whom had confirmed evidence of renal failure.[4] Most often, pericarditis is asymptomatic, with symptoms being reported in only 7–20% of patients.[1,2] Clinical disease is usually one of two different patterns. Some patients experience acute pericarditis with fever, chest pain and dyspnea. Others have a more chronic clinical picture with cardiomegaly, congestive heart failure, and sometimes pleural effusion. In this latter group, renal crisis may occur, although it remains unclear whether pericarditis heralds the renal failure and/or the treatment used for pericarditis, including diuretics and corticosteroids, may somehow induce scleroderma renal crisis. Massive effusion defined by an estimated volume > 200 mL carries with it a poor prognosis. As an example, Satoh et al. reported 5 cases with massive pericardial effusion that occurred mainly in patients in the diffuse cutaneous subset in association with flexion contractures (4/5 patients), pulmonary fibrosis (4/5 patients), and autoantibodies to topoisomerase I (3/5 patients). Four of the five cases died within 9 months of the diagnosis of pericarditis: two from renal failure, one from cardiac tamponade, and another had a sudden death.[5] Pericarditis may be a sign of overall disease activity and progression and may, therefore, herald renal involvement. On the other hand, a large pericardial effusion may interfere with cardiac output favoring renal hypoperfusion, thereby triggering renal crisis in high-risk patients (early diffuse SSc with autoantibodies directed to topoisomerase I or to RNA polymerase III). Although very rare in SSc, careful renal assessment and management is particularly critical in SSc patients with large pericardial effusions or reduced cardiac output due to cardiac tamponade.[6] If medical therapy is not successful then pericardiocentesis or a fenestration procedure may be considered and can give rapid and long-term hemodynamic benefit.

Echocardiography is the recommended tool to rapidly identify a pericardial effusion, the relationship between the effusion and cardiac structures, and the physiologic changes associated with tamponade. In addition, echocardiography may provide valuable information in the management of SSc patients, such as an estimate of left ventricular systolic and diastolic function, right ventricular systolic function, possible valvular damage, and in some cases an estimate of pulmonary arterial pressure. Recent echocardiographic data derived from various controlled clinical studies have provided additional information regarding the prevalence of pericardial effusion. Indeed, a study performed in Italy found pericardial effusion to be present in 33/77 (43%) SSc patients, but in only 11/77 (14%) was it deemed to be significant.[7] In another study performed by our group, pericardial effusion was found in 15/100 (15%) consecutive patients.[8] Therefore, using systematic echocardiography pericarditis is a quite common finding but typically it is not hemodynamically significant.

Our case study raises the question of a link between pericarditis and the presence of pulmonary hypertension. It should be noted that pericardial effusion associated with pulmonary hypertension is common, but usually represents a transudate and therefore is very unlikely to cause tamponade. In addition, effusions are generally relatively small in this context, as when the index case presented with dyspnea. Previous studies have reported a frequent association of pericardial effusion and pulmonary arterial hypertension in SSc patients,[9] as well as in patients with idiopathic pulmonary arterial hypertension, in which it is thought to be a marker of disease severity. The exact mechanism for such an association is unknown. As a consequence of increased pulmonary artery pressure, a transudative process from the right ventricule or possibly through cardiac veins to the pericardium has been proposed. In our patient, pulmonary arterial hypertension was not suspected after the first echocardiogram, until later in the course of disease. One may speculate that pulmonary artery pressure (PAP) increased after her initial evaluation, or that pulmonary arterial pressure was underestimated by earlier echocardiograms. In fact, the concordance between echocardiographically estimated PAP and direct measurement by right heart catheterization (RHC) is usually fair but varies among studies, and additionally a large pericardial effusion may lead to underestimation of the PAP. With a large pericardial effusion there might be invagination of the right atrium and right ventricular free wall possibly culminating in tamponade. Tricuspid regurgitation as well as RV output decreases (as a consequence of reduced RV filling), thus resulting in underestimation of PAP. Therefore, reassessment by echocardiography is recommended whenever a significant pericardial effusion is found in any patient suspected of having pulmonary hypertension. This was the case for our patient who had a very low DLco and also a low DLco/VA, the latter being less influenced by the presence of interstitial lung disease. Nevertheless, it remains unclear whether pulmonary hypertension existed at the outset in our patient (normal NTproBNP and clinical improvement after corticosteroids would argue against this), or whether the occurrence of pulmonary hypertension was a manifestation of progressive SSc.

Pericarditis is very common and does not require specific treatment in the large majority of cases. When symptomatic, acute pericarditis may be treated with nonsteroidal anti-inflammatory drugs and/or colchicine, and occasionally by brief treatment with corticosteroids. Although no trial has been performed in the context of SSc pericarditis, colchicine therapy (2 mg daily tapered to 1 or 0.5 mg daily) has significant benefit over conventional treatment by decreasing the recurrence rate in patients with an initial episode of acute and also recurrent pericarditis. On the other hand, corticosteroid treatment for the initial attack may favor recurrences.[10] Cardiac tamponade, while extremely rare, carries a poor prognosis; in such cases, corticosteroids at high dosage (1 mg/kg/day) may be used, together with pericardiocentesis if there is evidence of hemodynamic compromise. Cardiac monitoring is recommended during initial therapy of severe pericarditis because of the potential risk of malignant arrhythmias.

In conclusion, asymptomatic, mild pericarditis is common in SSc and does not require specific treatment in the large majority of patients. In the case of recurrent or severe effusion, anti-inflammatory drugs may be required. Renal as well as cardiac monitoring is critical in such cases since pericarditis may be associated with scleroderma renal crisis, cardiac arrhythmias, pulmonary arterial hypertension, and overall progression of the disease.

References

1. Kahan A, Allanore Y. Primary myocardial involvement in systemic sclerosis. *Rheumatology (Oxford)*. 2006;45(Suppl 4):iv14-iv17.
2. Champion HC. The heart in scleroderma. *Rheum Dis Clin North Am*. 2008;34:181-190.
3. Bulkley BH, Ridolfi RL, Salyer WR, Hutchins GM. Myocardial lesions of progressive systemic sclerosis. A cause of cardiac dysfunction. *Circulation*. 1976;53:483-490.
4. Byers RJ, Marshall DA, Freemont AJ. Pericardial involvement in systemic sclerosis. *Ann Rheum Dis*. 1997;56:393-394.
5. Satoh M, Tokuhira M, Hama N, et al. Massive pericardial effusion in scleroderma: a review of five cases. *Br J Rheumatol*. 1995;34:564-567.
6. Panchal P, Adams E, Hsieh A. Calcific constructive pericarditis: a rare complication of CREST syndrome. *Arthritis Rheum*. 1996;39:347-350.
7. Maione S, Cuomo G, Giunta A, et al. Echocardiographic alterations in systemic sclerosis: a longitudinal study. *Semin Arthritis Rheum*. 2005;34(5):721-727.
8. Meune C, Avouac J, Wahbi K, et al. Cardiac involvement in systemic sclerosis assessed by tissue-Doppler echocardiography in routine care: a controlled study of 100 consecutive patients. *Arthritis Rheum*. 2008;58:1803-1809.
9. Fischer A, Misumi S, Curran-Everett D, et al. Pericardial abnormalities predict the presence of echocardiographically defined pulmonary arterial hypertension in systemic sclerosis-related interstitial lung disease. *Chest*. 2007;131:988-992.
10. Imazio M, Bobbio M, Cecchi E, et al. Colchicine as first-choice therapy for recurrent pericarditis: results of the CORE (COlchicine for REcurrent pericarditis) trial. *Arch Intern Med*. 2005;165:1987-1991.

Chapter 15
A Patient with Systemic Sclerosis, Dyspnea on Exertion, Atypical Chest Pain, and Arrhythmia

André Kahan

Keywords Myocardium • Myocardial perfusion • Myocardial function • Small coronary arteries • Coronary vasospasm • Calcium channel blocker • Angiotensin-converting enzyme inhibitor • Endothelin receptor antagonist

Case Study

A 36-year-old woman presented with a 6-month history of Raynaud's phenomenon, arthralgia, heartburn, and rapid progression of diffuse thickening of the skin. She also complained of severe dyspnea on exertion and palpitations, with intermittent atypical chest pain at rest or after exercise. She never smoked and had no history of pulmonary or cardiac diseases.

Physical Examination

Temperature 37.2°C; pulse 92 bpm; blood pressure 125/80 mmHg; respirations 16 per min. Skin: diffuse thickening, including not only hands, feet, and face, with reduced oral aperture, but also proximal arms and legs, chest, and abdomen. Digital pitted scars were present on two fingerpads with flexion contractures of the fingers. The small joints in the hands were tender but not swollen. No edema of the extremities was noted. Cardiac examination was normal, with regular rhythm at rest. Chest, abdomen, and neurologic examinations were normal.

A. Kahan
Paris Descartes University, Department of Rheumatology A, Hôpital Cochin AP-HP,
27 rue du Faubourg Saint Jacques, Paris 75014, France

R.M. Silver and C.P. Denton (eds.), *Case Studies in Systemic Sclerosis*,
DOI: 10.1007/978-0-85729-641-2_15, © Springer-Verlag London Limited 2011

Fig. 15.1 Thallium-201
single photon emission
computerized tomography in
a patient with systemic
sclerosis: *upper part*: at
baseline, showing major
abnormalities in myocardial
perfusion; *lower part*: after
the oral administration of
40 mg nicardipine, showing
partial improvement in
myocardial perfusion

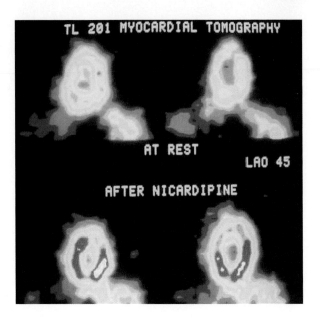

Laboratory Findings

Usual blood and urine analysis: normal (including normal serum creatinine, cholesterol, and triglyceride). Antinuclear antibody (ANA) by IIF: positive (titer 1:160); anti-topoisomerase I antibodies: positive. Hand radiographs: normal. Chest radiograph: clear lung fields and normal cardiac size. Pulmonary function test (PFTs): normal (FVC 90% predicted; FEV1 85% predicted; DLco 90% predicted). Echocardiogram: normal LV ejection fraction, normal RA and RV dimensions, no tricuspid regurgitation.

The unexplained symptom complex of severe dyspnea on exertion, palpitations, and atypical chest pain required further investigation. Chest CT scan: normal. EKG: normal. 24 h-Holter EKG: a few atrial premature beats, intermittent short atrial tachycardias. Thallium-201 single photon emission computerized tomography: diffuse abnormalities of myocardial perfusion, with significant improvement after oral administration of 40 mg nicardipine (Fig. 15.1). Radionuclide ventriculography: normal global left and right ventricular function; segmental left ventricular dysfunction, improved after oral administration of 40 mg nicardipine. Tissue Doppler echocardiography: decreased systolic and diastolic strain rates. Cardiac magnetic resonance imaging: abnormal heterogeneous myocardial perfusion, without coronary distribution and with significant partial improvement after oral administration of 40 mg nicardipine (Fig. 15.2). In addition, no abnormal enhancement suggestive of myocardial infarction was noticed on delayed gadolinium-enhanced acquisitions, more particularly in the area of early perfusion defects. Taking into account these

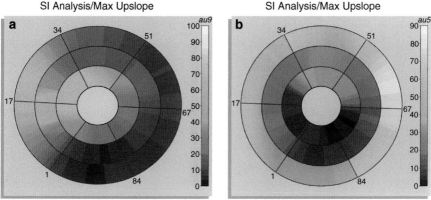

Phase range (1–50), min=6.35, max=91.01   Phase range (1–40), min=5.32, max=87.19

Fig. 15.2 Cardiac magnetic resonance imaging (MRI) in a patient with systemic sclerosis: parametric bull's eye of first-pass myocardial perfusion (maximum upslope of enhancement from yellow as high to dark brown as low) exhibiting: (**a**) at baseline, heterogeneous decreased myocardial perfusion; (**b**) partial improvement in myocardial perfusion after the oral administration of 40 mg nicardipine

results and the absence of other risk factors, the hypothesis of large coronary artery disease was unlikely: thus, coronary arteriography was not performed.

Course

A diagnosis of diffuse cutaneous systemic sclerosis was made based on the presence of the characteristic diffuse skin thickening, associated with Raynaud's phenomenon, digital pitted scars, esophageal involvement, arthralgia, and positive anti-topoisomerase I antibodies.

Baseline investigation revealed no evidence for lung or kidney involvement, nor was systemic or pulmonary arterial hypertension present. The myocardial perfusion and functional defects, reversible at least in part after the oral administration of the calcium channel blocker nicardipine, were consistent with primary scleroderma myocardial disease, with vasospastic or organic abnormalities of small coronary vessels; these abnormalities could explain the dyspnea after exertion, the palpitations, and the intermittent chest pain at rest or after exercise.

Long-term calcium-channel blocker therapy (40 mg nicardipine three times daily) strikingly improved the cardiac symptoms and the patient could resume her normal daily activities. Nicardipine also improved her Raynaud's phenomenon. Cold avoidance was strongly recommended. Proton pump inhibitor therapy significantly improved gastroesophageal reflux. Physical therapy hand exercises were prescribed. During the first years of the disease, close follow-up was recommended, including clinical assessment at least every 3 months and pulmonary function tests and cardiac evaluation every 6 months.

Discussion

"Primary" scleroderma myocardial disease may be defined as myocardial involvement in systemic sclerosis patients without pulmonary or systemic hypertension, and without significant renal or pulmonary involvement.

Primary myocardial involvement is common in systemic sclerosis and may be detected in up to 100% of patients.[1-5] Cardiac involvement is often clinically asymptomatic. Clinical symptoms may be considered as "late" events. EKG and chest X-ray are nonsensitive techniques; echocardiography is used for routine cardiac assessment; sensitive techniques such as single photon emission computerized tomography, radionuclide ventriculography, tissue Doppler echocardiography, and magnetic resonance imaging allow the early detection of functional or organic lesions.

When cardiac involvement appears clinically evident, it is recognized as a poor prognostic factor in systemic sclerosis patients.[3] A meta-analysis of pooled cohorts found heart involvement at any time in 10% of patients with systemic sclerosis (8–28% according to series).[6] A multivariate adjusted analysis showed the hazard ratio for cardiac mortality to be 2.8 (2.1–3.8).

Primary scleroderma myocardial involvement may be the consequence of the characteristic functional and organic vascular lesions of this disease. The frequency of atherosclerosis of the large coronary arteries appears to be similar to that of the general population. Some histological examinations demonstrated diffuse patchy fibrosis, with contraction band necrosis unrelated to epicardial coronary artery stenosis, and with concentric intimal hypertrophy associated with fibrinoid necrosis of intramural coronary arteries.[7,8] Angina pectoris and myocardial infarction were observed in patients with systemic sclerosis whose epicardial coronary arteries were normal. Repeated ischemia-reperfusion abnormalities may lead to the characteristic contraction band necrosis followed by irreversible myocardial fibrosis.

The coronary vasodilator reserve was strikingly reduced in clinically symptomatic systemic sclerosis patients[8]; endomyocardial biopsies showed fibrotic tissue and a typical systemic sclerosis vascular lesion with concentric intimal hypertrophy; these results, combined with myocardial metabolic evaluation, demonstrated that, despite normal epicardial coronary arteries, structural abnormalities of small coronary arteries or arterioles explained the reduced coronary reserve. Recent noninvasive studies confirmed the impaired coronary flow reserve in systemic sclerosis patients.[9] These fixed organic abnormalities of small coronary arteries and arterioles, inducing the reduced coronary reserve in systemic sclerosis patients, should be considered as "late" events.

In contrast, vasospasm of the small coronary arteries or arterioles plays a major role in the early myocardial abnormalities in patients with systemic sclerosis. These functional, reversible, abnormalities of myocardial perfusion were demonstrated using thallium-201 single photon emission computerized tomography at rest, or after exercise, or after cold stimulation.[1,2,10] Exercise-induced myocardial perfusion defects observed by scintigraphy were predictive of developing subsequent cardiac disease or death.[11]

The beneficial effect of vasodilator drugs on myocardial perfusion abnormalities was clearly demonstrated. Using thallium-201 single photon emission computerized tomography, improved myocardial perfusion was seen in systemic sclerosis patients after intravenous administration of dipyridamole,[12] as well as after treatment with nifedipine,[1] nicardipine,[13] or captopril.[14] Some myocardial perfusion defects were reversible, whereas others remained fixed, which is consistent with the coexistence of reversible vasopasm of small coronary arteries and irreversible lesions such as organic vessel disease or myocardial fibrosis. The beneficial effect of nifedipine on myocardial perfusion and metabolism in systemic sclerosis patients was also demonstrated using positron emission tomography.[15]

Cardiovascular magnetic resonance imaging is an accurate, quantitative, sensitive method for the noninvasive assessment of myocardial perfusion, coronary reserve, ventricular function, and parenchymal abnormalities (i.e., myocarditis or burden of fibrosis). High-resolution perfusion magnetic resonance imaging can be used to identify small subendocardial defects, which do not correspond to any epicardial coronary artery distribution, suggesting microvascular alteration. Nifedipine-induced improvement was confirmed using cardiac magnetic resonance imaging, with a mean 38% increase of the global perfusion index.[16] Using cardiac magnetic resonance imaging, similar results on myocardial perfusion in systemic sclerosis patients were observed with bosentan, an oral dual endothelin receptor antagonist.[17]

Thus, the beneficial effects of vasodilators, such as calcium channel blockers mostly of dihydropyridine type, angiotensin-converting enzyme inhibitors, and an endothelin receptor antagonist were clearly demonstrated in systemic sclerosis patients, inducing a striking improvement in the early reversible vasospastic component of the "primary" scleroderma myocardial disease.

Diffuse, patchy fibrosis, unrelated to large coronary artery distribution, is characteristic of late myocardial involvement in systemic sclerosis.[7,18] Although advanced myocardial fibrosis may lead to heart failure, systolic or diastolic dysfunction can occur early in the disease, many years before becoming clinically evident. Several studies, using radionuclide ventriculography, found a decreased global left ventricular ejection fraction in a minority of patients, although segmental dysfunction[19] or exercise-induced dysfunction[20] was more prevalent. Diastolic dysfunction in systemic sclerosis was reported using improved echocardiographic techniques.[21,22] In 42 systemic sclerosis patients with normal pulmonary arterial pressure and less than 5 years of disease duration, radionuclide ventriculography showed that 16 patients had reduced right ventricular ejection fraction, three had reduced left ventricular ejection fraction, and 10 had reduced peak filling rate, highlighting early right ventricular systolic and left ventricular diastolic dysfunction.[23] In systemic sclerosis patients, the group with thallium perfusion defect scores above the median had a significantly lower mean left ventricular ejection fraction than the other group, and all patients with abnormal resting left ventricular ejection fraction had thallium perfusion defect scores above the median.[2] The link between myocardial perfusion abnormalities and dysfunction suggests a similar mechanism for myocardial involvement.

The beneficial effect of vasodilators on myocardial dysfunction has also been demonstrated. Nicardipine was shown to acutely improve global left ventricular ejection fraction and segmental abnormalities.[19] Improvements in both left ventricular ejection fraction and right ventricular ejection fraction after oral treatment with nicardipine were confirmed, with a correlation between improvements in left and right ventricular ejection fractions.[23] These results provide further evidence for the same pathogenic pathway, with reversible vasospastic small coronary artery disease inducing heart dysfunction.

Tissue-Doppler echocardiography allows direct measurement of myocardial velocities and strain rate. Previous studies demonstrated that strain rate is a powerful indicator of myocardial contraction, independent of myocardial translational motion, and is far more sensitive than conventional echocardiography. Systemic sclerosis patients with normal cardiac examination, pulmonary artery pressure, and radionuclide left ventricular ejection fraction had lower systolic and lower diastolic strain rates than matched controls.[24]

Nifedipine significantly increased segmental (posterior wall) systolic and diastolic strain rates.[16] These results, together with the increased perfusion shown by magnetic resonance imaging, suggested that an increase in myocardial perfusion might be the main determinant in the observed increased contractility, emphasizing the global intrinsic beneficial effects of nifedipine.

The long-term beneficial effects of calcium channel blockers was demonstrated in a large series of 7,073 systemic sclerosis patients: age, male gender, digital ulcerations, myositis, and lung involvement were independently associated with increased prevalence of left ventricular dysfunction; in contrast, the use of calcium channel blockers appeared to be protective (OR 0.41; 95% CI 0.22–0.74).[25]

Conclusion

In summary, "primary" myocardial involvement is a frequent and early finding in systemic sclerosis patients. Primary myocardial involvement is likely to result from the general vasospastic mechanism which plays a major role in this disease. Reversible vasospasm of the small coronary arteries or arterioles would initially impair perfusion and function. This would be followed by a structural coronary arteriolar lesion leading to irreversible abnormalities. Early treatment with vasodilators, such as calcium channel blockers, angiotensin-converting enzyme inhibitors, and an endothelin receptor antagonist was shown to be beneficial for both myocardial perfusion and function. Long-term treatment with vasodilators, such as calcium channel blockers which appear to be protective against left ventricular dysfunction, might limit the progression of this major life-threatening complication of systemic sclerosis.

References

1. Kahan A, Devaux JY, Amor B, et al. Nifedipine and thallium-201 myocardial perfusion in progressive systemic sclerosis. *N Engl J Med*. 1986;314:1397-1402.
2. Follansbee WP, Curtiss EI, Medsger TA Jr, et al. Physiologic abnormalities of cardiac function in progressive systemic sclerosis with diffuse scleroderma. *N Engl J Med*. 1984;310:142-148.
3. Clements PJ, Lachenbruch PA, Furst DE, Paulus HE, Sterz MG. Cardiac score. A semiquantitative measure of cardiac involvement that improves prediction of prognosis in systemic sclerosis. *Arthritis Rheum*. 1991;34:1371-1380.
4. Ferri C, Emdin M, Nielsen H, Bruhlmann P. Assessment of heart involvement. *Clin Exp Rheumatol*. 2003;21(Suppl 29):S24-S28.
5. Steen VD, Medsger TA Jr. Severe organ involvement in systemic sclerosis with diffuse scleroderma. *Arthritis Rheum*. 2000;43:2437-2444.
6. Ioannidis JP, Vlachoyiannopoulos PG, Haidich AB, et al. Mortality in systemic sclerosis: an international meta-analysis of individual patient data. *Am J Med*. 2005;118:2-10.
7. Bulkley BH, Ridolfi RL, Salyer WR, Hutchins GM. Myocardial lesions of progressive systemic sclerosis: a cause of cardiac dysfunction. *Circulation*. 1976;53:483-490.
8. Kahan A, Nitenberg A, Foult JM, et al. Decreased coronary reserve in primary scleroderma myocardial disease. *Arthritis Rheum*. 1985;28:637-646.
9. Montisci R, Vacca A, Garau P, et al. Detection of early impairment of coronary flow reserve in patients with systemic sclerosis. *Ann Rheum Dis*. 2003;62:890-893.
10. Alexander EL, Firestein GS, Weiss JL, et al. Reversible cold-induced abnormalities in myocardial perfusion and function in systemic sclerosis. *Ann Intern Med*. 1986;105:661-668.
11. Steen VD, Follansbee WP, Conte CG, Medsger TA Jr. Thallium perfusion defects predict subsequent cardiac dysfunction in patients with systemic sclerosis. *Arthritis Rheum*. 1996;39:677-681.
12. Kahan A, Devaux JY, Amor B, et al. Pharmacodynamic effect of dipyridamole on thallium-201 myocardial perfusion in progressive systemic sclerosis with diffuse scleroderma. *Ann Rheum Dis*. 1986;45:718-725.
13. Kahan A, Devaux JY, Amor B, et al. Nicardipine improves myocardial perfusion in systemic sclerosis. *J Rheumatol*. 1988;15:1395-1400.
14. Kahan A, Devaux JY, Amor B, et al. The effect of captopril on thallium 201 myocardial perfusion in systemic sclerosis. *Clin Pharmacol Ther*. 1990;47:483-489.
15. Duboc D, Kahan A, Maziere B, et al. The effect of nifedipine on myocardial perfusion and metabolism in systemic sclerosis: a positron emission tomographic study. *Arthritis Rheum*. 1991;34:198-203.
16. Vignaux O, Allanore Y, Meune C, et al. Evaluation of the effect of nifedipine upon myocardial perfusion and contractility using cardiac magnetic resonance imaging and tissue Doppler echocardiography in systemic sclerosis. *Ann Rheum Dis*. 2005;64:1268-1273.
17. Allanore Y, Meune C, Vignaux O, Weber S, Legmann P, Kahan A. Bosentan increases myocardial perfusion and function in systemic sclerosis: a magnetic resonance imaging and tissue-Doppler echography study. *J Rheumatol*. 2006;33:2464-2469.
18. Follansbee WP, Miller TR, Curtiss EI. A controlled clinicopathologic study of myocardial fibrosis in systemic sclerosis (scleroderma). *J Rheumatol*. 1990;17:656-662.
19. Kahan A, Devaux JY, Amor B, et al. Pharmacodynamic effect of nicardipine on left ventricular function in systemic sclerosis. *J Cardiovasc Pharmacol*. 1990;15:249-253.
20. Follansbee WP, Zerbe TR, Medsger TA Jr. Cardiac and skeletal muscle disease in systemic sclerosis (scleroderma): a high risk association. *Am Heart J*. 1993;125:194-203.
21. Valentini G, Vitale DF, Giunta A. Diastolic abnormalities in systemic sclerosis: evidence for associated defective cardiac functional reserve. *Ann Rheum Dis*. 1996;55:455-460.
22. Maione S, Cuomo G, Giunta A, et al. Echocardiographic alterations in systemic sclerosis: a longitudinal study. *Semin Arthritis Rheum*. 2005;34:721-727.
23. Meune C, Allanore Y, Devaux JY, et al. High prevalence of right ventricular systolic dysfunction in early systemic sclerosis. *J Rheumatol*. 2004;31:1941-1945.

24. Meune C, Allanore Y, Pascal O, et al. Myocardial contractility is early affected in systemic sclerosis: a tissue Doppler echocardiography study. *Eur J Echocardiogr*. 2005;6: 351-357.
25. Allanore Y, Meune C, Vonk MC, et al. Prevalence and factors associated with left ventricular dysfunction in the EULAR Scleroderma Trial and Research group (EUSTAR) database of systemic sclerosis patients. *Ann Rheum Dis*. 2010;69:218-221.

Chapter 16
A Scleroderma Patient with Dysphagia and Reflux Who Experiences Worsening Cough

Romy Beatriz Christmann

Keywords Gastroesophageal reflux • Dysphagia • Diagnosis • Treatment

Case Study

A 57-year-old woman with a long history of limited cutaneous systemic sclerosis (lSSc) presented with dysphagia, heartburn, and nocturnal coughing that had increased in severity during the last 4 months. Initially, she noticed difficulty in swallowing solid foods that worsened over time such that she would choke when swallowing juice and soup.

The patient had a 30-year history of Raynaud's phenomenon that progressively worsened and became severe resulting in amputations of three phalanges during the past 10 years. Twelve years ago she noticed that her skin on the face and hands became thicker, her oral aperture decreased, and she was unable to make a full fist. At that time, her primary care provider made a diagnosis of limited cutaneous systemic sclerosis (lSSc) and referred her to a rheumatologist who prescribed vasodilators, physical therapy for her hand, facial exercises, and annual assessment of lung and heart involvement. She also complained of dysphagia and heartburn after meals, and a baseline esophagram showed aperistalsis (Figs. 16.1 and 16.2). Anti-reflux measures and medication (proton pump inhibitor twice daily) were prescribed in order to alleviate her gastroesophageal reflux (GER) complaints. Seven years later, a high resolution computed tomography (HRCT) scan of the lungs revealed interstitial lung disease, and pulmonary function tests (PFTs) revealed a decrease in forced vital capacity of more than 20% compared to baseline. Subsequently, cyclophosphamide

R.B. Christmann
Arthritis Center Rheumatology Division, University of Sao Paulo/Boston
University School of Medicine, 715, Albany Street, E5, Boston,
MA 02118-2531, USA

R.M. Silver and C.P. Denton (eds.), *Case Studies in Systemic Sclerosis*,
DOI: 10.1007/978-0-85729-641-2_16, © Springer-Verlag London Limited 2011

Fig. 16.1 Barium
esophagram of a systemic
sclerosis (SSc) patient with
gastroesophageal reflux.
Barium esophagram in
upright position showing
typical features of the SSc
esophageal involvement with
a dilated and atonic
esophagus. (Kindly provided
by Dr. Steven Schabel,
Medical University of South
Carolina)

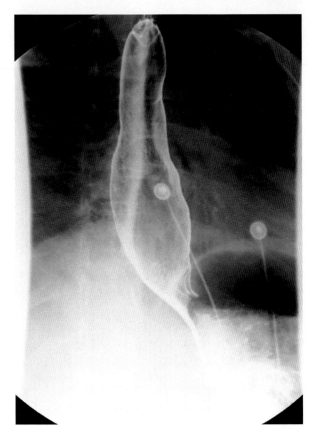

was prescribed for a year, administered intravenously once a month, which was associated with stabilization of her lung disease.

Physical Examination

Vitals: temperature 36°C; pulse 85 bpm; respirations 18 per min; blood pressure
110/80 mmHg. Skin: digital pitting scars on several fingerpads, loss of distal phalanges of second and third fingers on her right hand and the third finger on her left
hand. Skin thickness on her hands and face with microstomia, with normal skin
texture of the proximal arms and legs, chest, and abdomen. Chest: bilateral basilar
crackles. Cardiac: regular rate and rhythm with normal S1 and S2 heart sounds.
Abdomen: nondistended but mildly tender to palpation of the midgastric region.
Normal neurologic system. Musculoskeletal: no joint swelling and mild flexion
contractures of the fingers with inability to flatten her hand.

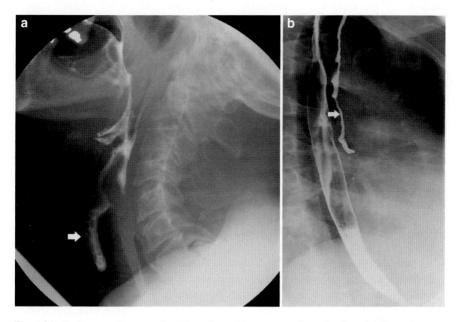

Fig. 16.2 Barium esophagram of a SSc patient with gastroesophageal reflux. (**a**) Extensive gastroesophageal reflux of the swallowed barium contrast into the upper airway (*arrow*) during the esophagram. (**b**) Spreading of the barium contrast into the bronchia (*arrow*) along with the dilated lower esophagus. (Kindly provided by Dr. Steven Schabel, Medical University of South Carolina)

Laboratory Findings

Chemistry panel and urinalysis: normal; mild hypochromic microcytic anemia (hemoglobin 10 g/dL). Antinuclear antibody (ANA) positive by IIF (titer 1:640; centromere pattern). Echocardiogram: normal LV ejection fraction, normal right atrial and right ventricular dimensions; no tricuspid regurgitation was detected and, therefore, estimate of the right ventricular systolic pressure (RVSP) was not possible. Lung HRCT: ground-glass pattern with reticular opacities associated with mild bronchiectasis in the lower lung zones. PFTs: FVC 2.0 L (70% predicted); FEV1 1.71 L (72% predicted); DLco 66% of predicted.

Course

The patient had a long history of lSSc with severe peripheral vascular involvement resulting in amputation of distal phalanges, as well as interstitial lung disease and chronic gastroesophageal reflux symptoms. She reported that despite medical recommendation for anti-reflux measures and PPI therapy, she had been noncompliant for the past 6 months. Esophagogastroduodenoscopy was performed and a distal esophageal ulcer was diagnosed. Therefore, proton pump inhibitors were increased to three times daily, and the rheumatologist emphasized the need for anti-reflux measures. After a month of treatment her GER complaints and nocturnal coughing disappeared and there was complete healing of the esophageal ulcer.

Discussion

The gastrointestinal tract is one of the most common organs involved in SSc, and esophageal involvement leads to symptoms in 75–90% of patients.[1-5] Usually, the distal two-thirds of the esophagus is affected resulting in abnormal esophageal motility with poor clearance of gastric acid. Therefore, gastroesophageal reflux and esophagitis are common problems in SSc patients.

The aspiration of gastric contents normally is avoided through a complex and multistep process involving a reflex mechanism consisting of sensory afferent and motor efferent processes. In SSc, the earliest lesion in the GI tract may be an innervation deficit, perhaps secondary to microvascular disease of the vasa nervorum or by compression of nerve fibers from the accumulation of collagen, causing an irreversible ischemic injury to the neural tissue.[1] The vascular dysfunction is manifested by an imbalance of the vascular tone, intimal proliferation, and vascular fibrosis that lead to luminal narrowing and ischemia. In addition, many immune cells activate the immune-inflammatory system[6] and, consequently, after a long period of ischemia, the smooth muscle will become atrophic and finally fibrotic resulting in motor dysfunction. Esophageal involvement is associated with significant morbidity in SSc resulting in erosive esophagitis, ulcers, as well as peptic stricture formation and Barrett's esophagus with its potential for adenocarcinoma transformation.

The most common symptom of GER in SSc patients is dysphagia, as illustrated by the index case. Other common symptoms include heartburn, regurgitation, nausea, vomiting, and poor eating that might result in malnutrition and severe weight loss. Interestingly, dysphagia and nausea/vomiting are the symptoms more frequently found in SSc patients with endoscopic Barrett's esophagus.[7] SSc patients with esophageal manifestations, though, can be asymptomatic; therefore, a high-index of suspicion is essential to establish a diagnosis. In addition, it is important to record the baseline esophageal involvement and its severity for future treatment decisions.

Many functional and morphological tests are used to investigate patients with complaints of dysphagia or esophageal/gastric symptoms. Esophageal manometry is considered the gold standard for documenting esophageal dysmotility. It is highly sensitive and specific for the detection of esophageal motility disorders and in SSc can demonstrate visceral involvement starting from very early stages of the disease.[8] A polyvinyl catheter is placed transnasally into the esophagus as the patient swallows, allowing physicians to assess peristalsis via shape, amplitude, and duration of the esophageal contractions. Multichannel intraluminal impedance-esophageal manometry evaluates the esophageal contractions by simultaneously measuring bolus transit.[9,10] A reduced pressure of LES, esophageal body aperistalsis, and a decrease in the amplitude of contraction in the distal two-thirds of the esophagus is characteristic of SSc.

Upper gastrointestinal radiography with barium contrast allows a dynamic examination of the esophagus, stomach, and duodenum, showing the barium boluses from the mouth through the entire esophagus. It provides little information regarding the presence, extent, and volume of the reflux material, although stricture, dilatation, and ulcers can be detected.[11] Esophageal scintigraphy has also been used in SSc esophageal involvement and can show a typical pattern of retention of radioactivity in the lower esophagus, with clearing after the patient drinks water. It is highly sensitive and might be an alternative for the barium contrast especially for sequential studies, such as to monitor treatment efficacy.[12] The patient in this case study had a baseline esophagram showing motor dysfunction with aperistalsis in the distal two-thirds of the esophagus, demonstrating severe involvement.

Esophagogastroduodenoscopy is frequently used to evaluate a patient with gastroesophageal disorders because it allows direct visualization of the esophageal, gastric, and duodenal mucosa, permitting also tissue biopsies of suspicious lesions.[13] The presence of esophagitis and Barrett's metaplasia can be easily visualized, although many SSc patients with GER-related symptoms do not have esophagitis. This invasive technique might not be well tolerated by some patients and also is operator dependent. The esophageal ulcer found in our patient was probably a consequence of several months of gastric acid reflux causing damage on the esophageal mucosa. It is recommended to repeat the exam after treatment to confirm esophageal healing.[14]

Esophageal exposure to gastric juice can be evaluated by ambulatory 24-h pH monitoring. A pH electrode is placed at the end of a catheter that will monitor the esophageal pH 5 cm above the LES. A combined impedance (esophageal motility) and pH monitoring allows the detection of GER independent of pH, detecting acid (reflux with $pH<4$) and nonacid (reflux with $pH>4$), as well as determining the proximal extent of reflux episodes.[9] This analysis was shown to be relevant in SSc patients with lung fibrosis (SSc-ILD), since patients with pulmonary involvement have more reflux episodes (acid and nonacid), thus enhancing their risk of microaspiration into the lungs.[15]

Lung aspiration of gastric fluids has been suggested to be an important cause of several fibrotic chronic lung diseases, including SSc-ILD. More recently, a novel lung pattern called "centrilobular fibrosis" (CLF) was described in SSc-ILD and is possibly caused by the reflux of gastric contents into the lungs.[16] In this study, 28 prospective SSc patients with confirmed lung fibrosis on HRCT underwent open lung biopsy. CLF was observed in 6 (21%) of the SSc-ILD patients. The CLF lung pattern is characterized by a bronchocentric distribution of lesions with intraluminal basophilic content, basement membrane exposure, and bronchiectasia (Fig. 16.3). Interestingly, foreign bodies were found within the airways in one third of the CLF patients, and the intraluminal basophilic content observed was similar

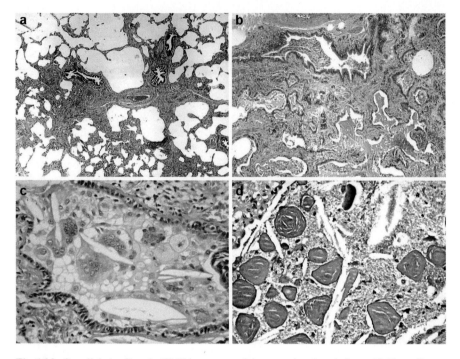

Fig. 16.3 Centrilobular fibrosis (CLF) lung pattern in a systemic sclerosis-interstitial lung disease (SSc-ILD) patient. (**a, b**) CLF lung pattern in patients with SSc. H&E staining with low-power magnification showing the typical combination of fibrosis around the small airways and interstitial fibrosis spreading away from the airways. Note the distortion of the lumens of the bronchioles caused by the peribronchiolar fibrous tissue. (**c**) H&E staining low-power view showing an amorphous substance with a basophilic staining present within the airways, similar to the characteristic peptic necrosis of gastric ulcers. (**d**) H&E staining with high-power magnification showing dense, amorphous, nonpolarizable blue to purple angular structures of kayexalate found within the basophilic material inside bronchioles. (Reprinted from de Souza RB[16] with permission from Karger Basel © 2009; kindly provided by Prof. Vera Capelozzi, University of Sao Paulo)

to the gastric contents seen with H&E staining. Tomographic images were strongly correlated with the lung tissue lesions with a predominantly central and patchy distribution (Fig. 16.4). Reinforcing this theory of cause and effect of GER and lung fibrosis, patients with isolated CLF were treated for 12 months with high-dose PPI and prokinetic medications, and their course was compared to an NSIP group treated with monthly intravenous cyclophosphamide. Surprisingly, after 1 year of treatment, lung function parameters were stable and comparable among the two groups.

In addition to the esophageal function analyses, histological and tomographic evidence strongly support a correlation and role of GER in the pathogenesis of SSc-ILD.[16-18] Supporting these findings, in this case study, after augmented compliance of the anti-GER measures and intensive anti-GER treatment, the patient's pulmonary symptoms improved promptly.

Fig. 16.4 High resolution computed tomography (HRCT) typical distribution of the lung injury in SSc-ILD patients with centrilobular fibrosis (CLF) and non-specific interstitial pneumonia (NSIP) lung pattern. (**a**) HRCT image from a systemic sclerosis-interstitial lung disease (SSc-ILD) patient with isolated CLF pattern. Note the predominant patchy and central distribution of the lung injury. (**b**) HRCT image from a SSc-ILD patient with NSIP pattern. Note the homogeneous and peripheral distribution of lung involvement. (Reprinted from de Souza RB[16] with permission from Karger Basel © 2009; kindly provided by Prof. Vera Capelozzi, University of Sao Paulo)

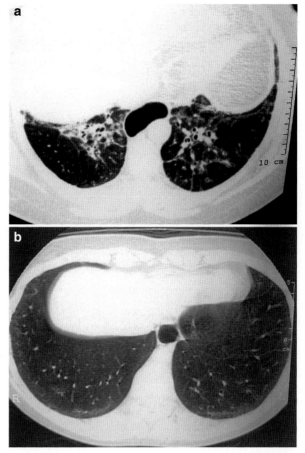

With regard to GER treatment, behavioral modifications are essential and include: avoidance of fatty and heavy meals, especially at night; discontinuing any medication or food that relaxes the LES such as chocolate and alcohol; avoidance of lying down right after eating; elevating the head of the bed during sleep; eating frequent small meals; sitting up during and after eating while taking liquids during the meal to help dislodge food stuck in the esophagus. These recommendations can be quite effective, although are frequently not rigorously followed by patients; therefore, focusing on preventive and behavioral modifications are of a great importance during routine medical appointments.

Medical therapy includes antisecretory and prokinetic agents. Proton pump inhibitors (PPI) are the mainstay of treatment and provide rapid relief of symptoms and esophageal healing. In patients with GER but without SSc, the healing rate of esophagitis was almost complete after 8 weeks of treatments.[19] Most patients are effectively controlled with a twice-daily dosing regime. Interestingly, a lower prevalence of Barrett's esophagus was observed in SSc patients who received PPI therapy at the time of diagnosis, compared to patients who had a delayed start of the treatment (at least 2 years later).[7] Increasing the dose and frequency of PPI therapy can be effective in refractory symptoms and addition of an H-2 antagonist such as ranitidine can be very helpful in cases where acid reflux symptoms persist despite full dose PPI.

Prokinetic medications are usually used in combination with other anti-reflux treatment, such as PPI. Metoclopramide, a dopaminergic antagonist and also a cholinergic agonist, promotes gastrointestinal motility. Its use though is limited because it might incite a number of neurologic and psychotropic side effects. It also has been shown that metoclopramide may improve LES pressure in patients with early diffuse SSc, but not in late disease.[20] Domperidone, a prokinetic agent with similar properties to those of metoclopramide, is commonly used 3–4 times a day and has the advantage of not crossing the blood–brain barrier. Cisapride facilitates the release of acetylcholine in the myenteric plexus and, similar to metoclopramide, increases LES pressure and esophageal peristalsis. It also can be used 3–4 times a day, although adverse reactions such as tachycardia, headache, and extrapyramidal effects might limit the daily dosage. Not all of these prokinetic agents are widely available; for example, in the USA, domperidone is not FDA-approved and cisapride was withdrawn.

A surgical approach in SSc is mainly the last option and reserved for those patients with the most severe and refractory GER. According to the published literature, postoperative dysphagia in SSc patients with severe GER is still high ranging from 29% to 75% with significant mortality.[21] Laparoscopic Roux-en-Y gastric bypass (RYGBP) or fundoplication are two surgical procedures that have been associated with improvement of dysphagia and reflux symptoms, whereas esophagectomy seems to have the highest postoperative complication rate.[21] Moreover, many SSc patients who might be candidates for such esophageal surgery will also have severe lung fibrosis, which considerably increases the mortality risk of the procedure.

In summary, esophageal involvement is highly prevalent in systemic sclerosis and confers high morbidity. It should be sought and detected early, and then treated in order to avoid complications or worsening of an already existing condition, such as Barrett's esophagus and lung fibrosis. Along with other chronic diseases, its treatment merits constant surveillance by both the rheumatologist and the gastroenterologist, and the relevance of its detection and management should always be addressed with the patient.

Acknowledgment The author sincerely thanks Prof. Eloisa Bonfa (University of Sao Paulo) for her invaluable contributions.

References

1. Sjogren RW. Gastrointestinal motility disorders in scleroderma. *Arthritis Rheum.* 1994;37(9): 1265-1282.
2. Clements PJ, Becvar R, Drosos AA, Ghattas L, Gabrielli A. Assessment of gastrointestinal involvement. *Clin Exp Rheumatol.* 2003;21(3 Suppl 29):S15-S18.

3. Ntoumazios SK, Voulgari PV, Potsis K, Koutis E, Tsifetaki N, Assimakopoulos DA. Esophageal involvement in scleroderma: gastroesophageal reflux, the common problem. *Semin Arthritis Rheum*. 2006;36(3):173-181.
4. Ebert EC. Esophageal disease in scleroderma. *J Clin Gastroenterol*. 2006;40(9):769-775.
5. Forbes A, Marie I. Gastrointestinal complications: the most frequent internal complications of systemic sclerosis. *Rheumatology (Oxford)*. 2009;48(Suppl 3):iii36-iii39.
6. Rohrmann CA Jr, Ricci MT, Krishnamurthy S, Schuffler MD. Radiologic and histologic differentiation of neuromuscular disorders of the gastrointestinal tract: visceral myopathies, visceral neuropathies, and progressive systemic sclerosis. *AJR Am J Roentgenol*. 1984;143(5): 933-941.
7. Marie I, Ducrotte P, Denis P, Hellot MF, Levesque H. Oesophageal mucosal involvement in patients with systemic sclerosis receiving proton pump inhibitor therapy. *Aliment Pharmacol Ther*. 2006;24(11–12):1593-1601.
8. Valentini G, Cuomo G, Abignano G, et al. Early systemic sclerosis: assessment of clinical and pre-clinical organ involvement in patients with different disease features. *Rheumatology (Oxford)*. 2011;50(2):317-323.
9. Tutuian R, Castell DO. Use of multichannel intraluminal impedance to document proximal esophageal and pharyngeal nonacidic reflux episodes. *Am J Med*. 2003;115(Suppl 3A):119S-123S.
10. Cho YK, Choi MG, Park JM, et al. Evaluation of esophageal function in patients with esophageal motor abnormalities using multichannel intraluminal impedance esophageal manometry. *World J Gastroenterol*. 2006;12(39):6349-6354.
11. Martin-Harris B, Logemann JA, McMahon S, Schleicher M, Sandidge J. Clinical utility of the modified barium swallow. *Dysphagia*. 2000;15(3):136-141.
12. Mariani G, Boni G, Barreca M, et al. Radionuclide gastroesophageal motor studies. *J Nucl Med*. 2004;45(6):1004-1028.
13. Moraes-Filho J, Cecconello I, Gama-Rodrigues J, et al. Brazilian consensus on gastroesophageal reflux disease: proposals for assessment, classification, and management. *Am J Gastroenterol*. 2002;97(2):241-248.
14. Liu JJ, Saltzman JR. Refractory gastro-oesophageal reflux disease: diagnosis and management. *Drugs*. 2009;69(14):1935-1944.
15. Savarino E, Bazzica M, Zentilin P, et al. Gastroesophageal reflux and pulmonary fibrosis in scleroderma: a study using pH-impedance monitoring. *Am J Respir Crit Care Med*. 2009;179(5):408-413.
16. de Souza RB, Borges CT, Capelozzi VL, et al. Centrilobular fibrosis: an underrecognized pattern in systemic sclerosis. *Respiration*. 2009;77(4):389-397.
17. Christmann RB, Wells AU, Silver RM. Gastroesophageal reflux incites interstitial lung disease in systemic sclerosis: clinical, radiologic, histopathologic, and treatment evidence. *Semin Arthritis Rheum*. 2010;40(3):241-249.
18. Gilson M, Zerkak D, Wipff J, et al. Prognostic factors for lung function in systemic sclerosis: prospective study of 105 cases. *Eur Respir J*. 2010;35(1):112-117.
19. Poh CH, Navarro-Rodriguez T, Fass R. Review: treatment of gastroesophageal reflux disease in the elderly. *Am J Med*. 2010;123(6):496-501.
20. Mercado U, Arroyo de Anda R, Avendano L, Araiza-Casillas R, Avendano-Reyes M. Metoclopramide response in patients with early diffuse systemic sclerosis. Effects on esophageal motility abnormalities. *Clin Exp Rheumatol*. 2005;23(5):685-688.
21. Kent MS, Luketich JD, Irshad K, et al. Comparison of surgical approaches to recalcitrant gastroesophageal reflux disease in the patient with scleroderma. *Ann Thorac Surg*. 2007; 84(5):1710-1715. discussion 1715–6.

Chapter 17
A Scleroderma Patient with Acute Drop in Hemoglobin and Occult Blood in Stool

Jayne Littlejohn and Chris T. Derk

Keywords Gastric antral vascular ectasia (GAVE) • Watermelon stomach • Scleroderma • Systemic sclerosis • Gastrointestinal bleeding

Case Study

A 52-year-old Caucasian female presented to the emergency department with fatigue and shortness of breath after a near syncopal episode. Her symptoms began approximately 3 months ago and have been progressive. She reports a general sense of feeling unwell, and she also notes dark stool in the past month but denies the presence of gross blood in her stool.

The patient was diagnosed with systemic sclerosis (SSc)18 months ago after referral from her primary care physician for a positive antinuclear antibody (ANA) and joint pain. On initial presentation, she described a 3-year history of Raynaud's phenomenon and a 1-year history of swelling of her hands and legs with painful joints and muscles. She has a long history of heartburn controlled with proton pump inhibitor therapy and essential hypertension treated with low-dose hydrochlorothiazide. She was found to have bilateral and symmetric swelling of her fingers, hands, and feet. No synovitis was noted. Laboratory tests were ordered. At 3-month follow-up, the patient continued to complain of arthralgia and myalgia, and her physical examination now showed bilateral and symmetric skin thickening of her fingers. She had developed thickening of her skin around her mouth, neck, anterior chest, and thighs. Her laboratory tests showed a positive ANA and negative anti-topoisomerase I antibody (anti-Scl-70 antibody). Other laboratory tests including

C.T. Derk (✉)
Department of Rheumatology, Thomas Jefferson University,
613 Curtis Bldg., 1015 Walnut Street, Philadelphia, PA 19107, USA

R.M. Silver and C.P. Denton (eds.), *Case Studies in Systemic Sclerosis,*
DOI: 10.1007/978-0-85729-641-2_17, © Springer-Verlag London Limited 2011

CBC, CMP, and PT/PTT were within normal limits. The patient was diagnosed with diffuse cutaneous systemic sclerosis (dSSc) with rapid progression of cutaneous disease.

Physical Examination

Temperature 36.9°C; pulse 104 bpm; respirations 16 per min; blood pressure 110/55 mmHg. Skin: scattered telangiectasias on the face and neck, thickening of the skin around the mouth, neck, and upper chest; areas of hyper- and hypopigmentation of the upper chest; edematous hands and fingers with skin thickening; periungual telangiectasia with nailbed pallor; palmar pallor; thickened skin of the proximal thighs. Head and neck examination revealed reduced oral aperture and pale palpebral conjunctivae. Chest: clear to auscultation. Cardiac: regular rate and rhythm with normal S1 and S2 heart sounds; II/VI systolic murmur heard best at the second right intercostal space. Abdomen: normal bowel sounds, soft, nondistended and nontender. Extremities: non-pitting edematous and erythematous feet. Musculoskeletal: no joint tenderness or swelling. Nailfold capillary microscopy revealed dilated capillary loops with few capillary hemorrhages and rare capillary dropout. Rectal: normal rectal tone, dark stool in rectal vault, no gross blood.

Laboratory Findings

CBC: WBC 8.3 K/µL, Hgb 6.4 g/dL, Hct 18%, Platelets 325 K/µL, MCV 75 femtoliter, reticulocytes 5%. Iron 12 mcg/dL, iron binding capacity 523 mcg/dL, iron saturation 3%, ferritin 7 ng/mL, B12 and folate normal. CMP, PT/PTT, and urinalysis normal. ANA by IIF positive (titer 1:640; fine speckled pattern). Anticentromere antibody negative, and anti-topoisomerase antibody (anti-Scl-70 antibody) negative. Stool positive for occult blood.

Course

The patient was admitted to the hospital and transfused 3 units of packed red blood cells. She had a normal colonoscopy and underwent esophagogastroduodenoscopy (EGD), which showed multiple parallel longitudinal stripes of red vessels radiating from the gastric antrum to the pylorus (Fig. 17.1). Pathology report of endoscopic biopsy showed superficial hyperplastic gastric antral mucosa with capillary ectasia and focal thrombosis (Fig. 17.2). A diagnosis of gastric antral vascular ectasia (GAVE) was made based on the clinical presentation, characteristic appearance on EGD, and pathological findings. Argon plasma coagulation was used on visible

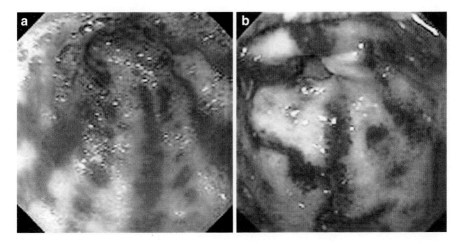

Fig. 17.1 Esophagogastroduodenoscopy (EGD) appearance of gastric antral vascular ectasia (GAVE) showing (**a**) parallel longitudinal rows of tortuous red vessels that traverse the gastric antrum and radiate in a spoke-like fashion to the pylorus and (**b**) stripes of ectatic vessels in the antrum

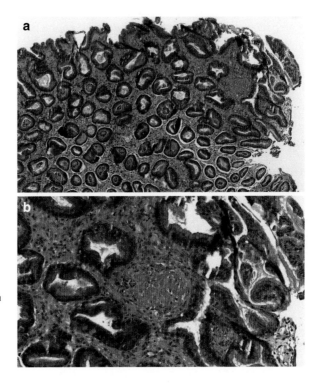

Fig. 17.2 Histopathologic appearance of gastric antral mucosa in GAVE showing (**a**) a large fibrin thrombus in a superficial capillary with adjacent dilated and ectatic capillaries. (**b**) Higher magnification of the fibrin thrombi

blood vessels for hemostasis. The patient was also treated with oral and parenteral iron therapy in addition to continuing a proton pump inhibitor for gastroesophageal reflux symptoms and gastric mucosal healing after the endoscopic procedure. Her hemoglobin stabilized at 10.3 g/dL during her hospitalization. The patient was followed for advancement of skin sclerosis, signs and symptoms of anemia, and regular laboratory testing of the hemoglobin and hematocrit.

Discussion

Gastric antral vascular ectasia (GAVE) is a rare but important to recognize cause of upper GI bleeding that can lead to iron deficiency anemia. The condition was described in case reports in the 1950s and 1960s, but it was not formally defined until 1984.[1-3] The largest study of GAVE has been 45 patients, where 62.2% of the cases were associated with autoimmune diseases[4] (Table 17.1). There have been three retrospective studies of GAVE associated with SSc in which the largest and most recent consisted of 28 patients.[5-7]

The typical patient affected by GAVE is usually a female 60 years of age, who presents with fatigue, shortness of breath, and sometimes congestive heart failure, and who is found to have occult blood in the stool and iron deficiency anemia.[1,4] Rarely do patients present with hematemesis or hematochezia. Greater than 50% of cases of GAVE are associated with autoimmune diseases, not only scleroderma but

Table 17.1 Medical conditions associated with GAVE

Autoimmune and connective tissue disorders	Nonautoimmune or connective tissue associated disorders
Autoimmune liver disease[a]	Cardiovascular disease[b]
Raynaud's phenomenon	Cirrhosis status post-jejunoileal bypass
Systemic sclerosis	Bone marrow transplant
Pernicious anemia	MGUS[d]
Hypothyroidism	COPD
Rheumatoid arthritis	Acute myeloid leukemia
Polymyalgia rheumatica	Sarcoidosis
	Parkinson disease
	Seizures
	Familiar Mediterranean Fever
	Chronic renal failure
	Diabetes
	Prior cancer[c]

Source: Adapted from Gostout[4] and Selinger[10]
[a]Primary biliary cirrhosis, autoimmune hepatitis
[b]Cardiovascular disease – coronary artery disease, hypertension, congestive heart failure, valvular disease, dysrhythmia
[c]Prior cancer – breast, colon, prostate, uterine
[d]Monoclonal gammopathy of undetermined significance

also including patients with primary biliary cirrhosis, pernicious anemia, hypothyroidism, or autoimmune hepatitis, and GAVE has also been observed in patients with chronic kidney or cardiovascular disease.[4]

Watermelon stomach affects patients with diffuse or limited cutaneous SSc. The development of GAVE varies significantly in relation to the initial diagnosis of scleroderma, but patients with diffuse cutaneous systemic sclerosis (dSSc) generally have earlier development of watermelon stomach, with the majority of cases developing within 18 months of the diagnosis of scleroderma. These patients also tend to have rapid progression of their cutaneous disease and a more severe anemia.[7] The development of GAVE is frequently more delayed in patients with limited cutaneous systemic sclerosis (lSSc), which could be a reflection of the more indolent nature of the disease, and these patient tend to present with less severe anemia.[7] Watermelon stomach and scleroderma have been diagnosed concomitantly, and some patients have developed GAVE years before the onset Raynaud's phenomenon and scleroderma.[5,8,9] Cutaneous telangiectasias and telangiectasias of other parts of the digestive tract including the esophagus and colon are commonly observed in patients with GAVE.[5,7]

The diagnosis of GAVE is simple, but its recognition is key. Any scleroderma patient with iron deficiency anemia and/or a positive test for occult fecal blood should undergo EGD for evaluation of possible watermelon stomach. The combination of the clinical, pathological, and endoscopic appearance of the stomach easily confirms the diagnosis.[7,10,11]

The striking endoscopic appearance strongly resembles the striped appearance of a watermelon rind, so the term watermelon stomach was coined to better describe GAVE. Visually the lesions consist of parallel rugal folds containing tortuous red vessels that traverse the gastric antrum and radiate in a spoke-like fashion to converge on the pylorus (Fig. 17.1). It is the appearance of longitudinal columns of red vessels parallel to normal appearing gastric mucosa that resembles the outside of a watermelon.[1,12]

The histological appearance of GAVE includes dilated capillaries, focal fibrin thrombi, and spindle cell proliferation on the mucosal surface with dilated tortuous submucosal vessels and fibromuscular hyperplasia within the lamina propria (Fig. 17.2).[1,11] These features are not necessary to diagnose GAVE but help differentiate it from severe antral gastritis and portal hypertensive gastropathy.[10,13]

The pathogenesis of GAVE remains unknown, and several theories have been proposed. Upon examining pathology specimens it was noted that the distal gastric mucosa was loosely attached to the underlying muscularis externa, which over time in combination with disordered motility, might possibly lead to antral mucosal prolapse through the pylorus.[1,4,5] In support of this theory are manometric studies in scleroderma patients showing high amplitude with uncoordinated gastric antral contractions, together with the histological findings of fibromuscular hyperplasia and dilated mucosal capillaries.[1,5,14] It has also been proposed that GAVE is part of the continuum of vascular alterations in scleroderma.[6] Studies have shown that up to 57% of patients with GAVE have telangiectasias of the skin, with a lesser percentage having telangiectasias in other gastrointestinal locations, including the esophagus, duodenum, ileum, colon, and rectum.[5] Supporting this theory are the similar histo-pathological changes seen in the dermis of scleroderma patients and in GAVE including capillary dilatation, small vessel fibrin deposits, and platelet thrombi.[5,6]

The management of GAVE lies first in its recognition and then may range from noninvasive measures to repeated endoscopic therapy. The mainstays of symptomatic therapy are proton pump inhibitors, iron supplementation and, as with our case study patient, transfusion, depending on the severity of anemia.[5,10] Endoscopic therapy utilizing Nd-YAG and argon plasma coagulation can be successful in achieving hemostasis, but a variable number of treatments may be required to eliminate transfusion dependence.[10,15] Surgical therapy with gastric antrectomy was the only long-term solution prior to the advent of endoscopic therapies and is rarely used now.

Several small trials have shown success in treating GAVE with methylpredniso-lone and cyclophosphamide, but additional controlled studies are needed to assess the potential benefit of immunosuppression which could spare patients multiple transfusions and endoscopic procedures.[16,17]

In summary, GAVE is an increasingly recognized cause of upper gastrointestinal bleeding in patients with scleroderma. The diagnosis of watermelon stomach can easily be made by EGD but is especially dependent on early clinical recognition. Watermelon stomach must always be suspected in the scleroderma patient who develops a sudden drop in hemoglobin or is found to have iron deficiency anemia. Although anemia is a strong clinical clue indicating a need for further evaluation for the presence of GAVE, certain serological tests may aid in disease prediction and earlier diagnosis. Patients with dSSc who have rapidly progressive skin disease, are negative for anti-Scl-70 antibody, and have a speckled pattern of their ANA appear to be at increased risk for the development of GAVE. These patients can also have earlier development of watermelon stomach in addition to rapid progression of their cutaneous disease and a more severe anemia. It is important to keep in mind, however, that watermelon stomach can develop at any time during the course or even before the diagnosis of dSSc or lSSc.

References

1. Jabbari M, Cherry R, Lough JO, Daly DS, Kinnear DG, Goresky CA. Gastric antral vascular ectasia: the watermelon stomach. *Gastroenterology*. 1984;87:1165-1170.
2. Holt JM, Wright R. Anaemia due to blood loss from the telangiectases of scleroderma. *Br Med J*. 1967;3:537-538.
3. Rider AJ et al. Gastritis with venocapillary ectasia as a source of massive gastric hemorrhage. *Gastroenterology*. 1953;24:118-123.
4. Gostout CJ, Viggiano TR, Ahlquist DA, Wang KK, Larson MV, Balm R. The clinical and endoscopic spectrum of the watermelon stomach. *J Clin Gastroenterol*. 1992;15:256-263.
5. Marie I, Ducrotte P, Antonietti M, Herve S, Levesque H. Watermelon stomach in systemic sclerosis: its incidence and management. *Aliment Pharmacol Ther*. 2008;28:412-421.
6. Watson M, Hally RJ, McCue PA, Varga J, Jiménez SA. Gastric antral vascular ectasia (watermelon stomach) in patients with systemic sclerosis. *Arthritis Rheum*. 1996;39:341-346.

7. Ingraham KM, O'Brien MS, Shenin M, Derk CT, Steen VD. Gastric antral vascular ectasia in systemic sclerosis: demographics and disease predictors. *J Rheumatol*. 2010;37(3):603-607.
8. Yamamoto M, Takahashi H, Akaike J, et al. Gastric antral vascular ectasia (GAVE) associated with systemic sclerosis. *Scand J Rheumatol*. 2008;37:315-316.
9. Taylor A, Sanders DS, Lobo AJ, Snaith ML. Gastric antral vascular ectasia as the only presenting feature of limited cutaneous systemic sclerosis. *J Clin Gastroenterol*. 2002;34:490-491.
10. Selinger CP, Aug YS. Gastric antral vascular ectasia (GAVE): an update on clinical presentation, pathophysiology and treatment. *Digestion*. 2008;77:131-137.
11. Gilliam JH, Geisinger KR, Wu WC, Weidner N, Richter JE. Endoscopic biopsy is diagnostic in gastric antral vascular ectasia the "watermelon stomach". *Dig Dis Sci*. 1989;34:885-888.
12. Brumit M, Carter E. Patient with systemic sclerosis and anemia. *Arch Pathol Lab Med*. 2002;126:375-376.
13. Burak KW, Beck PL. Portal hypertension gastropathy and gastric antral vascular ectasia (GAVE) syndrome. *Gut*. 2001;49:866-872.
14. Sjogren RW. Gastrointestinal features of scleroderma. *Curr Opin Rheum*. 1996;8:569-575.
15. Shibukawa G, Irisawa A, Sakamoto N, et al. Gastric antral vascular ectasia (GAVE) associated with systemic sclerosis: relapse after endoscopic treatment by argon plasma coagulation. *Intern Med*. 2007;46:279-283.
16. Lorenzi AR, Johnson AH, Davies G, Gough A. Gastric antral vascular ectasia in systemic sclerosis: complete resolution with methylprednisolone and cyclophosphamide. *Ann Rheum Dis*. 2001;60:796-798.
17. Schullz SW, O'Brien M, Maqsood M, Sandorfi N, Del Galdo F, Jimenez SA. Improvement of severe systemic sclerosis-associated gastric antral vascular ectasia following immunosuppressive treatment with intravenous cyclophosphamide. *J Rheumatol*. 2009;36:1653-1656.

Chapter 18
A 62-Year-Old Woman with Scleroderma and Severe Weight Loss

Geneviève Gyger and Murray Baron

Keywords Scleroderma • Gastrointestinal • Small bowel • Small bowel intestinal bacterial overgrowth • Malnutrition • Motility disorders

Case Study

A 62-year-old female computer teacher was first seen in the rheumatology clinic in March 2010 and diagnosed with scleroderma (SSc) in April 2010. Her illness began 3 years prior when she developed severe gastro-esophageal reflux disease (GERD) with a 50 lb weight loss in 1 year. In October 2009, she started to develop diarrhea, up to 6 times per day, alternating with periods of constipation. In December 2009, she noticed shortness of breath. Her family doctor noticed Raynaud's phenomenon of both hands, and lung fibrosis was diagnosed on the chest radiograph. She was then referred to the rheumatology clinic.

When seen in March 2010, her alternating constipation and diarrhea had worsened. She had severe bloating, nausea, occasional vomiting, and a further 7 lb weight loss. Her medication included domperidone 10 mg three times daily, metoclopramide 10 mg hs, and a polyethylene glycol electrolyte solution (GoLYTELY®) when needed.

Physical Examination and Investigations

Physical examination revealed sclerodactyly as well as skin thickening on forearms and hypopigmentation around the neck. Crackles were audible at the lung bases, and her abdomen was distended. Her body mass index (BMI) was 21.3.

M. Baron (✉)
Department of Rheumatology, Jewish General Hospital, 3755, Cote St. Catherine Rd., Suite A216, Montreal H3T 1E2, QC, Canada

R.M. Silver and C.P. Denton (eds.), *Case Studies in Systemic Sclerosis*, DOI: 10.1007/978-0-85729-641-2_18, © Springer-Verlag London Limited 2011

Fig. 18.1 Supine radiography. There is significant dilatation of the transverse and distal colon with the transverse colon measuring 11.6 cm in diameter (normal is less or equal to 5 cm). There is also probably air-filled dilated small bowel loops

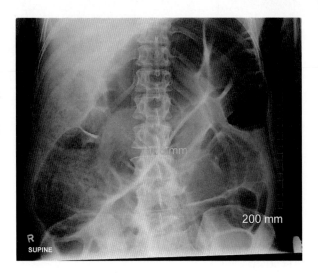

Standard abdominal series showed significant dilatation of the transverse and distal colon as well as small bowel dilatation (Fig. 18.1). A chest and abdominal CT scan showed interstitial lung fibrosis and an atonic, dilated small intestine starting at the duodenum and extending as far as the ileum without signs of obstruction. There was a mild anemia with a normal serum ferritin and slightly elevated erythrocyte sedimentation rate. C-reactive protein, homocysteine, folate, vitamin B12, and INR were all normal. Zinc, magnesium, and 25-OH vitamin D levels were low. Serum calcium was normal as was albumin and total protein. Colonoscopy was normal but a biopsy revealed an excess of subepithelial collagen.

Course

The domperidone was increased to 20 mg three times daily, metoclopramide 10 mg hs continued, and octreotide 50 mcg subcutaneous injection was started at bedtime. Magnesium, vitamin D supplement, and a multiple vitamin were also added, and a referral to a nutritionist was made. The rheumatology team worked closely with the gastroenterologist and nutritionist to plan her care. Her GI symptoms improved initially but rapidly recurred, and we added a 10 day trial of antibiotic for suspected bacterial overgrowth. She improved in 48 h but unfortunately, 2 days after discontinuing the antibiotic, she relapsed again with abdominal cramps and vomiting and had to be admitted to the hospital. Standard abdominal series showed marked distension of the small bowel with air–fluid levels compatible with pseudo-obstruction (Fig. 18.2). A nasogastric tube was installed and the antibiotic for suspected bacterial overgrowth was restarted. The dosage of octreotide was doubled to 100 mcg subcutaneous daily, erythromycin was added and metoclopramide was increased to four times daily. Total parenteral nutrition (TPN) was started. After 4 weeks of bowel rest and TPN, the patient could start to eat normally again and was discharged home on the same medications.

Fig. 18.2 Upright radiography. There is marked distension of the small bowel with air–fluid levels in keeping with pseudo-obstruction

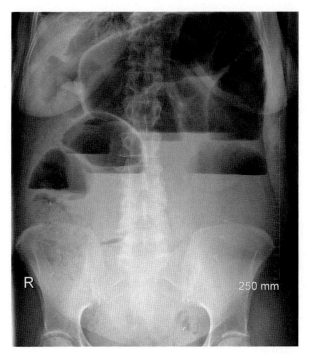

Discussion

Weight loss in SSc may be an ominous finding, usually due to severe intestinal disease. Although severe gastrointestinal (GI) involvement affects only 8% of scleroderma patients, mortality is high, with only 15% of such patients alive after 9 years.[1] Moreover, low BMI is one of the few variables able to predict mortality in patients with early SSc.[2] Small bowel involvement has been found in 48% of cases in an autopsy study,[3] in 22–66% of cases in radiologic studies[3,4], and in nearly 88% of cases in manometric studies.[5,6] Approximately 20% of patients are symptomatic[7] but small bowel involvement is often noticed only when severe complications have already occurred and are difficult to manage.[8,9]

The pathophysiology of the GI tract involvement in SSc is not completely understood and few studies have looked at the intestinal pathology.[3,10-20] Sjogren proposed a four-stage process similar to that in the skin.[21] The first is an early vascular lesion that manifests as mild changes in intestinal permeability, transport, and absorption. The second stage is neural dysfunction and is responsible for the earliest symptomatic lesion. This neural dysfunction could be in part secondary to circulating autoantibodies to myenteric neurons, which have been demonstrated in a considerable number of patients with scleroderma, and suggests an autoimmune etiology in the pathophysiological process of GI disease.[22,23] The third stage is smooth muscle atrophy and the end-stage lesion is muscle fibrosis, when pharmacological restoration of function is no longer possible.[10]

The end result of intestinal disease is altered peristaltic activity with multiple secondary problems including pseudo-obstruction, pneumatosis cystoides intestinalis, small intestine bacterial overgrowth (SIBO), malabsorption, and ultimately malnutrition.

Various degrees of intestinal pseudo-obstruction may occur in as many as 40% of patients with SSc.[24] Pneumatosis cystoides intestinalis (PCI), a rare condition characterized by the presence of air-filled cysts in the intestinal wall, is a poor prognostic sign.[8,9,24-29] More commonly, stasis of the intestinal contents leads to SIBO,[27,30-33] which may affect 33–43% of SSc patients.[31,34-37] It can be clinically asymptomatic[38] or manifest as abdominal distension and pain, diarrhea, or steatorrhea, and, in some cases, obstipation causing intestinal pseudo-obstruction.[27] SIBO can also lead to malabsorption[10,27,30,34,39,40] by competition for essential nutrients (such as vitamin B12) and deconjugation of bile acids, leading to fat malabsorption.[8,24,33,36] Malabsorption has been found in 10–25%[25,41] of patients and presents with diarrhea and weight loss. It is a poor prognostic factor with a 50% mortality rate at 8.5 years.[24,39] It is probably a multifactorial disorder[9] although it is mainly caused by SIBO.[10,27,30,34,39,40] Other causes include surface exchange disturbances,[9,42] dysfunction of epithelial absorptive epithelial cells,[20] lymphatic drainage disturbance,[10,14,16] reduced intestinal permeability secondary to submucosa and mucosa fibrosis[10,24,27], as well as chronic intestinal ischemia.[14,16,35] Pancreatic dysfunction[7,24,43] and primary biliary cirrhosis[7,24] are other potential causes.

Malnutrition usually refers to protein-energy malnutrition.[44] A recent study on malnutrition in SSc showed that 10.8% of the SSc patients were at medium risk for malnutrition and 17.4% were at high risk.[44] Poor appetite, early satiety, nausea, constipation, and diarrhea were associated with malnutrition. Decreased food intake secondary to anorexia, diminution of mouth aperture, xerostomia (dry mouth), gingival recession, and periodontal disease may also contribute to weight loss (see Chap. 32).[7]

Diagnosis of Small Bowel Intestine Involvement

Radiographic Assessment

Plain radiography can show small intestinal dilatation[45] with air fluid levels[27] and pneumoperitoneum if there is a pneumatosis cystoides intestinalis complication.[26] Barium studies may show several abnormalities which are fairly specific for scleroderma.[27] The duodenum and proximal jejunum seem to be more affected[24,33,40] with a "hide-bound" small bowel, a characteristic mucosal fold pattern with diffuse dilatation of the small bowel with closely packed valvulae conniventes.[17,46] Large, wide-necked diverticula may be seen in the small bowel.[17,47] Prolonged transit may be seen,[17] with a barium meal remaining from 2.5 to 24 h.[45] One should be cautious performing barium studies in patients with clinical evidence of severe intestinal disease because life-threatening impaction may occur.[48]

Manometric Study

Manometry is the gold standard test for motility disturbances of the small intestine[9,24] but is not convenient because it usually requires intubation of the stomach and small intestine for periods ranging from 5 to 24 h.[24] Manometric study can reveal asymptomatic small bowel dysfunction in SSc[5] and also more clearly characterize the dysmotility pattern in the small bowel, with early neuropathic and later myopathic dysfunction.[49]

Diagnosis of SIBO

Many tests can be used to diagnose SIBO including jejunal culture ("gold standard"), breath tests[24,50] and Schilling tests.[24] None has been validated[51] but the hydrogen breath test is probably the most widely used and is noninvasive[24,39,50]. The patient ingests a nonabsorbable carbohydrate such as lactulose, and breath hydrogen levels are determined every 15 min for 3 h. Normally the carbohydrate takes 2–3 h to reach the cecum where bacteria degrade the carbohydrate, releasing hydrogen which is picked up as a rise in hydrogen in the expired air. A premature rise in hydrogen suggests bacterial overgrowth more proximally.[24] Absorbable carbohydrates like glucose can also be used. As they are absorbed within the first 3 ft of small bowel, there should not be any hydrogen production at all. Thus, detecting hydrogen in this test implies SIBO in a very proximal location.[51] A limitation of hydrogen breath tests is that 20% of humans do not have any detectable hydrogen production from their intestinal flora and a breath test could miss non-hydrogen-producing bacteria (such as methane producers).[51,52] Methane can be added to the glucose to overcome this.[34,38] For SSc, one should note that results of breath tests are difficult to interpret in the case of advanced lung disease.[38]

Finally, when a patient with clinical and/or radiologic evidence of gastrointestinal hypomotility responds to an antibiotic trial, SIBO is likely.[38]

Malabsorption

The following tests should also be considered for further confirmation of malabsorption: hemoglobin level, vitamin B12, serum methylmalonic acid, iron, folic acid (elevated in SIBO because folates can be synthesized by intestinal bacterial flora,[24,27,53]) carotene,[54] selenium,[54] zinc, 25-OH vitamin D levels, and vitamin K (usually normal or increased owing to its bacterial overproduction)[38] or prothrombin time (PT).

Malnutrition

Weight loss is a very sensitive marker of a patient's nutritional status. As a general rule of thumb, significant weight loss is recognized as follows: 1–2% in the previous week, >5% in the previous month, >7.5% in the previous 3 months, and >10% in the previous year.[55] An easy-to-use screening tool such as the "Malnutrition Universal Screening Tool" (MUST) can also be utilized to rule out malnutrition.[56-58] Although serum albumin is commonly used to screen for malnutrition, it is neither sensitive nor specific for malnutrition. In SSc, serum albumin is probably not helpful in diagnosing malnutrition.[59] Serum prealbumin (transthyretin) is useful to monitor improvement in nutritional status if a treatment is instituted, especially if it is abnormally low at baseline.[60-62]

Management

Malabsorption

A North American panel recently reviewed the work-up and management of weight loss and malabsorption in SSc.[59] Patients with small bowel disease and malnutrition should be referred to a dietitian and a gastroenterologist. Use of dietary supplements including commercial meal replacement products may be included into a comprehensive nutritional plan. If SIBO is suspected, irrespective of the results of breath testing, a 10-day course of a selective antibiotic should be tried.[59,63] Ciprofloxacin 500 mg twice daily, Amoxicillin/clavulanic acid 875 mg twice daily, tetracycline 250 mg four times daily, and doxycycline 100 mg twice daily are among the most frequently used. If there is a clinical response but the patient quickly relapses, options include use of this antibiotic for the first 10 days of each of 4 consecutive months, or restart the antibiotic as soon as symptoms relapse. For those who continue to relapse whenever antibiotics are stopped, continuous antibiotic therapy may be required. In that situation, rotational antibiotics with two different antibiotics is used, alternating every 15 days. Alternatively, adding a probiotic when antibiotics are withdrawn may be considered.[64] When started, the probiotics are usually permanently continued. When malabsorption is severe, not responding to antibiotics and dietary supplements, and patients are unable to maintain their nutritional status, total parenteral nutrition may be needed.[27] Long-term intermittent overnight home parenteral nutrition has been proven effective and safe for systemic sclerosis-related intestinal failure, and life saving.[65,66] Enteral nutrition via a jejunostomy[32] should always be attempted first as parenteral nutrition can be associated with complications including catheter-related sepsis, vascular thrombosis, and liver failure. This decision should be tailored to the patient's clinical status and should depend on close communication between the rheumatologist, gastroenterologist, and dietician.[64]

Pseudo-Obstruction and Motility Disturbance

Metoclopramide is inconsistently effective, but it[22,38,62] and domperidone[40] may be tried.[24,40,67] With refractory small bowel symptoms, consider therapy with octreotide 50–100 mcg subcutaneous at bedtime.[68-71] Long-acting-release octreotide 20 mg intramuscular each month seems to limit short relapse.[72] Possible disadvantages include inhibitory effects on gastric emptying, pancreatic secretions, gallbladder contractions[64,73], and increased incidence of cholelithiasis.[24] Octreotide at bedtime, in association with erythromycin, may provide relief of abdominal pain and nausea in pseudo-obstruction.[74] For situations which do not respond to the above therapies, parenteral[27,65,75] or enteral nutrition via a jejunostomy[32] may be considered, as discussed above.

Surgical intervention in intestinal pseudo-obstruction should be avoided as the disease is almost always generalized, surgical options are very limited and healing and postoperative recovery is likely to be poor. Moreover, comorbidity often increases anesthetic and operative risk and the risk of perforation is much lower than in mechanical obstruction due to much lower intraluminal pressures. Recurrence is the rule and operative manipulation of scleroderma bowel tends to result in a prolonged ileus.[8,48]

In summary, small bowel involvement is frequent in scleroderma and can lead to serious morbidity. Severe weight loss is often a sign of malabsorption or decreased oral intake because of intestinal involvement. Unfortunately, small bowel disease is often diagnosed when involvement is already quite severe and irreversible. None of the treatments used have been shown to reverse GI involvement related to scleroderma. They may, however, relieve the patient's symptoms and improve quality of life. Complications of small bowel involvement predict a poor prognosis. Supporting the patient through difficult times, and team work between rheumatologist, nutritionist, and gastroenterologist, are essential for this very complicated problem.

References

1. Steen VD, Medsger TA Jr. Severe organ involvement in systemic sclerosis with diffuse scleroderma. *Arthritis Rheum*. 2000;43:2437-2444.
2. Assassi S, Del Junco D, Sutter K, et al. Clinical and genetic factors predictive of mortality in early systemic sclerosis. *Arthritis Rheum*. 2009;61:1403-1411.

3. D'Angelo WA, Fries JF, Masi AT, Shulman LE. Pathologic observations in systemic sclerosis (scleroderma). A study of fifty-eight autopsy cases and fifty-eight matched controls. *Am J Med.* 1969;46:428-440.

4. Bluestone R, Macmahon M, Dawson JM. Systemic sclerosis and small bowel involvement. *Gut.* 1969;10:185-193.

5. Marie I, Levesque H, Ducrotte P, et al. Manometry of the upper intestinal tract in patients with systemic sclerosis: a prospective study. *Arthritis Rheum.* 1998;41:1874-1883.

6. Greydanus MP, Camilleri M. Abnormal postcibal antral and small bowel motility due to neuropathy or myopathy in systemic sclerosis. *Gastroenterology.* 1989;96:110-115.

7. Attar A. Atteintes digestives au cours de la sclérodermie. *Ann Med Interne Paris.* 2002;153:260-264.

8. Lock G, Holstege A, Lang B, Scholmerich J. Gastrointestinal manifestations of progressive systemic sclerosis. *Am J Gastroenterol.* 1997;92:763-771.

9. Marie I, Lévesque H, Ducrotté P, Courtois H. Atteinte de l'intestin grêle au cours de la sclérodermie systémique. *Rev Méd Interne.* 1999;20:504-513.

10. Sjogren RW. Gastrointestinal features of scleroderma. *Curr Opin Rheumatol.* 1996;8: 569-575.

11. Cobden I, Rothwell J, Axon AT, Dixon MF, Lintott DJ, Rowell NR. Small intestinal structure and passive permeability in systemic sclerosis. *Gut.* 1980;21:293-298.

12. Schuffler MD, Beegle RG. Progressive systemic sclerosis of the gastrointestinal tract and hereditary hollow visceral myopathy: two distinguishable disorders of intestinal smooth muscle. *Gastroenterology.* 1979;77:664-671.

13. Ebert EC, Ruggiero FM, Seibold JR. Intestinal perforation. A common complication of scleroderma. *Dig Dis Sci.* 1997;42:549-553.

14. Greenberger NJ, Dobbins WO 3rd, Ruppert RD, Jesseph JE. Intestinal atony in progressive systemic sclerosis (scleroderma). *Am J Med.* 1968;45:301-308.

15. Bevans M. Pathology of Scleroderma, with special reference to the changes in the gastrointestinal tract. *Am J Pathol.* 1945;21:25-51.

16. Hoskins LC, Norris HT, Gottlieb LS, Zamcheck N. Functional and morphologic alterations of the gastrointestinal tract in progressive systemic sclerosis (scleroderma). *Am J Med.* 1962;33:459-470.

17. Rohrmann CA Jr, Ricci MT, Krishnamurthy S, Schuffler MD. Radiologic and histologic differentiation of neuromuscular disorders of the gastrointestinal tract: visceral myopathies, visceral neuropathies, and progressive systemic sclerosis. *AJR Am J Roentgenol.* 1984;143: 933-941.

18. DeSchryver-Kecskemeti K, Clouse RE. Perineural and intraneural inflammatory infiltrates in the intestines of patients with systemic connective-tissue disease. *Arch Pathol Lab Med.* 1989;113:394-398.

19. Lortat-Jacob JL, Giuli R, Duperrat B, Conte-Marti J. Arguments en faveur de l'origine nerveuse de la sclérodermie. *Ann Dermatol Syphiligr Paris.* 1974;101:121-134.

20. Hendel L, Kobayasi T, Petri M. Ultrastructure of the small intestinal mucosa in progressive systemic sclerosis (PSS). *Acta Pathol Microbiol Immunol Scand A.* 1987;95:41-46.

21. Prescott RJ, Freemont AJ, Jones CJ, Hoyland J, Fielding P. Sequential dermal microvascular and perivascular changes in the development of scleroderma. *J Pathol.* 1992;166:255-263.

22. Howe S, Eaker EY, Sallustio JE, Peebles C, Tan EM, Williams RC Jr. Antimyenteric neuronal antibodies in scleroderma. *J Clin Invest.* 1994;94:761-770.

23. Eaker EY, Kuldau JG, Verne GN, Ross SO, Sallustio JE. Myenteric neuronal antibodies in scleroderma: passive transfer evokes alterations in intestinal myoelectric activity in a rat model. *J Lab Clin Med.* 1999;133:551-556.

24. Sjogren RW. Gastrointestinal motility disorders in scleroderma. *Arthritis Rheum.* 1994;37:1265-1282.

25. Stafford-Brady FJ, Kahn HJ, Ross TM, Russell ML. Advanced scleroderma bowel: complications and management. *J Rheumatol.* 1988;15:869-874.

26. Bloch F, Leport J, Mallet L, Fiessinger J-N, Housset E, Petite J-P. Pneumopéritoine spontané au cours de la sclérodermie. *Gastroentérol Clin Biol*. 1984;8:557-559.
27. Cohen S. The gastrointestinal manifestations of scleroderma: pathogenesis and management. *Gastroenterology*. 1980;79:155-166.
28. Ponge T, Bruley des Varannes S. Atteintes digestives sclérodermiques. *La Revue du Praticien*. 2002;52:196-200.
29. Abu-Shakra M, Guillemin F, Lee P. Gastrointestinal manifestations of systemic sclerosis. *Semin Arthritis Rheum*. 1994;24:29-39.
30. Kahn IJ, Jeffries GH, Sleisenger MH. Malabsorption in intestinal scleroderma. Correction by antibiotics. *N Engl J Med*. 1966;274:1339-1344.
31. Kaye SA, Lim SG, Taylor M, Patel S, Gillespie S, Black CM. Small bowel bacterial overgrowth in systemic sclerosis: detection using direct and indirect methods and treatment outcome. *Br J Rheumatol*. 1995;34:265-269.
32. Forbes A, Marie I. Gastrointestinal complications: the most frequent internal complications of systemic sclerosis. *Rheumatology (Oxford)*. 2009;48(Suppl 3):iii36-iii39.
33. Olmsted WW, Madewell JE. The esophageal and small-bowel manifestations of progressive systemic sclerosis. A pathophysiologic explanation of the roentgenographic signs. *Gastrointest Radiol*. 1976;1:33-36.
34. Marie I, Ducrotte P, Denis P, Menard JF, Levesque H. Small intestinal bacterial overgrowth in systemic sclerosis. *Rheumatology (Oxford)*. 2009;48:1314-1319.
35. Kaye SA, Seifalian AM, Lim SG, Hamilton G, Black CM. Ischaemia of the small intestine in patients with systemic sclerosis: Raynaud's phenomenon or chronic vasculopathy? *QJM*. 1994;87:495-500.
36. Ebert EC. Gastric and enteric involvement in progressive systemic sclerosis. *J Clin Gastroenterol*. 2008;42:5-12.
37. Cobden I, Axon AT, Ghoneim AT, McGoldrick J, Rowell NR. Small intestinal bacterial growth in systemic sclerosis. *Clin Exp Dermatol*. 1980;5:37-42.
38. Bures J, Cyrany J, Kohoutova D, et al. Small intestinal bacterial overgrowth syndrome. *World J Gastroenterol*. 2010;16:2978-2990.
39. Jaovisidha K, Csuka ME, Almagro UA, Soergel KH. Severe gastrointestinal involvement in systemic sclerosis: report of five cases and review of the literature. *Semin Arthritis Rheum*. 2005;34:689-702.
40. Modigliani R. Localisations digestives de la sclérodermie. *Ann Méd Interne*. 1984;135:601-605.
41. Poirier TJ, Rankin GB. Gastrointestinal manifestations of progressive systemic scleroderma based on a review of 364 cases. *Am J Gastroenterol*. 1972;58:30-44.
42. Leparco J, Chemaly A, Bader J, Martin E, Lambling A. Localisation digestive de la sclérodermie et malabsorption. *Sem Hôp Paris*. 1972;42:2057-2067.
43. Scudamore HH, Green PA, Hofman HN, 2nd, Rosevear JW, Tauxe WN. Scleroderma (progressive systemic sclerosis) of the small intestine with malabsorption. Evaluation of intestinal absorption and pancreatic function. *Am J Gastroenterol*. 1968;49:193-208.
44. Baron M, Hudson M, Steele R. Malnutrition is common in systemic sclerosis: results from the Canadian scleroderma research group database. *J Rheumatol*. 2009;36:2737-2743.
45. Heinz ER, Steinberg AJ, Sackner MA. Roentgenographic and pathologic aspects of intestinal scleroderma. *Ann Intern Med*. 1963;59:822-826.
46. Horowitz AL, Meyers MA. The "hide-bound" small bowel of scleroderma: characteristic mucosal fold pattern. *Am J Roentgenol Radium Ther Nucl Med*. 1973;119:332-334.
47. Queloz JM, Woloshin HJ. Sacculation of the small intestine in scleroderma. *Radiology*. 1972;105:513-515.
48. Medsger TA Jr. Treatment of systemic sclerosis. *Ann Rheum Dis*. 1991;50(Suppl 4): 877-886.
49. Marie I, Ducrotte P, Denis P, Hellot MF, Levesque H. Outcome of small-bowel motor impairment in systemic sclerosis – a prospective manometric 5-yr follow-up. *Rheumatology (Oxford)*. 2007;46:150-153.

50. Gasbarrini A, Corazza GR, Gasbarrini G, et al. Methodology and indications of H2-breath testing in gastrointestinal diseases: the Rome Consensus Conference. *Aliment Pharmacol Ther*. 2009;29(Suppl 1):1-49.
51. Khoshini R, Dai SC, Lezcano S, Pimentel M. A systematic review of diagnostic tests for small intestinal bacterial overgrowth. *Dig Dis Sci*. 2008;53:1443-1454.
52. Khin Maung U, Tin A, Ku Tin M, et al. In vitro hydrogen production by enteric bacteria cultured from children with small bowel bacterial overgrowth. *J Pediatr Gastroenterol Nutr*. 1992;14:192-197.
53. Camilo E, Zimmerman J, Mason JB, et al. Folate synthesized by bacteria in the human upper small intestine is assimilated by the host. *Gastroenterology*. 1996;110:991-998.
54. Lundberg AC, Akesson A, Akesson B. Dietary intake and nutritional status in patients with systemic sclerosis. *Ann Rheum Dis*. 1992;51:1143-1148.
55. Blackburn GL, Bistrian BR, Maini BS, Schlamm HT, Smith MF. Nutritional and metabolic assessment of the hospitalized patient. *JPEN J Parenter Enteral Nutr*. 1977;1:11-22.
56. Stratton RJ, Hackston A, Longmore D, et al. Malnutrition in hospital outpatients and inpatients: prevalence, concurrent validity and ease of use of the 'malnutrition universal screening tool' ('MUST') for adults. *Br J Nutr*. 2004;92:799-808.
57. Godfrey K. Implementation of the malnutrition universal screening tool. *Nurs Times*. 2004;100:61.
58. Stratton RJ, King CL, Stroud MA, Jackson AA, Elia M. 'Malnutrition universal screening tool' predicts mortality and length of hospital stay in acutely ill elderly. *Br J Nutr*. 2006;95: 325-330.
59. Baron M, Bernier P, Cote LF, et al. Screening and therapy for malnutrition and related gastrointestinal disorders in systemic sclerosis: recommendations of a North American expert panel. *Clin Exp Rheumatol*. 2010;28:S42-S46.
60. Beck FK, Rosenthal TC. Prealbumin: a marker for nutritional evaluation. *Am Fam Physician*. 2002;65:1575-1578.
61. Devoto G, Gallo F, Marchello C, et al. Prealbumin serum concentrations as a useful tool in the assessment of malnutrition in hospitalized patients. *Clin Chem*. 2006;52:2281-2285.
62. Kuszajewski ML, Clontz AS. Prealbumin is best for nutritional monitoring. *Nursing*. 2005;35:70-71.
63. Toskes P. In: Warrell D, Cox T, Firth J, Benz E, eds. Oxford Textbook Of Medicine: Oxford University Press; 2003:580-4.
64. Baron M, Bernier P, Côté L-F, et al. Screening and therapy for malnutrition and related gastrointestinal disorders in systemic sclerosis: Recommendations of a North American expert panel. *Semin Arthritis Rheum*. 2010;in PRESS.
65. Brown M, Teubner A, Shaffer J, Herrick AL. Home parenteral nutrition – an effective and safe long-term therapy for systemic sclerosis-related intestinal failure. *Rheumatology (Oxford)*. 2008;47:176-179.
66. Grabowski G, Grant JP. Nutritional support in patients with systemic scleroderma. *JPEN J Parenter Enteral Nutr*. 1989;13:147-151.
67. Rees WD, Leigh RJ, Christofides ND, Bloom SR, Turnberg LA. Interdigestive motor activity in patients with systemic sclerosis. *Gastroenterology*. 1982;83:575-580.
68. Perlemuter G, Cacoub P, Chaussade S, Wechsler B, Couturier D, Piette JC. Octreotide treatment of chronic intestinal pseudoobstruction secondary to connective tissue diseases. *Arthritis Rheum*. 1999;42:1545-1549.
69. Soudah HC, Hasler WL, Owyang C. Effect of octreotide on intestinal motility and bacterial overgrowth in scleroderma. *N Engl J Med*. 1991;325:1461-1467.
70. Owyang C. Octreotide in gastrointestinal motility disorders. *Gut*. 1994;35:S11-S14.
71. Descamps V, Duval X, Crickx B, Bouscarat F, Coffin B, Belaich S. Global improvement of systemic scleroderma under long-term administration of octreotide. *Eur J Dermatol*. 1999;9:446-448.

72. Nikou GC, Toumpanakis C, Katsiari C, Charalambopoulos D, Sfikakis PP. Treatment of small intestinal disease in systemic sclerosis with octreotide: a prospective study in seven patients. *J Clin Rheumatol.* 2007;13:119-123.
73. Domsic R, Fasanella K, Bielefeldt K. Gastrointestinal manifestations of systemic sclerosis. *Dig Dis Sci.* 2008;53:1163-1174.
74. Verne GN, Eaker EY, Hardy E, Sninsky CA. Effect of octreotide and erythromycin on idiopathic and scleroderma-associated intestinal pseudoobstruction. *Dig Dis Sci.* 1995;40:1892-1901.
75. Levien DH, Fiallos F, Barone R, Taffet S. The use of cyclic home hyperalimentation for malabsorption in patients with scleroderma involving the small intestines. *JPEN J Parenter Enteral Nutr.* 1985;9:623-625.

Chapter 19
A Patient with Diffuse Systemic Sclerosis with Hypertension and Acute Renal Failure

Ulf Müller-Ladner

Keywords Scleroderma renal crisis (SRC) • Angiotensin converting enzyme inhibitors (ACE-I) • Diffuse scleroderma • Corticosteroids

Case Study

A 57-year-old female was referred from a county hospital to the Cardiology Department for management of uncontrollable hypertension and azotemia. The patient, a worker in the logistics center of a courier service, had a 40-year history of moderate smoking (20 pack-years) and had suffered from Raynaud's phenomenon during winter months and upon exposure to cold. A visit to a rheumatologist several years ago for wrist pain had led to a diagnosis of suspected Raynaud's phenomenon which was felt to be associated with an undifferentiated connective tissue disease with ANA positivity. The patient was lost to follow-up, but in the years leading up to the recent presentation the family doctor had treated her joint pain repeatedly with intermittent courses of prednisone (20–30 mg daily for 2–4 weeks) with good success. Thickening of the skin on the hands and the arms had been attributed to long-term hands-on work handling packages in the courier service. Aside from intermittent mild heartburn, the patient felt well until 6 months ago, when she began to note a decrease in physical capabilities, and which initially had been thought to result from her age and long-term smoking. After emergency treatment for hypertension, an urgent rheumatology consultation was arranged. This confirmed the presence of skin thickening and the patient was referred to the Rheumatology Department with suspected SSc-associated multiorgan involvement.

U. Müller-Ladner
Department of Rheumatology & Clinical Immunology, Kerckhoff-Clinic,
Justus-Liebig-University Giessen, Benekestr. 2-8, D-61231 Bad Nauheim, Germany

R.M. Silver and C.P. Denton (eds.), *Case Studies in Systemic Sclerosis*,
DOI: 10.1007/978-0-85729-641-2_19, © Springer-Verlag London Limited 2011

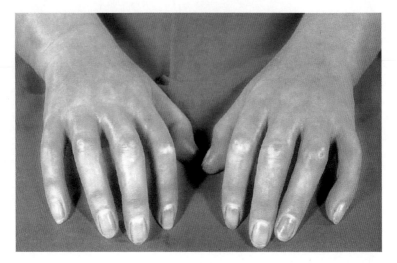

Fig. 19.1 Typical sclerodactyly of the hands without digital ulcers or pitting scars and swelling of metacarpophalangeal joints due to SSc-associated arthritis

Physical Examination

Temperature 37.3°C; pulse 105 bpm; respirations 18/min; blood pressure 190/130 mmHg. Skin: sclerodactyly also with sclerosis of the skin over the proximal and distal areas of all four extremities and the anterior chest (modified Rodnan Skin Score 35/51). Perioral skin furrowing with reduced oral aperture. No pitting scars or digital ulcers. Chest: moderate crackles during inspiration with reduced breath sounds. Cardiac: tachycardia, regular rhythm with normal S1 and S2 heart sounds. Abdomen: nondistended and nontender. Extremities: in addition to scleroderma, there was significant edema in both lower legs. Neurologic: all reflexes normal, no loss in sensation. Musculoskeletal: moderate swelling of the MCP joints of both hands (Fig. 19.1). Moderate flexion contractures of the fingers, tender flexion, and moderate swelling of wrists with inability to flatten hand.

Laboratory Findings

CBC remarkable for Hgb 10.5 g/dL and hematocrit 33%. CMP normal except serum creatinine 3.2 mg/dL and elevated potassium of 5.5 mmol/L, GFR 25 mL/min, Urine analysis: 70 mg/L protein; no casts. ANA by IIF was positive (titer 1:2,560) and anti-Scl-70 /topoisomerase-1 antibodies were strongly positive. Antineutrophil cytoplasmic antibodies (ANCA) and anti-cardiolipin antibodies were negative. Hand radiographs: small erosions at each ulnar styloid. Chest radiograph: bilateral moderate-sized pleural effusions, slight basal fibrosis, normal cardiac size. PFTs: FVC

Fig. 19.2 Typical late pattern in nailfold capillaroscopy showing several giant capillaries and substantial reduction of vasculature including avascular areas

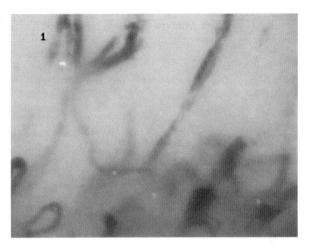

1.9 1 (60% predicted); FEV1 2.9 L (95% predicted); DLco 19.5 (80% predicted). Echocardiogram: tachycardia, no pericardial effusion, normal LV ejection fraction, normal RA, RV moderate hypertrophy. Nailfold capillary microscopy showed SSc late pattern (few giant capillaries and microhemorrhage, severe loss of capillaries with extensive avascular areas).

Course

With respect to the general underlying disease, a diagnosis of diffuse systemic sclerosis (dSSc) was made based on the following findings: diffuse cutaneous scleroderma involving not only the distal areas but also extending to involve the proximal extremities and the chest with a MRSS of >30/51. The diagnosis was supported by the presence of positive ANA together with Scl-70 autoantibodies and abnormal nailfold capillary morphology (Fig. 19.2). In addition, rapidly evolving scleroderma renal crisis (SRC) was suspected owing to uncontrolled hypertension, increasing azotemia, pleural effusions, and severe edema of the lower legs. Immediate high-dose treatment with an ACE inhibitor was started by prescribing captopril 200 mg daily po in four divided doses in combination with moderate doses of a loop diuretic, torasemide 10 mg twice daily po. In the next days, azotemia worsened with serum creatinine rising to 4.5 mg/dL and GFR falling to 15 mL/min. Supportive dialysis in the ICU was discussed. However, after 5 days renal function began to improve. Pleural effusions decreased down to a minimum over the following 3 weeks without requiring dialysis, and renal function remained stable with a creatinine of 1.4 mg/dL and a GFR of 50 mL/min for the next 15 months. Despite being maintained on daily ACE inhibitor therapy without the need for diuretics, renal function began to decrease slowly and constantly at a rate of about −0.1 mg/dL for serum creatinine every 2 months, until recently when in addition to the SRC a diagnosis of secondary amyloidosis with only slightly elevated serum amyloid A levels based on the long-term connective tissue disease was made.

Discussion

Scleroderma renal crisis (SRC) is the most acute and life-threatening manifestation of SSc, occurring predominantly in patients who have diffuse cutaneous involvement (dSSc). Patients at greatest risk of developing SRC are those having diffuse cutaneous or rapidly progressive SSc and (repeated) treatments with high doses of corticosteroids.[1-4] Owing to the clinically overt phenotype of SSc patients, differential diagnosis of kidney failure is not too difficult; however, other significant renal conditions, for example, thrombotic thrombocytopenic purpura (TTP), hemolytic uremic syndrome (HUS) and ANCA-associated pauci-immune glomerulonephritis, need to be considered as well. In conditions such as TTP, neurologic symptoms such as seizures and coma are more prominent than in SRC. TTP may be diagnosed when the typical pentad is present: microangiopathic hemolytic anemia, thrombocytopenia, renal dysfunction, fever, and neurologic symptoms and signs. HUS is usually a childhood disease and usually is not easily confused with SRC. Another important cause of renal failure in SSc patients is an ANCA-associated, pauci-immune glomerulonephritis. Such patients are usually normotensive, may have massive proteinuria with renal insufficiency, and do not have a microangiopathic hemolytic anemia or thrombocytopenia (see Chap. 20). In contrast, SRC patients often report headaches and can present with hypertensive retinopathy associated with visual disturbances and encephalopathy, seizures, fever, and general malaise. Pulmonary edema is also common, resulting from water and salt retention due to oliguria and often the co-occurrence of cardiac disease. Myocarditis and pericarditis with associated arrhythmia may indicate an overall poorer outcome.[5]

In general, laboratory tests demonstrate elevated levels of serum creatinine, microangiopathic hemolytic anemia, thrombocytopenia, and hyperreninemia. Renal crisis is also linked to a positive ANA with a speckled pattern, antibodies to RNA polymerase III, and the absence of anti-centromere antibodies. Anti-fibrillarin or anti-U3-RNP antibodies can also be found in young patients at risk of developing internal organ manifestations of SSc, including SRC.[6] ANCA is negative; if ANCA is present, then a pauci-immune glomerulonephritis should be considered (see Chap. 20).

The increased synthesis of renin, although not shown to be a predictive biomarker of SRC, facilitates hypertension which is usually accompanied by mild proteinuria, hematuria, and granular casts. Secondary phenomena include hypertensive vascular damage, glomerular ischemia, thrombotic vascular occlusion and fibrosis, and proliferation of intimal cells. Renal histology shows mucin accumulation in the arcuate and interlobular arteries, mucoid intimal thickening, and fibrinoid necrosis of arterioles with fibrin thrombi.[7] Figure 19.3 shows a typical histopathologic picture of a patient with SSc-associated renal complications. In general, renal biopsy is not necessary to confirm the diagnosis of SRC, especially if waiting for the

Fig. 19.3 Histopathologic findings in a patient with SSc-associated renal involvement showing fibrinoid vascular alterations with obstruction of the affected vessels. (Generously provided courtesy of Prof. Dr. Jörg Kriegsmann, Trier, Germany)

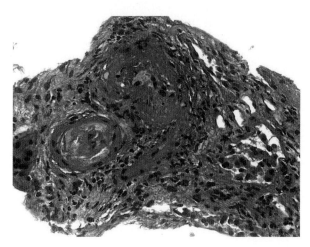

result of the biopsy would hinder the immediate treatment with antihypertensive treatment. However, when SSc occurs as an overlap syndrome with other connective tissue diseases, persistent inflammation, and/or overt vasculitis and signs for glomerulonephritis such as casts, renal biopsy may be necessary to exclude or confirm other reasons for the deterioration of renal function.

Until the availability of ACE-I therapy in 1979, SRC resulted usually in malignant hypertension, rapidly progressive renal failure, and early mortality.[8] However, during the following decades, the proportion of deaths in SSc patients attributed to SRC decreased from 42% to 6%.[9] Despite this progress, long-term mortality in SRC still remains high.[1,10] In a recent worldwide survey, 76 incident cases of SRC were identified in only the first 15 months of the survey. Of these, 66 (87%) had a hypertensive SRC and remarkably 10 (13%) a normotensive SRC. This is in line with the observation that in about 20% of patients the diagnosis of SRC may precede diagnosis of SSc.[1] Twenty-two percent (22%) of the patients were on an ACE-I therapy immediately prior to the onset of the SRC. Of the patients (30% of the initial population) that were reported in the 1-year follow-up data, over 50% have died or remain on dialysis at 1 year, which underlines the fact that SRC continues to be an emergency situation for SSc patients in the twenty-first century.[11] In this context, it needs to be noted that prophylactic therapy with ACE-I has not (yet) proven to prevent SRC in controlled clinical trials but when on ACE-I for other reasons, it does not need to be terminated.

Renal Protection

In a study addressing the therapeutic effect of ACE–I therapy, patients with SRC not receiving ACE-I had a 1-year survival of 15% and a 5-year survival of 10%, even in the face of aggressive antihypertensive treatment with minoxidil, hydralazine and alpha-methyldopa. In contrast, patients receiving ACE-I had an impressive 1-year survival of 76% and a 5-year survival of 65%. Therefore, ACE-I therapy should be administered immediately in any SSc patient with high blood pressure, especially with new-onset hypertension. With or without overt evidence of renal injury, these patients should be treated and maintained on a maximum tolerable dose of an ACE-I, even if deterioration of renal function develops.[8,12] In general, treatment should be started with a short-acting ACE-I such as captopril, especially in an ICU setting when continuous adaptation of the medication to the actual clinical status is required. In a more stable situation or when renal function is stabilized, captopril can be exchanged for a long-acting ACE-I if desired. Angiotensin receptor blockers (ARB) should only be used if side effects preclude use of ACE-I, as the increase in vasodilatory metabolites following ACE-I therapy is not induced by ARB. However, similar to the addition of calcium channel blockers (CCB) and diuretics, combination therapy with an ARB may be beneficial for patients with inadequate blood pressure reduction on ACE-I therapy alone. Intravenous iloprost may also help to reverse microvascular changes. Additional oral antihypertensive agents (e.g., labetalol), together with nitrate infusion if there is pulmonary edema, can be used if required. Plasma exchange needs to be considered if there is evidence of significant thrombotic microangiopathy. Support of renal function can be provided by intermittent hemodialysis or continuous venous-venous hemofiltration. Inhibiting endothelin overactivity, which has been implicated in the pathogenesis of SRC, may be an additional future therapeutic approach. This idea is based on the observation of increased levels of endothelin-1 (ET-1) in SSc patients with SRC[13] and increased expression of both ET-1 and ET-1 receptors in the small renal arteries of SRC patients.[14] In vivo studies also suggest that organ-specific activation of the endothelin system is responsible for the development of hypertensive nephropathy in renin-angiotensin-mediated hypertension.[15]

It should be noted that some authors recommend a rather gradual reduction in blood pressure to avoid excessive pressure decrease and subsequent reduced renal perfusion. If renal protection is sufficient, median time to recovery is 1 year and typically occurs within the first 3 years. Prognosis is worse for males. For those patients who fail to recover adequate renal function, renal transplantation may need to be discussed. However, owing to the possibility of (partial) renal recovery for a period of up to 2 years after onset of SRC with renal failure, it is recommended that one wait at least 1 year before listing a SSc patient for renal transplantation. Similar to other disease entities that require renal transplantation and due to the multiorgan involvement in SSc, the long-term outcome of transplanted SSc patients can be poor with a graft survival rate as low as 25%.[16] As in our case, additional sequelae secondary to the main disease, such as (renal) amlyoidosis (Fig. 19.4a, b) can develop later in the course[17] even without high serum amyloid values.[18] Such complications must be taken into account when monitoring the "renal survivors" for an extended period of time.

Fig. 19.4 Histopathologic findings of (peri)vascular amyloidosis in the kidney showing (**a**) Congo red staining of amyloid in glomeruli and the vessel walls and (**b**) polarized light microscopy highlighting amyloid as green deposits. (Generously provided courtesy of Prof. Dr. Jörg Kriegsmann, Trier, Germany)

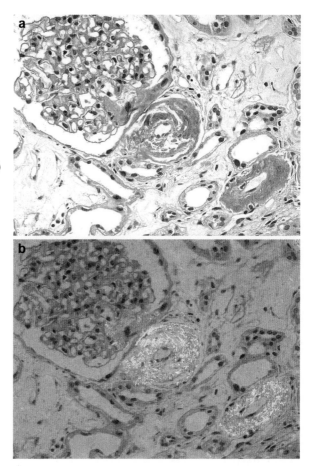

Table 19.1 Suggested criteria for SRC based on a recent international survey

Hypertensive SRC:

Systolic blood pressure >140 mmHg

Diastolic blood pressure >90 mmHg

Rise in systolic blood pressure >30 mmHg compared to baseline

Rise in diastolic blood pressure >20 mmHg compared to baseline

AND

One of the following features:

(a) Increase in serum creatinine >50% over baseline OR serum creatinine >120% of upper limit of normal for local laboratory,

(b) Proteinuria: >2+ by dipstick and confirmed by protein: creatinine ratio >upper limits of normal (ULN),

(c) Hematuria: >2+ by dipstick or >10 RBCs/HPF (without menstruation),

(d) Thrombocytopenia: <100,000 plts/mm^3,

(e) Hemolysis: by blood smear or increased reticulocyte count,

(f) Hypertensive encephalopathy.

(continued)

Table 19.1 (continued)

Normotensive SRC:
Increase in serum creatinine >50% over baseline OR serum creatinine >120% of upper limit of normal for local laboratory
AND
One of the following features:
(a) Proteinuria: >2+ by dipstick and confirmed by protein: creatinine ratio > upper limits of normal (ULN),
(b) Hematuria: >2+ by dipstick or >10 RBCs/HPF (without menstruation),
(c) Thrombocytopenia: ≤100,000 plts/mm³,
(d) Hemolysis: by blood smear or increased reticulocyte count,
(e) Hypertensive encephalopathy.

Reproduced with permission from the Creative Commons Attribution License: Hudson et al.[11]

Table 19.2 EULAR recommendations for management of scleroderma renal crisis

Recommendations	
#10	Despite the lack of RCTs, experts believe that ACE inhibitors should be used in the treatment of scleroderma renal crisis
#11	Four retrospective studies suggest that steroids are associated with a higher risk of scleroderma renal crisis. Patients on steroids should be carefully monitored for blood pressure and renal function

Reproduced from Kowal-Bielecka et al.[12] with permission from BMJ Publishing Group Ltd.

SRC has become a relatively infrequent yet critical event in the course of a patient with SSc. SRC requires immediate diagnosis, for example, by defined criteria as suggested recently (Table 19.1),[11] and emergent treatment to optimize outcomes. Considerable additional research is needed to supplement the currently available evidence-based recommendations (Table 19.2).

References

1. Penn H, Howie AJ, Kingdon EJ, et al. Scleroderma renal crisis: patient characteristics and long-term outcomes. *Q J Med*. 2007;100:485-494.
2. Teixeira L, Mouthon L, Mahr A, et al. Mortality and risk factors of scleroderma renal crisis: a French retrospective study in 50 patients. *Ann Rheum Dis*. 2008;67:110-116.
3. Steen VD, Medsger TA Jr, Osial TA, et al. Factors predicting development of renal involvement in progressive systemic sclerosis. *Am J Med*. 1984;76:779-786.
4. Steen VD, Medsger TA Jr. Case-control study of corticosteroids and other drugs that either precipitate or protect from the development of scleroderma renal crisis. *Arthritis Rheum*. 1998;41:1613-1619.
5. Steen VD, Medsger TA Jr. Long-term outcomes of scleroderma renal crisis. *Ann Intern Med*. 2000;133:600-603.

6. Tormey VJ, Bunn CC, Denton CP, et al. Anti-fibrillarin antibodies in systemic sclerosis. *Rheumatology.* 2001;40:1157-1162.
7. Lee S, Lee S, Sharma K. The pathogenesis of fibrosis and renal disease in scleroderma: recent insights from glomerulosclerosis. *Curr Rheumatol Rep.* 2004;6:141-148.
8. Steen VD, Costantino JP, Shapiro AP, Medsger TA Jr. Outcome of renal crisis in systemic sclerosis: relation to availability of angiotensin converting enzyme (ACE) inhibitors. *Ann Intern Med.* 1990;113:352-357.
9. Steen VD, Medsger TA. Changes in causes of death in systemic sclerosis, 1972–2002. *Ann Rheum Dis.* 2007;66:940-944.
10. DeMarco PJ, Weisman MH, Seibold JR, et al. Predictors and outcome of scleroderma renal crisis: the high-dose versus low-dose D-penicillamine in early diffuse systemic sclerosis trial. *Arthritis Rheum.* 2002;46:2983-2989.
11. Hudson M, Baron M, Lo E, et al. An international, web-based, prospective cohort study to determine whether the use of ACE inhibitors prior to the onset of scleroderma renal crisis is associated with worse outcomes – methodology and preliminary results. *Int J Rheumatol.* 2010;2010:347-402.
12. Kowal-Bielecka O, Landewé R, Avouac J, et al. EULAR recommendations for the treatment of systemic sclerosis: a report from the EULAR Scleroderma Trials and Research group (EUSTAR). *Ann Rheum Dis.* 2009;68:620-628.
13. Vancheeswaran R, Magoulas T, Efrat G, et al. Circulating endothelin-1 levels in systemic sclerosis subsets – a marker of fibrosis or vascular dysfunction? *J Rheumatol.* 1994;21: 1838-1844.
14. Kobayashi H, Nishimaki T, Kaise S, et al. Immunohistological study of endothelin-1 and endothelin-A and B receptors in two patients with scleroderma renal crisis. *Clin Rheumatol.* 1999;18:425-427.
15. Maki S, Miyauchi T, Kakinuma Y, et al. The endothelin receptor antagonist ameliorates the hypertensive phenotypes of transgenic hypertensive mice with renin-angiotensin genes and discloses roles of organ specific activation of endothelin system in transgenic mice. *Life Sci.* 2004;74:1105-1118.
16. Batal I, Domsic RT, Medsger TA, Bastacky S. Scleroderma renal crisis: a pathology perspective. *Int J Rheumatol.* 2010;2010:543-704.
17. Pamuk GE, Pamuk ON, Altiparmak MR, et al. Secondary amyloidosis in progressive systemic sclerosis. *Clin Rheumatol.* 2001;20:285-287.
18. Tennent GA, Dziazhio M, Triantafillidou E, et al. Normal circulating serum amyloid P component concentration in systemic sclerosis. *Arthritis Rheum.* 2007;56:2013-2017.

Chapter 20
A 34-Year-Old Woman with Limited Cutaneous Scleroderma Who Develops Normotensive Renal Failure with Pulmonary Hemorrhage

Hirahito Endo

Keywords Renal failure • Glomerulonephritis • Antineutrophil cytoplasmic autoantibodies (ANCA) • Pulmonary hemorrhage

Case Study

A 34-year-old Japanese woman presented with a 15-year history of Raynaud's phenomenon with stiffness and swelling of the hands. Limited cutaneous systemic sclerosis (lSSc) and rheumatoid arthritis overlap syndrome had been diagnosed 5 years previously, treated with D-penicillamine and corticosteroids. She was admitted to our hospital after she developed hemoptysis with progressive dyspnea and was found to have acute renal failure. She had a low-grade fever 2 weeks before admission along with erythema of the legs. Hemoptysis and dyspnea began 3 days before admission. She required intubation and was placed on a ventilator while her renal failure was treated by hemodialysis.

Antineutrophil cytoplasmic autoantibodies in a perinuclear distribution (P-ANCA) were detected by indirect immunofluorescence (IIF). This ANCA was shown to be an anti-myeloperoxidase (MPO) antibody when tested by confirmatory ELISA, suggesting a diagnosis of ANCA-associated vasculitis complicating limited SSc.

H. Endo
Division of Rheumatology, Department of Internal Medicine,
Toho University School of Medicine, 6-11-1, Ohmori-nishi,
Otaku, Tokyo 143-8541, Japan

R.M. Silver and C.P. Denton (eds.), *Case Studies in Systemic Sclerosis*,
DOI: 10.1007/978-0-85729-641-2_20, © Springer-Verlag London Limited 2011

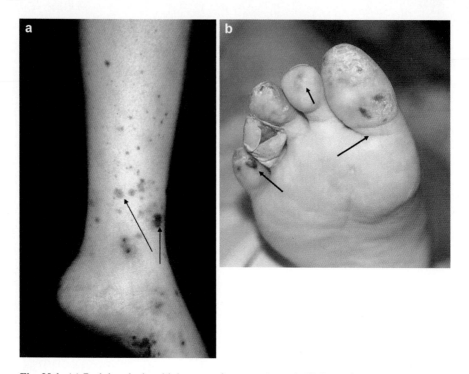

Fig. 20.1 (a) Both legs had multiple areas of purpura (*arrow*). (b) Purpuric lesions on a toe and planter surface of foot (*arrow*)

Physical Examination

Body weight was 58 kg, temperature was 37.6°C, pulse rate was 98 bpm, respiration rate was 32/min, and blood pressure was 148/80 mmHg. Her fingers were puffy with loss of skin creases on the dorsum of the distal fingers. There were shallow digital pitted scars on two finger pads as well as nailfold infarcts. Telangiectasias were present on the fingers and hands. The proximal arms, chest, and the abdomen had apparently normal skin. Both legs showed erythema with signs of cutaneous hemorrhage. There was perioral skin furrowing with reduced oral aperture. Chest examination revealed moist crackles that were audible in all lung fields. Cardiac examination revealed regular rate and rhythm with normal S1 and S2 heart sounds. Examination of the abdomen was normal. Examination of the extremities revealed edematous and erythematous lesions with purpura (Fig. 20.1a, b). Neurological examination was normal. There were mild flexion contractures of the fingers with inability to flatten the hands, as well as joint tenderness and swelling of the wrist joints. Dilated capillary loops were seen at the nailfold margins with extensive cuticular hemorrhage, while the toes showed multiple purpuric lesions (Fig 20.1b).

Laboratory Findings

The CBC showed WBC $12,300/mm^3$ with 84% neutrophils, RBC $292 \times 10^4/mm^3$ with hemoglobin concentration 8.8 g/dL, and hematocrit 26%, platelet count $20.2 \times 10^4/mm^3$. Serum chemistry analysis revealed SGOT 85 U/mL, SGPT 35 U/mL, LDH 1,285 U/mL, creatinine 3.0 mg/dL, blood urea nitrogen 38 mg/dL, uric acid 11.2 mg/dL, and C-reactive protein 24.9 mg/mL. Blood gas examination showed PaO_2 55, $PaCO_2$ 25.1. ANA was positive by IIF (titer 1:1,280; speckled pattern). Anti U1-RNP antibody was positive, but anti-topoisomerase and anti-centromere antibodies were negative. Rheumatoid factor was positive (642 U), P-ANCA was 224 EU, and C-ANCA was negative. CH50 was <5U, C3 was 37 mg/dL, C4 was 15.2 mg/dL. Urinalysis revealed the following: protein 2+, hematuria 3+, hyaline casts +, cellular casts 3+. Radiographs of the hands revealed focal calcification in the soft tissues of multiple distal fingers, joint erosions of the carpal bones, and joint space narrowing of both wrists. A chest radiograph showed diffuse consolidation of bilateral lungs and cardiomegaly (Fig. 20.2a). Chest CT revealed diffuse consolidation in all lung fields (Fig. 20.2b). Echocardiography showed a normal left ventricular (LV) ejection fraction, normal RA, and RV dimensions, and no tricuspid regurgitation.

Course

A diagnosis of ANCA-associated vasculitis was made based on the following clinical and laboratory findings: high MPO-ANCA titer, pulmonary hemorrhage and renal failure. Concurrent limited SSc (lSSc) was confirmed by Raynaud's phenomenon with digital pitted scars, sclerodactyly, telangiectasias, and esophageal dysmotility. Also supporting the diagnosis was ANA positivity with U1-RNP pattern, radiographic findings, anemia consistent with pulmonary hemorrhage, and progressive renal failure. Laboratory data showed a high MPO-ANCA titer consistent with a diagnosis of MPO-ANCA-associated vasculitis, or microscopic polyangiitis, complicating her history of lSSc. After admission to the intensive care unit, she was supported by mechanical ventilation and treated with methylprednisolone pulse therapy (1,000 mg daily for 3 days). Then prednisolone (80 mg daily) was administrated and she received intravenous cyclophosphamide (500 mg). Daily plasma exchange was performed for 3 days. Her serum P-ANCA titer decreased, but renal function gradually worsened and she needed hemodialysis on the 7th hospital day. Proton pump inhibitor therapy was continued to manage gastroesophageal reflux. Pulmonary findings did not improve despite full active management in the ICU, and she died of acute respiratory distress syndrome on the 20th hospital day. Autopsy showed diffuse alveolar hemorrhage with neutrophil infiltration in the alveolar septae in both lungs and crescentic

Fig. 20.2 (a) Chest
radiograph showing bilateral
diffuse consolidation.
(b) Chest CT scan also
shows diffuse consolidation
of bilateral lungs

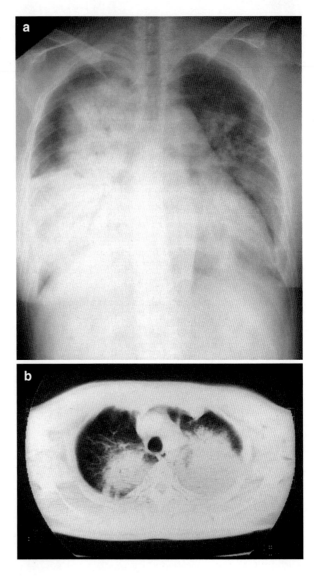

glomerulonephritis (Fig. 20.3a, b). Pathological assessment of cutaneous vasculitis was done by biopsy of an area of erythema on the legs (Fig. 20.4a, b).

Discussion

In SSc patients, renal involvement is classically characterized by malignant hypertension, elevated plasma renin activity, and rising serum creatinine due to worsening
renal function, a constellation of findings known as scleroderma renal crisis[1] (see

Fig. 20.3 (a) Light microscopic examination of a lung autopsy specimen showing massive hemorrhage with neutrophil infiltration in the alveolar septa. (b) Light microscopic examination of a renal biopsy specimen showing a circumferential cellular crescent surrounding a glomerular tuft, indicating crescentic glomerulonephritis (hematoxylin and eosin stain, ×200)

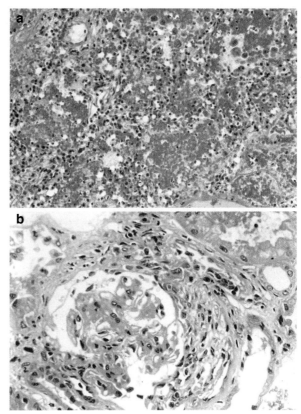

Chap. 19). Helfrich et al.[2] reported 11 patients who had normotensive renal failure accompanied by microangiopathic hemolytic anemia, thrombocytopenia, and pulmonary hemorrhage. These patients were initially felt to represent a subtype of scleroderma renal crisis. On the other hand, we reported a series of six patients who presented with normotensive, rapidly progressive renal failure in association with ANCA.[3] Of the three who underwent renal biopsy, all were found to have a pauci-immune crescentic glomerulonephritis and, as with the case study, two of them also had pulmonary hemorrhage.[3] Several similar cases from various countries also suggest an association between normotensive progressive renal failure with MPO-ANCA–positive crescentic glomerulonephritis and SSc.[4-10] These cases emphasize the need to carefully evaluate every SSc patient who develops renal insufficiency for non-scleroderma causes of renal disease. Patients with this type of glomerulonephritis are usually normotensive, may have massive proteinuria and renal insufficiency, and do not have a microangiopathic hemolytic anemia or thrombocytopenia. Thus, they are quite different from the usual patient with scleroderma renal crisis. Progressive renal insufficiency can occur and treatment with steroids and immunosuppressive agents may be helpful, as in classic cases of microscopic polyangiitis.[9,10] A PubMed search revealed 31 reports of ANCA-associated vasculitis with scleroderma (>60 cases),[11] including several case reports and small series of SSc

Fig. 20.4 (**a**) Light microscopic examination of the skin biopsy specimen showing a thickened dermis due to collagen deposition and inflammatory cell (especially neutrophil) infiltration in small arteries of the dermis. These findings indicate cutaneous vasculitis (hematoxylin and eosin stain, ×100). (**b**) Immunofluorescent staining of the skin biopsy specimen showing IgG deposition in the dermal vessels and vasculitis (×100)

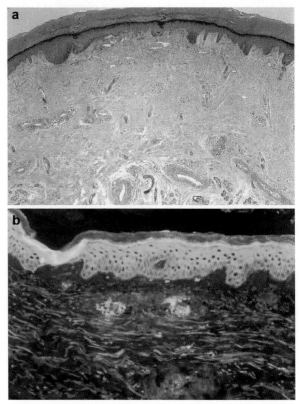

patients developing a MPO-ANCA-associated necrotizing, crescentic glomerulonephritis.[4-10] These SSc patients have pulmonary hemorrhage with acute renal failure due to crescentic glomerulonephritis, that is, a pulmonary-renal syndrome.[12,13] A patient who had diffuse cutaneous SSc (dSSc) and microscopic polyangiitis presenting with diffuse alveolar hemorrhage and crescentic glomerulonephritis has also been reported. Thus, pulmonary-renal syndrome in SSc patients should be classified together with MPO-ANCA associated vasculitis or microscopic polyangiitis.[12,13] A much smaller number of cases with anti-PR3 ANCA have been reported in SSc, and this may also be associated with potentially aggressive pauci-immune glomerulonephritis.

Some examples of this condition were previously reported as occurring due to drug toxicity, for example, in patients receiving D-penicillamine as treatment for SSc. More recently, several cases were reported in patients with lSSc who had not been exposed to any drugs known to cause glomerulonephritis or pulmonary hemorrhage.[14,15] Our patient had received D-penicillamine for 5 years. In a 104-week trial of D-penicillamine for early SSc, serum ANCA was measured and no evidence of ANCA seroconversion was observed, nor was vasculitis noted.[16] Adverse effects of D-penicillamine include proteinuria, which is usually reversible on withdrawal of the drug, and glomerulonephritis occurs in less than 1% of treated subjects. Membranous nephropathy is the most common type of glomerulonephritis seen in association with D-penicillamine.[14,15] In contrast, crescentic glomerulonephritis (sometimes with positive P-ANCA, particularly with anti-myeloperoxidase antibodies) is a very uncommon complication of D-penicillamine therapy.[14,15] However, drug withdrawal is not associated with resolution of this complication because only patients who received immunosuppressive therapy had a good outcome.

In the present case, there was histologically proven angiitis with crescentic glomerulonephritis and cutaneous vasculitis. According to previous reports, ANCA-associated vasculitis led to pulmonary involvement in 75% of the patients and renal involvement occurred in 82%.[11] There does not appear to be an association between SSc subtype and the development of ANCA-associated vasculitis, that is, it is observed in diffuse or limited SSc. Anti-topoisomerase I antibody was associated with ANCA-associated vasculitis (70%), while anti-centromere antibody was less frequently detected (14%).[11]

In conclusion, when a SSc patient presents with atypical features such as high fever, elevated inflammatory markers, or normotensive renal failure with glomerulonephritis, it is prudent to test for ANCA by IIF and ELISA. If ANCA is detected in such a situation, it should not be ascribed to coincidence. Patients with an ANCA-associated vasculitis in association with SSc should be managed with supportive measures and a therapeutic strategy to treat small vessel vasculitis.[17]

References

1. Steen VD. Scleroderma renal crisis. *Rheum Dis Clin North Am*. 2003;29:315-333.
2. Helfrich DJ, Banner B, Steen VD, Medsger TA Jr. Normotensive renal failure in systemic sclerosis. *Arthritis Rheum*. 1989;32:1128-1134.
3. Endo H, Hosono T, Kondo H. Antineutrophil cytoplasmic antibodies in 6 patients with renal failure and systemic sclerosis. *J Rheumatol*. 1994;21:864-870.
4. Huong DL, Papo T, Gatfosse M, Frances C, Godeau P, Beaufils H. Antineutrophil cytoplasmic autoantibodies in systemic sclerosis with renal failure. *J Rheumatol*. 1995;22:791-792.
5. Omote A, Muramatsu M, Sugimoto Y, et al. MPO-ANCA-related scleroderma renal crisis treated with double-filtration plasmapheresis. *Intern Med*. 1997;36:508-513.
6. Anders HJ, Wiebecke B, Haedecke C, Sanden S, Combe C, Schlondorff D. MPO-ANCA-Positive crescentic glomerulonephritis: a distinct entity of scleroderma renal disease. *Am J Kid Dis*. 1999;33:E3.
7. Villaverde V, Balsa A, Cabezas JA, Fernandez-Prada M, Torre A, Mola EM. Normotensive renal failure in a patient with systemic sclerosis and a p-antineutrophil cytoplasmic autoantibodies which developed into Paget's disease of bone after immunosuppressive therapy. *Rheumatology (Oxford)*. 1999;38:190-191.
8. Katrib A, Strugess A, Bertouch JV. Systemic sclerosis and antineutrophil cytoplasmic autoantibody-associated renal failure. *Rheumatol Int*. 1999;19:61-63.
9. Carvajal I, Bernis C, Sanz P, Garcia A, Garcia-Vadillo A, Traver JA. Antineutrophil cytoplasmic autoantibodies (ANCA) and systemic sclerosis. *Nephrol Dial Transplant*. 1997;12:576-577.
10. Maes B, Van Mieghem A, Messiaen T, Kuypers D, Van Damme B, Vanrenferghem Y. Limited cutaneous systemic sclerosis associated with MPO-ANCA positive renal small vessel vasculitis of the microscopic polyangitis type. *Am J Kidney Dis*. 2000;36:E16.

11. Rho YH, Choi SJ, Lee YH, Ji JD, Song GG. Scleroderma associated with ANCA-associated vasculitis. *Rheumatol Int*. 2006;26:369-375.
12. Wutzl AL, Foley RN, O'Driscoll BR, Reeve RS, Chisholm R, Herrick AL. Microscopic polyangiitis presenting as pulmonary-renal syndrome in a patient with long-standing diffuse cutaneous systemic sclerosis and antibodies to myeloperoxidase. *Arthritis Rheum*. 2001;45: 533-536.
13. Bar J, Ehrenfeld M, Rozenman J, Perelman M, Sidi Y, Gur H. Pulmonary-renal syndrome in systemic sclerosis. *Semin Arthritis Rheum*. 2001;30:403-410.
14. Hillis GS, Khan IH, Simpson JG, Rees AJ. Scleroderma, D-penicillamine treatment and progressive renal failure associated with positive antimyeloperoxidase antineutrophil cytoplasmic antibodies. *Am J Kidney Dis*. 1997;30:279-281.
15. Karpinski J, Jothy S, Radoux V, Levy M, Baran D. D-penicillamine-induced crescentic glomerulonephritis and antimyeloperoxidase antibodies in a patient with scleroderma. Case report and review of the literature. *Am J Nephrol*. 1997;17:528-532.
16. Choi HK, Slot MC, Pan G, Weissbach CA, Niles JL, Merkel PA. Evaluation of antineutrophil cytoplasmic antibody seroconversion induced by minocycline, sulfasalazine, or penicillamine. *Arthritis Rheum*. 2000;43:2488-2492.
17. Mukhtyar C, Guillevin L, Cid MC, et al. EULAR recommendations for the management of primary small and medium vessel vasculitis. *Ann Rheum Dis*. 2009;68:310-317.

Chapter 21
A Scleroderma Patient Inquires About Pregnancy

Virginia Steen

Keywords Pregnancy • Scleroderma renal crisis (SRC)

Case Study

A 35-year-old Caucasian woman with a 3-year history of diffuse systemic sclerosis (dSSc) felt well, but had mild arthralgia and difficulty with hand function. Raynaud's phenomenon was well controlled with nifedipine, and gastroesophageal reflux was controlled with omeprazole. She denied any shortness of breath. She worked as a social worker and went for consultation to help determine if she can safely have a child. On examination, her blood pressure was 100/75 mmHg, lung and heart examinations were normal, her skin was thickened on the fingers, hands, forearms, and chest, she had no tendon friction rubs or digital ulcers, but she had moderate contractures of her hands. Her medications include 60 mg nifedipine daily, 500 mg naproxen twice daily, 20 mg omeprazole twice daily, and 2.5 g mycophenolate mofetil daily. Her laboratory studies revealed a normal CBC, sedimentation rate, chemical profile, and a positive Scl-70 autoantibody. Pulmonary function tests (PFTs) demonstrated a forced vital capacity (FVC) of 72% predicted and a DLco of 75% predicted, both of which were stable over the past 3 years. Echocardiogram was normal.

After discussion she was advised to taper the mycophenolate mofetil over the course of the next year and to have her tests repeated. She tapered and discontinued the medication without difficulty. She returned in 1 year feeling very well and had even been able to switch the naproxen to acetaminophen as needed. Repeat PFTs showed an FVC of 78% predicted and a DLco of 72% predicted, and a high resolution CT chest scan showed only mild interstitial fibrosis unchanged from 2 years prior. She was told she could go ahead and try to become pregnant.

V. Steen
Department of Rheumatology & Clinical Immunology, Georgetown University,
3800 Reservoir Road, PHC 3, Washington, DC 20007, USA

R.M. Silver and C.P. Denton (eds.), *Case Studies in Systemic Sclerosis*,
DOI: 10.1007/978-0-85729-641-2_21, © Springer-Verlag London Limited 2011

She returned 4 months later at which time she was 8 weeks pregnant and very excited. She had met with her obstetrician, who specialized in high-risk pregnancy, prior to becoming pregnant and was told to stop the nifedipine and omeprazole when she became pregnant. At this point, she had some mild reflux symptoms at night and some heartburn for which she was taking TUMS® and elevating the head of her bed. Over the next 6 months she continued to do well although she had more heartburn and the usual pregnancy symptoms. She was thrilled that she was not having any symptoms of Raynaud's phenomenon. The baby was growing well. She was being followed very closely and there was no sign of any problems.

At 36 weeks gestation, she noted that her home blood pressure readings were elevated (140/86 mmHg), which was definitely a change for her. She immediately notified her rheumatologist and was admitted to the hospital, at which time she was found to have had a decrease in plasma hemoglobin, a fall in platelet count to 100,000/mm^3, 2+ proteinuria, and a serum creatinine of 0.8 mg/dL. The serum uric acid was normal. There was much discussion as to whether she had preeclampsia or scleroderma renal crisis (SRC), and because she was already 36 weeks in gestation and the baby was of good size, it was decided to perform a Cesarean section. This went well without any complications and she had a healthy baby girl weighing 5 lb 10 oz with good APGAR score. Within 3 h after delivery the patient's blood pressure had improved to 120/78 mm/Hg, and a repeat CBC showed a platelet count of 120,000/mm^3 and a serum creatinine of 0.7 mg/dL. The decision was made to hold off on the use of an angiotensin converting enzyme (ACE) inhibitor and watch the blood pressure very closely. Over the next 2 days her blood pressure returned to its normal level of 100/75 mmHg and she went home with her baby girl.

Discussion

Systemic sclerosis is a connective tissue disease that occurs in women 3–5 times more frequently than in men. The interrelationships of SSc and pregnancy are important from both the effects of SSc on pregnancy and the effects of pregnancy on SSc. With the mean age of onset of symptoms in the early 40s, almost half of the women with this illness have the potential of becoming pregnant after the onset of their disease. Until recently, most women would have completed their pregnancies prior to this age, but at this point, women are frequently delaying pregnancy. Thus, there is an increased likelihood for a concurrent pregnancy in women who develop SSc in their adult life.

Fertility

One of the first questions a patient asks is whether she can become pregnant. The issue of fertility in women with SSc is difficult to determine because there are many factors, both physical and psychological, that affect the ability and desire to become pregnant. Early studies suggested there was decreased fertility but that was most likely because most women had completed their pregnancies prior to getting SSc or were too sick to even want to become pregnant. More recent studies have not identified decreased overall fertility, but little attempt has been made to relate the timing of pregnancy to the onset of SSc.[1,2]

We surveyed 214 SSc patients, 167 rheumatoid arthritis (RA) patients, and 105 healthy women with questions about the occurrence of pregnancy and any delays in conception.[3] There was a significantly larger number of women with SSc or RA who had never been pregnant (21% SSc, 23% RA, and 12% healthy control subjects, $p < 0.05$). When this was adjusted for factors such as the number of women who had never married, who were sexually inactive, or who had chosen not to have children, there was no difference between the three groups. Only 2–5% of patients in each group had ever attempted to become pregnant but were unsuccessful. Also, the percentage of women with at least a 1-year delay in conception was not significantly different in the three groups (12–15%). During infertility evaluations, SSc patients were more likely to be told of possible causes of infertility such as fallopian tube obstruction or endometriosis. However, no unique cause of infertility was found among SSc patients. The overall successful pregnancy rate in those patients with a prior period of infertility was similar in all three groups, 37%, 40%, and 43%, respectively. Curiously, the SSc patients' partners were more likely to have fertility problems than the controls' partners.

When in Illness to Get Pregnant

The next question is when in the course of their illness is the best time for a patient to become pregnant. Patients with a recent onset of Raynaud's phenomenon and diagnosis of SSc should be counseled not to get pregnant until the course of their disease is established and stabilized. In patients with less than 2 years of any symptoms, it may be difficult to determine whether a patient will ultimately have limited or diffuse SSc. If a patient has an anti-centromere antibody one can be very confident that she will not develop diffuse SSc or serious pulmonary fibrosis, and thus could become pregnant at that time. However, most patients who have an anti-Scl-70 antibody, nucleolar pattern ANA or an anti-RNA Polymerase III antibody are at high risk for developing serious internal organ involvement early in their disease. Even if such patients do not initially have diffuse cutaneous disease, they still are at high risk for developing renal crisis, pulmonary fibrosis, cardiomyopathy, and other poor prognostic signs. They need to be followed carefully and treated aggressively during that time. Patients should be discouraged from becoming pregnant during the first 4 years of their illness and until they clearly have had no progression of skin thickening, no tendon friction rubs, and stable PFTs and echocardiograms for 1 year. However, patients with pulmonary arterial hypertension (PAH) should be strongly discouraged from ever becoming pregnant because of the major risk of death to both mother and fetus. Reports estimate a 36–50% maternal death rate in women with PAH,[4,5] although a more recent study suggested it might be lower (17–33%), but still unacceptably high.[6]

The decision to become pregnant for the woman who has previously had renal crisis and is taking ACE-inhibitors is particularly challenging. After an episode of renal crisis, ACE inhibitors are required to maintain normal blood pressure and renal function. Patients have had successful pregnancy outcomes while on ACE-inhibitors,[3,7] but the use of these drugs during the third trimester of pregnancy is associated with an increased risk of serious kidney problems in the baby. However, stopping the ACE inhibitor in such patients could also be disastrous for both mother and baby. There are several possible approaches that a patient can take if she desires a pregnancy after renal crisis, but they each carry significant risk. I encourage the patient to try to taper the ACE-inhibitor before getting pregnant to see if the blood pressure and kidney function can be controlled with other medications. In our experience with a small series of patients, the worst outcomes occurred in patients who had very poor blood pressure control off ACE-inhibitor therapy. Another possible way of managing the pregnancy would be to use a small dose of ACE-inhibitor along with non-ACE-inhibitor medication to control blood pressure, along with close monitoring for oligohydramnios or other signs of fetal abnormalities. In any situation, the patient and her spouse have to seriously consider a variety of options and potential outcomes before deciding whether to become or continue a pregnancy. There are no easy answers.

Pregnancy Outcomes

Patients are very eager to know the possible outcomes of pregnancy and the risks for miscarriage and other problems. The reports of pregnancy outcomes in women with SSc have been quite variable. Early literature is filled with case reports of negative outcomes to the mother and/or the baby.[8-10] Several case-control studies identified an increased frequency of miscarriages per pregnancy,[2,11] or in women prior to the onset of SSc.[11-13] In our retrospective case-control study, the frequency of miscarriage in SSc patients was only 9%, which is not different than the frequency of 7.5% in healthy women.[3] In our prospective scleroderma pregnancy study, there were 91 pregnancies in 59 women.[7] We divided the patients into SSc subsets, that is, limited and diffuse scleroderma as well as early and late disease (less than or greater than 4 years of symptoms, respectively). Miscarriage occurred with similar frequency to historical controls except in the group of patients with late diffuse SSc, who had a surprisingly high frequency: 42% of the 15 women with late diffuse SSc had miscarriages compared to 13% in all of the other groups. Renal insufficiency and severe gastrointestinal malabsorption were present in two of the seven women who had miscarriages. Only one woman with limited SSc was a habitual aborter, experiencing four miscarriages (two after disease onset) and never having a healthy child.

Prematurity has not been specifically addressed in most studies, although several early series noted more than the expected number of premature infants.[8,10]

Our series identified a marked increase in the frequency of premature infants in SSc patients and RA patients compared to healthy women.[3] Interestingly, prematurity was more common in SSc patients before the onset of their illness compared to after onset of the disease. Fortunately, the premature infants in our series did well. They were small and had the usual prematurity complications, but there was only one fetal death related to prematurity. It is likely that having a chronic disease, for example, SSc or RA, is the common denominator for the increased occurrence of prematurity. In our prospective study, prematurity again was much increased compared to historical controls, 29% versus 5%. In 65% of the pregnancies in women with early diffuse SSc, the pregnancy ended before 38 weeks (the American Obstetrical Association definition of premature births). In 13 of the 23 preterm births, the babies were born at 36 or 37 weeks and weighed a mean of 5.7 lb. Eight of these 13 pregnancies were induced for non-emergent issues. There was only one neonatal death, which was of a 25-week fetus, although several small babies required prolonged hospital stays. Interestingly, unlike our retrospective study, none of the full-term babies were small for dates, and all weighed more than 5.5 lb (mean 7.1 lb). Thus, although the frequency of mildly premature infants was increased, the overall success rate, that is, a live birth, was 84% for limited SSc women and 77% for diffuse SSc women, compared with 84% for historical controls.

Infant deaths are quite commonly noted in individual case reports. Many were associated with an acute exacerbation of SSc complications in the mother. Neonatal deaths occasionally were noted in the series and case-control studies including our own, but none found a statistically or clinically excessive number compared with controls. Thus, although women with SSc may have increased risks of miscarriage or premature infants, these risks are not so excessive as to discourage women from becoming pregnant. Recent studies from Spain, India, and Brazil have confirmed these findings.[14-16]

Effects of Pregnancy on Systemic Sclerosis

Patients are also very concerned whether pregnancy will make their scleroderma worse. Table 21.1 describes what is known about how pregnancy specifically affects scleroderma. Once again, the early literature described individual cases of bad maternal outcomes, particularly with regard to renal crisis. In both our retrospective and prospective studies, we carefully looked at the effects of pregnancy on the course of scleroderma and its symptoms. It is difficult to determine the definite changes that pregnancy has on SSc, because so many symptoms of pregnancy are similar to symptoms of SSc (e.g., edema, arthralgia, and gastrointestinal reflux). The consensus from reports describing overall effects of pregnancy on SSc is that there are no significant changes in disease status during pregnancy.[8,10] The 10-year cumulative survival for women suffering from SSc with and without a pregnancy is similar.[3]

Table 21.1 Effects of pregnancy on systemic sclerosis (SSc)

SSc involvement	Change during pregnancy
Overall	Disease generally stable
Raynaud's phenomenon	Improves during pregnancy, worsens after or during complicated deliveries
Skin	Can have onset during pregnancy and some diffuse SSc patients have progression of skin thickening postpartum
Joints	Worsening arthralgia, similar to non-scleroderma pregnancy
Gastrointestinal	Worsening reflux, similar to non-scleroderma pregnancy
Cardiopulmonary	Shortness of breath from SSc aggravated as in other diseases and managed as they would be in any pregnancy with compromised cardiopulmonary status
Kidney	Renal crisis may occur in early diffuse scleroderma with or without pregnancy. Management must be with ACE-inhibitors inspite of potential risks to baby

Many patients volunteer that Raynaud's phenomenon is noticeably improved during pregnancy, only to worsen postpartum. This is not surprising with the increased blood flow during pregnancy. There have been a few cases of acute gangrenous changes developing late in pregnancy. However, this has been associated with the use of beta-blockers or with other problems including complicated deliveries and sepsis.[17,18] There were no reported changes in skin disease during pregnancy in any of the studies. In our prospective series, the disease was stable in 61% of pregnancies, whereas 20% experienced some improvement and another 20% experienced some worsening.[7]

Typical pregnancy symptoms may occur with greater frequency. Musculoskeletal complaints during pregnancy in general are common, including carpal tunnel syndrome,[19] muscle leg cramps,[20] arthralgia, and back pain.[21] SSc patients are not immune to any of these problems and it is difficult to say whether they occur with more than expected frequency. Likewise, gastrointestinal symptoms, particularly reflux, but also constipation, occur with increased frequency during pregnancy,[22] so it is not surprising that patients complain of increased pyrosis, early satiety, or constipation. In a normal pregnancy, the tone of the lower half of the esophagus becomes profoundly depressed during the second and third trimesters.[23,24]

Pregnancy complications in any woman with serious cardiopulmonary problems occur with very high frequency, but women with SSc do not seem to be at greater risk than other pregnant patients having similar cardiopulmonary problems.[25-28] As these complications are common in SSc, all patients should have PFTs and an echocardiogram prior to becoming pregnant. Patients with significant SSc-ILD can have an uneventful pregnancy, particularly if they are not hypoxic.[29,30] Patients should be carefully monitored for oxygen desaturation with exercise, and when present, should be treated with supplemental oxygen. In two recent SSc-ILD patients whose FVC was in the 60% predicted range, successful pregnancy outcomes were observed. One had a full-term healthy infant without complications; the other had mildly increased blood pressure and delivered a small but healthy baby at 34 weeks. Both had previously received 1 year of treatment with cyclophosphamide. Other than increased shortness of breath (typical in most pregnant women), there is no evidence that pregnancy causes any worsening of pulmonary function. However, patients who have PAH should be strongly discouraged from becoming pregnant because of the major risk of death to both mother and fetus. Patients with diffuse SSc who have mild or silent myocardial damage could theoretically develop problems from the cardiovascular changes of pregnancy and particularly during treatment of preterm labor with beta-agonists, but this has not been well documented.[31]

Scleroderma renal crisis (SRC) is the most serious complication of SSc and the cause of the most maternal deaths in SSc pregnancies. Pregnancy itself has been hypothesized to be a precipitant of SRC.[32,33] The appearance of hypertension and proteinuria related to preeclampsia of pregnancy can be easily confused with SRC. The more recent pregnancy series and case–control studies found far fewer episodes of SRC than were seen in the individual anecdotal case reports. Our retrospective series included two patients with classic SRC developing during pregnancy.[3] Both had early diffuse SSc and were at high risk for developing SRC independent of their pregnancy. Comparing these pregnant SSc patients with a subset of women with early diffuse SSc without a pregnancy, we were unable to identify any increased occurrence of SRC in the pregnant patients. Prior to the advent of ACE-inhibitors, one of our two patients and her premature infant survived following nephrectomy, which was required for management of her refractory malignant hypertension. The other mother died during the renal crisis, but her premature infant survived.

In 91 SSc pregnancies followed prospectively, there were three early diffuse SSc patients who developed SRC during pregnancy. All had early disease (mean 2.2 years). This is similar to the 10–20% of diffuse SSc patients who develop SRC independent of pregnancy.[34] One woman was forced to abort her pregnancy at 20 weeks. In the other two cases, SRC was treated successfully with ACE inhibitors, although each woman required dialysis for a short time. These two women had premature infants (29 and 34 weeks) who survived, although they had prolonged hospitalizations.

There have been several recent case reports of SRC during pregnancy that were successfully treated with ACE-inhibitors.[35-38] These drugs have dramatically changed the outcome of SRC[39,40] and, in spite of their contraindications during pregnancy, they MUST be used if other antihypertensive medications do not control the blood pressure or when the serum creatinine is rising. The best option, if possible, is delivery of the fetus (see below).

The complete spectrum of pregnancy complications has been reported in SSc, including preeclampsia, abruptio placentae, premature rupture of membranes, placenta previa, and excessive bleeding.[10] Neither our retrospective case–control study nor a prospective study found evidence for an increased frequency of any pregnancy complication, including preeclampsia.[3] However, in a recent population-based study employing hospital discharge databases (504 pregnancies in women with SSc during a 3-year period),[41,42] there was a 22.9% rate of hypertensive disorders, including preeclampsia with a fourfold increased odds compared to the general population.

Pregnancy Management

Women with SSc who become pregnant should be considered to be at high risk for problems related to the pregnancy, since they are at increased risk of having premature and small full-term infants. They should be followed by an obstetrician experienced in high-risk pregnancies. At the onset of pregnancy (preferably even prior to pregnancy) the SSc patient should be carefully evaluated to determine the type of disease and duration of symptoms as well as the extent and severity of visceral involvement. Women having less than 4 years of symptoms, those who have diffuse cutaneous SSc, or those who test positive for anti-topoisomerase (Scl-70) or RNA polymerase III autoantibodies are at greater risk of having more active, aggressive disease than are those who have more longstanding disease or centromere autoantibodies and need to be followed very closely.[43] Table 21.2 summarizes some of the special management required during pregnancy to monitor for problems and optimize outcomes.

When organs are severely damaged, for example, in cases of severe cardiomyopathy (ejection fraction <30%), pulmonary hypertension, severe restrictive lung disease (forced vital capacity <50% of predicted), malabsorption, or renal insufficiency,

Table 21.2 Management of scleroderma patients during pregnancy, labor, and delivery

1. Early evaluation of the extent of scleroderma organ involvement and autoantibody analysis
2. Discontinue use of disease-remitting drugs (i.e., D-penicillamine, Methotrexate, etc.) before pregnancy
3. High-risk obstetric care
4. Minimal use of proton pump inhibitors, histamine blockers, or calcium-channel blockers for gastrointestinal and vascular problems
5. Avoidance of corticosteroids
6. More frequent monitoring of fetal size and uterine activity
7. Frequent blood pressure monitoring
8. Aggressive treatment of any hypertension (preeclampsia or other)
9. Close observation and treatment for premature labor (avoid beta-adrenergic agonists)
10. Epidural anesthesia preferred
11. Special warming of delivery room, intravenous fluids, patients themselves (e.g., extra blankets, thermal socks, gloves)
12. Venous access before delivery
13. Careful attention to the episiotomy and Cesarean section incisions, which generally heal without difficulty
14. No significant worry for hereditary neonatal scleroderma
15. Continued careful monitoring postpartum, with early reinstitution of medication and aggressive treatment of hypertension if it is present (do not assume it will resolve following delivery)

decisions concerning the continuation of the pregnancy must be based on the risks to the mother and the infant. This decision should be made based on the specific abnormalities found and independent of the fact that SSc is the cause of the problem. Patient, partner, and all physicians involved in her care will need to make this difficult decision together.

Although it is not clear whether preeclampsia occurs with increased frequency in SSc,[3,10,41] patients who have diffuse SSc in particular should have their blood pressure monitored very closely. We recommend home monitoring at least three to five times a week. The presence of even a slight elevation in blood pressure compared with previous levels should be considered potentially very serious. Evidence of elevated serum creatinine, proteinuria, or microangiopathic hemolytic anemia should be sought promptly. Differentiating SRC, preeclampsia and HEELP syndrome can be very difficult. However, if the patient is at high-risk for SRC, that is, early diffuse SSc, presence of Scl-70 or RNA polymerase III autoantibody, then control of the blood pressure is absolutely necessary. Other antihypertensive medications can be tried, but if the blood pressure is not controlled or the serum creatinine is increasing, an ACE inhibitor should be started. Allowing uncontrolled blood pressure to continue or watching the creatinine increase without using an ACE-inhibitor could make the difference between life and death of the mother and the fetus. One can start treating with low doses in combination with other antihypertension medications, but the key is to decrease the blood pressure to normal levels, that is, 120–140/80 mmHg. If the fetus is viable, giving steroid to mature the lungs is appropriate in order to deliver a premature infant and it may be the best option if the blood pressure cannot be controlled. Even though ACE-inhibitors can cause significant fetal abnormalities including anhydramnios, renal atresia, pulmonary hypoplasia, and fetal death, particularly when used in the latter half of pregnancy,[44] the frequency of this deadly problem, or fetopathy, as it is known, is unclear.[45] However, if the patient has SRC, there is no question that management of the hypertension without ACE inhibitors would have an unacceptably high risk for maternal problems which would outweigh the risk of toxicity to the fetus.

Successful use of captopril or other ACE-inhibitors during pregnancy has been documented.[7,35,36] In one series, non-scleroderma pregnant women with refractory hypertension were given low-dose captopril (total 25 mg/day), which improved their blood pressure and cardiac function. No fetal or neonatal complications were noted in the ten patients.[37] This was reassuring considering the degree of hypertension in these patients. In a recent review of the literature (85 patients) and 20 other prospective patients treated with ACE-inhibitors,[38] the frequency of complications was very high but dependent on the number of patients studied. Twenty-one percent of patients in series of fewer than ten patients had complications, compared with only 1.4% in series of larger numbers of patients, including their own prospective study. No abnormal events occurred with the use of ACE-inhibitors early in pregnancy. All the complications were seen after exposure in the second and third trimesters.[38]

Ten women from our cohort have had 12 pregnancies after an episode of SRC.[46] Five healthy babies were born to four women who remained on ACE-inhibitors throughout the pregnancy. Two women discontinued ACE-inhibitors prior to or early in pregnancy and their hypertension was successfully managed with other medications including calcium-channel blockers. Their three pregnancies were not associated with maternal problems and they had premature but healthy babies. Three other women who discontinued ACE-inhibitors prior to pregnancy had major problems with hypertension off ACE-inhibitors. Even with aggressive non-ACE-inhibitor treatment their hypertension was not easily controlled and several had major increases in their serum creatinine. One woman had a 29-week still-birth after blood pressure remained in the 150/100 mmHg range in spite of other medications. Another woman was restarted on captopril during the 20th week of pregnancy in as low a dose as necessary, along with other medications to control her hypertension. At 31 weeks, when she developed oligohydramnios, there was concern for the fetus and labor was induced. The 2.8 lb infant had some hypotension but did well. The third patient had very poor control of her high blood pressure. Even though a very small dose of captopril was added in the 24th week, her hypertension was still inadequately controlled. When her creatinine reached 2.9 mg/dL, labor was induced. The 1.3 lb infant died after a 2 month struggle for life, but he did not have any renal problems. None of these infants had any significant evidence of ACE-inhibitor toxicity. Pregnancy in patients after SRC may be successful, but potentially disastrous outcomes both to the mother as well as the infant are possible.

Management of Delivery

The pregnant SSc patient is both a potential anesthetic challenge and nightmare, and thus anesthetic considerations need to be carefully discussed before delivery.[28,47,48] Taut skin can lead to difficult venous access. Vaginal constriction, taut abdominal skin and joint contractures may interfere with monitoring of blood pressure and with positioning during delivery. All of these potentially can complicate the delivery. Regional anesthesia, particularly an epidural block, can be useful for delivery by providing adequate anesthesia while also providing peripheral vasodilatation and increased skin perfusion of lower extremities.[28,47] Eisele suggests using smaller-than-normal doses of regional anesthesia because SSc patients may exhibit prolonged motor and sensory blockade after delivery. General anesthesia should be avoided because of the potentially difficult intubation in a SSc patient who has a reduced oral aperture, as well as because of concerns about aspiration.

Venous access, even if it requires a central line and consideration of a Swan-Ganz catheter, may be necessary if cardiopulmonary problems, hypertension, or renal dysfunction are present. Measures that could prevent problems related to Raynaud's phenomenon during delivery should be routinely used, including warming the delivery room, warming intravenous fluids and blood products, thermal socks, and warm external compresses.[10] Severe abdominal skin thickening is not a contraindication for Cesarean section because even the tightest skin usually heals if care is taken in the surgical repair of the incision. Care also should be taken with the episiotomy incision.

Postnatal care should include continued attentiveness to monitoring disease activity, particularly progressive skin changes or new hypertension, so that therapeutic intervention can begin immediately. There are no data on postpartum depression being greater in SSc mothers, but if the pregnancy was stressful, the baby is particularly fussy, or the mother has more difficulty caring for the infant than she anticipated, she may be at greater risk for depression. Close observation and early therapeutic intervention are indicated. Medications that had been disrupted specifically because of the pregnancy should be reinstituted promptly rather than waiting to see it they will or will not be needed.

Summary

Pregnancy in SSc may be uneventful with good maternal and fetal outcomes. SSc is a multisystem disease and complications do occur and thus, careful antenatal evaluations, discussion of potential problems, and participation in a high-risk obstetric monitoring program is very important to optimize the outcome. Women who have diffuse SSc are at a greater risk for developing serious cardiopulmonary and renal problems early in the course of their disease, so they should be encouraged to delay pregnancy until the disease has stabilized. All patients who become pregnant during this high-risk time should be monitored extremely carefully, particularly for renal crisis.

Although there are some suggestions that infertility and miscarriages are increased, recent studies show that these issues do not have major impact in women with established SSc. The high risk of premature and small infants may be minimized with specialized obstetric and neonatal care. Scleroderma renal crisis is the only truly unique aspect of these pregnancies. The malignant hypertension of SRC must be treated aggressively with ACE inhibitors. Other pregnancy problems may not be unique, but because SSc is a chronic illness, any complication carries higher risks for both mother and child. Careful planning, close monitoring, and aggressive management should allow women with SSc to have a high likelihood of a successful pregnancy.

References

1. Ballou SP, Morley JJ, Kushner I. Pregnancy and systemic sclerosis. *Arthritis Rheum.* 1984;27(3):295-298.
2. Giordano M, Valentini G, Lupoli S, Giordano A. Pregnancy and systemic sclerosis. *Arthritis Rheum.* 1985;28(2):237-238.
3. Steen VD, Medsger TA Jr. Fertility and pregnancy outcome in women with systemic sclerosis. *Arthritis Rheum.* 1999;42(4):763-768.

4. Madden BP. Pulmonary hypertension and pregnancy. *Int J Obstet Anesth.* 2009;18(2):156-164.
5. Huang S, DeSantis ER. Treatment of pulmonary arterial hypertension in pregnancy. *Am J Health Syst Pharm.* 2007;64(18):1922-1926.
6. Bedard E, Dimopoulos K, Gatzoulis MA. Has there been any progress made on pregnancy outcomes among women with pulmonary arterial hypertension? *Eur Heart J.* 2009;30(3):256-265.
7. Steen VD. Pregnancy in women with systemic sclerosis. *Obstet Gynecol.* 1999;94(1):15-20.
8. Black CM, Stevens WM. Scleroderma. *Rheum Dis Clin North Am.* 1989;15(2):193-212.
9. Maymon R, Fejgin M. Scleroderma in pregnancy. *Obstet Gynecol Surv.* 1989;44(7):530-534.
10. Weiner SR. Organ function: sexual function and pregnancy. In: Clements PJ, Furst D, eds. *Systemic Sclerosis.* New York: Williams and Wilkins; 1995:483-499.
11. Siamopoulou-Mavridou A, Manoussakis MN, Mavridis AK, Moutsopoulos HM. Outcome of pregnancy in patients with autoimmune rheumatic disease before the disease onset. *Ann Rheum Dis.* 1988;47(12):982-987.
12. Englert H, Brennan P, McNeil D, Black C, Silman AJ. Reproductive function prior to disease onset in women with scleroderma. *J Rheumatol.* 1992;19(10):1575-1579.
13. Silman AJ, Black C. Increased incidence of spontaneous abortion and infertility in women with scleroderma before disease onset: a controlled study. *Ann Rheum Dis.* 1988;47(6):441-444.
14. Jimenez FX, Simeon CP, Fonollosa V, et al. Scleroderma and pregnancy: obstetrical complications and the impact of pregnancy on the course of the disease. *Med Clin (Barc).* 1999;113(20):761-764.
15. Wanchu A, Misra R. Pregnancy outcome in systemic sclerosis. *J Assoc Physicians India.* 1996;44(9):637-640.
16. Sampaio-Barros PD, Samara AM, Marques Neto F. Gynaecologic history in systemic sclerosis. *Clin Rheumatol.* 2000;19(3):184-187.
17. Avrech OM, Golan A, Pansky M, Langer R, Caspi E. Raynaud's phenomenon and peripheral gangrene complicating scleroderma in pregnancy—diagnosis and management. *Br J Obstet Gynaecol.* 1992;99(10):850-851.
18. Smith CA, Pinals RS. Progressive systemic sclerosis and postpartum renal failure complicated by peripheral gangrene. *J Rheumatol.* 1982;9(3):455-458.
19. Gould JS, Wissinger HA. Carpal tunnel syndrome in pregnancy. *South Med J.* 1978;71(2):144-145, 154.
20. Hammar M, Larsson L, Tegler L. Calcium treatment of leg cramps in pregnancy. Effect on clinical symptoms and total serum and ionized serum calcium concentrations. *Acta Obstet Gynecol Scand.* 1981;60(4):345-347.
21. Fast A, Shapiro D, Ducommun EJ, Friedmann LW, Bouklas T, Floman Y. Low-back pain in pregnancy. *Spine.* 1987;12(4):368-371.
22. Calhoun BC. Gastrointestinal disorders in pregnancy. *Obstet Gynecol Clin North Am.* 1992;19(4):733-744.
23. Ulmsten U, Sundstrom G. Esophageal manometry in pregnant and nonpregnant women. *Am J Obstet Gynecol.* 1978;132(3):260-264.
24. Van Thiel DH, Gavaler JS, Joshi SN, Sara RK, Stremple J. Heartburn of pregnancy. *Gastroenterology.* 1977;72(4 Pt 1):666-668.
25. Fortin F, Wallaert B. Interstitial pathology and pregnancy. *Rev Mal Respir.* 1988;5(3):275-278.
26. Raymond R, Underwood DA, Moodie DS. Cardiovascular problems in pregnancy. *Cleve Clin J Med.* 1987;54(2):95-104.
27. Sullivan JM, Ramanathan KB. Management of medical problems in pregnancy—severe cardiac disease. *N Engl J Med.* 1985;313(5):304-309.
28. Thompson J, Conklin KA. Anesthetic management of a pregnant patient with scleroderma. *Anesthesiology.* 1983;59(1):69-71.
29. Hoshino T, Kita M, Takahashi T, Nishimura T, Yamakawa M. Management of two pregnancies in a woman with mixed connective tissue disease, pulmonary fibrosis, frequent pneumothorax and oxygen inhalation therapy along with a published work review. *J Obstet Gynaecol Res.* 2008;34(4 Pt 2):613-618.

30. Ratto D, Balmes J, Boylen T, Sharma OP. Pregnancy in a woman with severe pulmonary fibrosis secondary to hard metal disease. *Chest.* 1988;93(3):663-665.
31. Katz M, Gill PJ, Newman RB. Detection of preterm labor by ambulatory monitoring of uterine activity for the management of oral tocolysis. *Am J Obstet Gynecol.* 1986;154(6):1253-1256.
32. Karlen JR, Cook WA. Renal scleroderma and pregnancy. *Obstet Gynecol.* 1974;44(3):349-354.
33. Traub YM, Shapiro AP, Rodnan GP, et al. Hypertension and renal failure (scleroderma renal crisis) in progressive systemic sclerosis. Review of a 25-year experience with 68 cases. *Medicine (Baltimore).* 1983;62(6):335-352.
34. Steen VD. Scleroderma renal crisis. *Rheum Dis Clin North Am.* 1996;22(4):861-878.
35. Altieri P, Cameron JS. Scleroderma renal crisis in a pregnant woman with late partial recovery of renal function. *Nephrol Dial Transplant.* 1988;3(5):677-680.
36. Watson MA, Radford NJ, McGrath BP, Swinton GW, Agar JW. Captopril-induced agranulocytosis in systemic sclerosis. *Aust N Z J Med.* 1981;11(1):79-81.
37. Easterling TR, Carr DB, Davis C, Diederichs C, Brateng DA, Schmucker B. Low-dose, short-acting, angiotensin-converting enzyme inhibitors as rescue therapy in pregnancy. *Obstet Gynecol.* 2000;96(6):956-961.
38. Burrows RF, Burrows EA. Assessing the teratogenic potential of angiotensin-converting enzyme inhibitors in pregnancy. *Aust N Z J Obstet Gynaecol.* 1998;38(3):306-311.
39. Steen VD, Costantino JP, Shapiro AP, Medsger TA Jr. Outcome of renal crisis in systemic sclerosis: relation to availability of angiotensin converting enzyme (ACE) inhibitors. *Ann Intern Med.* 1990;113(5):352-357.
40. Steen VD. Organ involvement: renal. In: Clements PJ, Furst D, eds. *Systemic Sclerosis.* New York: Williams and Wilkins; 1995:425-440.
41. Chakravarty EF, Khanna D, Chung L. Pregnancy outcomes in systemic sclerosis, primary pulmonary hypertension, and sickle cell disease. *Obstet Gynecol.* 2008;111(4):927-934.
42. Chakravarty EF. Vascular complications of systemic sclerosis during pregnancy. *Int J Rheumatol.* 2010. doi: 10.1155/2010/287248.
43. Steen VD. The many faces of scleroderma. *Rheum Dis Clin North Am.* 2008;34(1):1-15.
44. Mehta N, Modi N. ACE inhibitors in pregnancy. *Lancet.* 1989;2(8654):96-97.
45. Pryde PG, Barr M Jr. Low-dose, short-acting, angiotensin-converting enzyme inhibitors as rescue therapy in pregnancy. *Obstet Gynecol.* 2001;97(5 Pt 1):799-800.
46. Steen VD. Pregnancy in scleroderma. *Rheum Dis Clin North Am.* 2007;33(2):345-358.
47. Eisele JH, Reitan JA. Scleroderma, Raynaud's phenomenon, and local anesthetics. *Anesthesiology.* 1971;34(4):386-387.
48. Younker D, Harrison B. Scleroderma and pregnancy. Anaesthetic considerations. *Br J Anaesth.* 1985;57(11):1136-1139.

Chapter 22
A 38-Year-Old Man with Systemic Sclerosis and Erectile Dysfunction

Edward V. Lally

Keywords Male scleroderma • Erectile dysfunction • Impotence • Scleroderma in men

Case Study

A 38-year-old man presented for rheumatologic evaluation with a 6-month history of stiffness and swelling in his hands, wrists, and forearms; Raynaud's phenomenon; dry mouth; and dysphagia for solid foods. During his evaluation, he was noted to have sclerodactyly, proximal cutaneous sclerosis of the forearms, neck, face, lower legs, and feet. No digital ulcers or tendon friction rubs were present. He had an abnormal nailfold capillary examination that showed capillary dilatation as well as capillary dropout. His antinuclear antibody titer was 1:2,560 (speckled pattern). Antibodies to topoisomerase I (anti-Scl-70) were negative. A diagnosis of systemic sclerosis was made.

The patient also noted that he had developed erectile dysfunction within 3 months of the onset of his arthralgias and Raynaud's phenomenon. He had been married for 10 years with two children. He previously had had no problems with impotence or sexual function. He noted that his libido was normal but he was totally unable to achieve erections after onset of his other symptoms. The patient worked as an insurance salesman and had no relevant exposure to toxic environmental agents. There was no prior history of neurologic or psychiatric illness.

Subsequently, the patient was found to have progressive interstitial lung disease. He was treated with cyclophosphamide and subsequently mycophenolate mofetil. The patient was also seen by a psychiatrist who found no evidence of clinical depression.

E.V. Lally
Department of Medicine, Rhode Island Hospital,
The Warren Alpert Medical School of Brown University,
593 Eddy St., 2 Dudley St., Providence, RI 02905, USA

R.M. Silver and C.P. Denton (eds.), *Case Studies in Systemic Sclerosis*,
DOI: 10.1007/978-0-85729-641-2_22, © Springer-Verlag London Limited 2011

His testosterone level was normal. He was subsequently treated with sildenafil 50 mg as needed and there was slight improvement in his ability to achieve erection.

Discussion

Systemic sclerosis (SSc) is an acquired disorder of connective tissue manifested by cutaneous sclerosis, fibrosis of visceral organs, and characteristic clinical and pathologic vascular lesions.[1,2] Damage to the endothelial lining of small blood vessels or altered vasomotor control of the capillary circulation have been proposed as early lesions leading to vascular compromise, tissue hypoxia, and widespread deposition of collagen and other connective tissue components. The vasculopathy of SSc includes intimal proliferation, medial hypertrophy, and adventitial fibrosis in the absence of true vasculitis. Depending on which vascular bed is involved, clinical disease typically results from ischemia and fibrosis.

The major sexual problem attributed directly to SSc in male patients is impotence. Erectile failure in men with SSc was first described in 1981.[3] In the five male patients described in this initial report, impotence was an early feature of SSc. Primary gonadal failure was not found in any of these patients. Impotence was felt to be due to vascular and/or neurogenic dysfunction associated with SSc. Subsequently, several reports have described erectile dysfunction (ED) in male patients with scleroderma.[4-10] The prevalence of ED in SSc has been estimated to be between 27% and 81%.[5,6,11]

In order to determine if ED is more common in SSc than in other chronic rheumatic diseases, Hong and colleagues,[11] in a case control manner, studied men with SSc and rheumatoid arthritis (RA). These authors found that 81% of men with SSc had ED. ED occurred in SSc three times more commonly than in RA. In both SSc and RA, ED was associated with the presence of Raynaud's phenomenon (80% of men with RP vs 50% of men without RP). The same report noted that ED frequently developed within the first 3 years of the onset of disease and was a prominent symptom in these involved patients.

The etiology of ED is not well understood. Factors attributed to ED in SSc, similar to those prevalent in the disease itself, include microvascular abnormalities and fibrosis. Nowlin and colleagues[6] reported that microvascular insufficiency was significant in male patients with ED and SSc. They studied ten SSc patients for sexual function. Five of the patients reported complete impotence and three partial potence. Endocrinological evaluation including measurements of serum testosterone, prolactin, estradiol, follicle-stimulating hormone, and luteinizing hormone levels were normal in all patients. Penile blood flow, evaluated by the Doppler technique, was abnormal in all five impotent and one partially potent patient. None of the age-matched controls with RA was impotent and none had reduced penile blood flow. Another study of the penile vasculature in SSc used the duplex ultrasound technique in 15 male patients.[12] Nine of these 15 patients had moderate to severe erectile dysfunction. Severely impaired mean peak systolic velocities in the presence of mild venous leakage were found in these patients. Penile cutaneous temperature was evaluated in a study by Merla and colleagues[13] using noncontact thermal imaging. This study compared ten male patients with SSc to ten healthy controls. Penile thermal abnormalities were demonstrated in almost all SSc patients and were not seen in the control group.

Vascular changes in the circulation to the penis may impede the distending pressure required for penile erection. Granchi and colleagues[14] reported that penile smooth muscle cells synthesized endothelin-1 (ET-1), one of the main regulators of microvascular contractility. ET-1 is a major vasoactive peptide causing vasoconstriction. ET-1 levels have been shown to be elevated in patients with SSc[15] and exert both vascular and profibrotic effects in this disorder.[15,16] Autonomic nervous system alterations may interfere with neurogenic control of penile vascular tone and contribute to ED. Autonomic dysfunction has been demonstrated in patients with SSc.[17-19] Neurogenic dysfunction that occurs in patient with diabetes and ED may play a similar role in ED associated with SSc.

Penile fibrosis may also contribute to ED in SSc and may impede penile arterial and smooth muscle relaxation. In a clinicopathological study by Nehra and colleagues,[20] hemodynamic testing on a patient who underwent a penile implant revealed diffuse corporeal veno-occlusive dysfunction. The excised corporeal tissue documented severe fibrosis. It is likely that ED in SSc has a multifactorial etiology.[21]

The evaluation of ED in men with SSc should systematically include attention to medications known to be associated with ED, symptoms of depression, and awareness of comorbidities including diabetes, hypertension, smoking, and peripheral vascular disease. An endocrinologic evaluation should also be carried out including testosterone levels, which may contribute to ED in some patients with SSc.

Pharmacologic management of ED and SSc has received little attention. In small series, it does not appear that calcium channel blockers or vasodilators have a beneficial role to play in this condition. Phosphodiesterase inhibitors (PDEIs) such as sildenafil or tadalafil may improve ED. However, on demand PDEIs generally have been ineffective in producing improvement.[21,22] Certainly, medications in this category given on a daily or every other daily basis might improve symptoms, although this has not been specifically studied.[21,22]

Given the role of ET-1 in the penile vasculature it is possible that endothelin receptor antagonists may have a role to play in treating patients with ED.[22,23] However, there have not been any formal studies to evaluate this or to explore whether there could be synergy between PDEIs and endothelin receptor antagonists. If patients do not respond to medication in these categories they should be referred to a urologist for other treatments including intracorporeal prostaglandin, mechanical suction devices or penile implants.[21]

ED is a common manifestation of SSc in men. The symptom often develops early and is a major cause of morbidity in such patients. Careful consideration should be given to other causes of ED in this population including medications, comorbidities, and clinical depression. Vasodilator therapy may be beneficial but doses required to achieve clinical improvement are often much higher than in other types of ED. This is an important nonlethal complication of SSc that needs to be explored sensitively and in context. Collaborative management with urogenital and endocrinology specialists is likely to achieve the best outcome.

References

1. Seibold JR. Scleroderma. In: Harris ED, Budd RC, Firestein GS, Genovese MC, Serger JS, Ruddy S, Sledge CB, eds. *Kelley's Textbook of Rheumatology*. 7th ed. Philadelphia: Elsevier/Saunders; 2005:1279-1308.
2. Gabrielli A, Avvedimento EV, Kreig T. Scleroderma [review article]. *N Engl J Med*. 2009;1989–2003.
3. Lally EV, Jimenez SA. Impotence in progressive systemic sclerosis. *Ann Intern Med*. 1981;95(2):150-153.
4. Klein LE, Posner MS. Progressive systemic sclerosis and impotence. Letter to the Editor. *Ann Intern Med*. 1981;95:658.
5. Lally EV, Jimenez SA. Impotence in progressive systemic sclerosis. Letter to the Editor. *Ann Intern Med*. 1982;96:125.
6. Nowlin NS, Brick JE, Weaver DJ, et al. Impotence in scleroderma. *Ann Intern Med*. 1986;104(6):794-798.
7. Nowlin NS, Brick JE, Weaver DJ, Wilson DA, Judd HL, Lu JK, Carlson HE. Impotence in scleroderma. Letter to the Editor. *Ann Intern Med*. 1987;106:910.
8. Nowlin NS, Brick JE, Weaver DJ, Wilson DA, Judd HL, Lu JK, Carlson HE. Impotence in scleroderma. Letter to the Editor. *Ann Intern Med*. 1988;109:148.
9. Sukenik S, Abarbanel JM, Buskila D, Potashnik G, Horowitz J. Impotence, carpal tunnel syndrome and peripheral neuropathy as presenting symptoms in progressive systemic sclerosis. Letter to the Editor. *J Rheumatol*. 1987;14:641-643.
10. Rossman B, Zorgniotti AW. Progressive systemic sclerosis (scleroderma) and impotence. *Urology*. 1989;33(3):189-192.
11. Hong P, Pope JE, Ouimet JM, Rullan E, Seibold JR. Erectile dysfunction associated with scleroderma: a case-control study of men with scleroderma and rheumatoid arthritis. *J Rheumatol*. 2004;31(3):508-513.
12. Aversa A, Proietti M, Bruzziches R, Salsano F, Spera G. The penile vasculature in systemic sclerosis: a duplex ultrasound study. *J Sex Med*. 2006;3(3):554-558.
13. Merla A, Romani GL, Tangherlini A, et al. Penile cutaneous temperature in systemic sclerosis: a thermal imaging study. *Int J Immunopathol Pharmacol*. 2007;20(1):139-144.
14. Granchi S, Vannelli GB, Vignozzi L, et al. Expression and regulation of endothelin-1 and its receptors in human penile smooth muscle cells. *Mol Hum Reprod*. 2002;8(12):1053-1064.
15. Vancheeswaran R, Magoulas T, Efrat G, et al. Circulating endothelin-1 levels in systemic sclerosis subsets–A marker of fibrosis or vascular dysfunction? *J Rheumatol*. 1994;21(10):1838-1844.
16. Lagares D, García-Fernández RA, Jiménez CL, et al. Endothelin 1 contributes to the effect of transforming growth factor beta1 on wound repair and skin fibrosis. *Arthritis Rheum*. 2010;62(3):878-889.
17. Dessein PH, Joffe BI, Metz RM, Millar DL, Lawson M, Stanwix AE. Autonomic dysfunction in systemic sclerosis: sympathetic overactivity and instability. *Am J Med*. 1992;93(2):143-150.
18. Morelli S, Piccirillo G, Fimognari F, et al. Twenty-four hour heart period variability in systemic sclerosis. *J Rheumatol*. 1996;23(4):643-645.
19. Malandrini A, Selvi E, Villanova M, et al. Autonomic nervous system and smooth muscle cell involvement in systemic sclerosis: ultrastructural study of 3 cases. *J Rheumatol*. 2000;27(5):1203-1206.
20. Nehra A, Hall SJ, Basile G, et al. Systemic sclerosis and impotence: a clinicopathological correlation. *J Urol*. 1995;153(4):1140-1146.
21. Walker UA, Tyndall A, Ruszat R. Erectile dysfunction in systemic sclerosis. *Ann Rheum Dis*. 2009;68(7):1083-1085.
22. Proietti M, Aversa A, Letizia C, et al. Erectile dysfunction in systemic sclerosis: effects of longterm inhibition of phosphodiesterase type-5 on erectile function and plasma endothelin-1 levels. *J Rheumatol*. 2007;34(8):1712-1717.
23. Aversa A, Caprio M, Rosano GM, Spera G. Endothelial effects of drugs designed to treat erectile dysfunction. *Curr Pharm Des*. 2008;14(35):3768-3778.

Chapter 23
A Female Scleroderma Patient with Sexual Dysfunction

Patricia E. Carreira

Keywords Genital tract • Vaginal dryness • Dyspareunia • Sexual dysfunction • Quality of life

Case Study

A 36-year-old woman presented with a 4-year history of systemic sclerosis with diffuse cutaneous involvement (dSSc). She wanted advice to plan a pregnancy, and she complained of vaginal dryness and dyspareunia.

SSc onset was at 32 years of age, beginning with puffy hands and rapidly progressing skin induration over her hands, arms, buttocks, face, chest, and abdomen, together with the development of joint contractures in her fingers. During the cold season she began to notice Raynaud's phenomenon, but she denied painful lesions or sores on the fingerpads. She complained of intermittent nocturnal heartburn, without vomiting or regurgitation. She was seen by a rheumatologist who diagnosed dSSc. Blood pressure was normal. Chest radiograph, high resolution CT scan, PFT with DLco, echocardiography, and electrocardiogram were also normal. A barium swallow exam showed mild dysmotility of the distal esophagus with gastroesophageal reflux. Complete blood count, ESR, serum chemistry, and urinalysis were normal. Antinuclear antibody (ANA) was positive by IIF, and she had anti-Scl-70 (anti-topoisomerase-1) antibodies. She was treated with a proton pump inhibitor and calcium-channel blocker during the winter months. She was also treated with low-dose prednisolone (6 mg daily) and methotrexate, 15 mg weekly. After 3 months of this therapy, she noted significant improvement in her skin stiffness. Over the past 2 years skin induration has been limited to the hands and fingers, causing only mild functional hand impairment. Raynaud's phenomenon persisted in very cold weather,

P.E. Carreira
Rheumatology Department, Hospital Universitario 12 de Octubre,
Avda. De Cordoba s/n, Madrid 28041, Spain

R.M. Silver and C.P. Denton (eds.), *Case Studies in Systemic Sclerosis*,
DOI: 10.1007/978-0-85729-641-2_23, © Springer-Verlag London Limited 2011

without development of digital ulcers. She was able to maintain her own business, a clothing boutique, without fatigue or other problems related to her disease.

From the onset of SSc, she complained of mouth dryness and especially of vaginal dryness, accompanied by intense dyspareunia, which severely interfered with her sexual activity, mainly vaginal penetration. This had worsened in the first months of her illness due to skin pain, more pronounced in the abdomen and buttocks, and by joint mobility impairment in her hands, arms, and legs. She had developed on three separate occasions superficial vaginal ulcerations that prevented sexual intercourse because of excruciating pain. She had tried several lubricating preparations with only minor relief. At the onset of her disease she also reported a sensation of vaginal tightness, which improved as her skin induration and joint mobility improved. She reported having somewhat less sexual desire and mild difficulties in arousal and orgasmic response, which she attributed to the pain associated with skin tightness and to the distress caused by the fear of having scleroderma. As her disease began to improve, she recovered normal desire and orgasmic response. She had normal menstruation, and she did not report menstrual abnormalities even when her skin disease was at its worst, or during the years she was taking methotrexate.

Methotrexate had been discontinued 9 months earlier, without worsening of skin induration. Since her disease had remained stable, she wanted to have children. She asked advice about pregnancy, and she was afraid of possible complications of pregnancy and labor because of vaginal and/or uterus involvement from scleroderma.

Physical Examination

General examination was normal, with BP 110/70 mmHg and heart rate 72 bpm. There was tight skin over the dorsum of the fingers, hands, distal forearms, and the face. Skin appeared normal elsewhere. No pitted scars were seen over the fingerpads. Small telangiectasias could be seen over the cheeks, and the oral aperture was slightly reduced. Cardiac and pulmonary examination was normal. Abdomen was not tender, nor painful to palpation, and no masses were palpated. Lower extremities were normal and in the upper extremities she had mild contractures in the fingers with preserved motility. Musculoskeletal examination was otherwise normal.

Gynecologic examination performed by a gynecologist revealed a normal sized uterus, normal adnexa, and absence of vaginal fissures or ulcerations. Breast examination was also normal.

Laboratory Findings

CBC, serum chemistry panel, and urinalysis were normal. ESR was 6 mm/h. ANA and anti-Scl-70 antibodies were positive, but SS-A (Ro), SS-B (La) and RF autoantibodies were negative. Serum C3 and C4 complement levels were normal. PFT, chest radiograph and electrocardiogram were normal. Echocardiogram with Doppler showed normal cardiac cavities without evidence of pulmonary hypertension.

Papanicolaou smear and mammogram were also normal.

Course

The diagnosis of dSSc was confirmed. Although the actual skin involvement was limited to the hands and distal forearms, her history of truncal involvement was unequivocal and consistent with a diagnosis of dSSc. Lung, heart, and kidney investigations did not show evidence of visceral organ involvement, so her disease was considered stable at that moment. She was maintained on a proton pump inhibitor. Calcium-channel blocker therapy was also prescribed during cold months, in order to improve Raynaud's phenomenon. Annual assessment including PFT, electrocardiogram, and Doppler echocardiography was also advised.

Secondary sicca syndrome was also diagnosed, based on her symptoms of mouth and vaginal dryness. Although an overlap between SSc and Sjögren's syndrome might have been suspected, the absence of serological markers (SS-A, SS-B, and RF) characteristic of the latter disease did not provide evidence for Sjögren's syndrome and so sicca symptoms are attributable to SSc. She continued using lubricating vaginal gels with acceptable control of dryness, allowing her to have regular and satisfactory sexual relationship.

Since gynecologic study was absolutely normal and there were no significant renal or cardiorespiratory impairment that might have been problematic, pregnancy and eventually breastfeeding were not contraindicated. She was advised to be carefully monitored during pregnancy, both by obstetrician and rheumatologist, with frequent assessment of blood pressure, creatinine levels, and urinalysis (see Chap. 21).

Discussion

Scleroderma, a chronic autoimmune disease characterized by vascular involvement and fibrosis in multiple organs, can have a major impact on numerous aspects of life, including sexuality. Sexual dysfunction is common in both male (see Chap. 22) and female patients with systemic sclerosis.[1,2] The disease affects women about three times more frequently than men; however, most studies about the effects of scleroderma on sexuality have been conducted exclusively in men.[1,2] Although sexuality is an integral part of human nature and clearly associated with quality of life, until recently, investigation of sexual issues in female SSc patients has been relegated to fertility, pregnancy, or contraception, while very little attention has been paid to sexual function. In fact, before 2009, besides case studies[3] and a clinical review,[1] only one study had documented the negative impact of scleroderma on sexual health.[4]

Recently, diverse aspects of sexual function have been addressed by different means in four series of female scleroderma patients.[5-8] The results of these studies indicate that sexual dysfunction and sexual distress are overall higher in females with systemic sclerosis than in healthy controls,[6,8] or in some other groups of females suffering chronic diseases, such as HIV-positive or gynecological cancer patients.[7] Some scleroderma-related symptoms are reported by patients as factors contributing to sexual dysfunction. The most frequently cited are vaginal dryness, dyspareunia, fatigue, body pain, skin tightness, reflux and heartburn, and muscle weakness.[4,5] Sexual dysfunction seems to be more related to psychological factors, such as marital distress, depressive symptoms, or antidepressant therapies, than to physical function or disease duration,[5,6] and only one study suggested that patients with dSSc are more severely affected than those who have lSSc.[7] On the other hand, scleroderma did not seem to affect the desire or frequency of sexual activity in one cross-sectional study,[6] although another group reported that more than 50% of scleroderma patients reported diminished sexual desire and decreased number and intensity of orgasms after disease onset compared with before.[4]

Since sexuality is a complex aspect of life, and goes far beyond the act of sexual intercourse, both physical and psychological aspects may contribute to altered sexuality in female scleroderma patients[1] (Table 23.1).

Table 23.1 The causes potentially contributing to sexual dysfunction in scleroderma females

Physical

- General: malaise, fatigue, weakness
- Skin and mucosa: hardness, pain, stiffness, limited mobility, shrinking mouth, constricted vaginal introitus
- Sicca symptoms: vaginal dryness and ulcers, dyspareunia, mouth dryness
- Vascular: Raynaud's phenomenon, digital ischemic ulcers, less intense orgasms?
- Calcinosis
- Joints: pain, stiffness, limited mobility, joint contractures
- Muscles: myalgia, muscular weakness
- Gastrointestinal: reflux, diarrhea, constipation, fecal incontinence, abdominal pain
- Pulmonary: dyspnea, cough, exercise intolerance
- Cardiac: palpitations
- Adverse effects of therapies

Psychological

- Depression
- Fear
- Emotional distress
- Change in body and face appearance
- Decrease in sexual desire

Vaginal dryness is reported by more than 70% of scleroderma patients, and dyspareunia is described by 35–50% in several studies.[4,5,9] Both symptoms are frequent in primary Sjögren's syndrome,[10] characterized by widespread exocrine gland lymphocytic infiltration, which can also involve the genital tract. Typical sicca symptoms, for example, oral or ocular dryness, are present in over 60% of scleroderma patients,[11,12] in patients classified as either the limited or diffuse subset. Although the physiopathology of sicca syndrome in SSc is not fully understood, it is thought to be secondary to fibrotic involvement of the exocrine glands, rather than glandular inflammation. In fact, histological analysis of salivary glands from SSc patients with xerostomia has revealed fibrotic involvement in more than half of these patients. Histological features of inflammation characteristic of Sjögren's syndrome were present only in 14%, mainly in those with lSSc and in association with anticentromere antibodies.[11]

Dyspareunia is defined as painful sexual intercourse and is mainly attributed to pelvic disorders, for example, vaginal dryness or vaginal infection. It may be superficial when pain occurs with attempted penetration or deep, which is associated with pelvic thrusting. In SSc superficial dyspareunia is more common than deep. Vaginal lubrication is not related to the production of fluids from the local glands, but is mostly a transudate through the vaginal wall, and is also derived from the cervical mucous.[10] The cause of insufficient vaginal lubrication is usually multifactorial, most commonly related to an estrogen deficiency, lack of adequate sexual stimulation, or both.[10,13] In primary Sjögren's syndrome, dyspareunia has been associated in premenopausal patients with a histology showing nonkeratinized stratified squamous epithelia, and a mild to moderate inflammatory lymphocytic infiltration of the underlying stroma, more prominent around the thin-walled vessels and capillaries.[10] It has been suggested that this lymphocytic vasculitis could be involved in the pathogenesis of dyspareunia through impaired vaginal wall transudation and inadequate lubrication during sexual intercourse.[13] The pathophysiology of dyspareunia in SSc may be similar to that of primary Sjögren's syndrome in a small percentage of patients, as happens with xerostomia.[11] However, it is also possible that vascular or fibrotic changes, characteristic of SSc in other organ systems, may also be involved.

Physical changes associated with SSc such as skin tightness around the vaginal introitus may also contribute to sexual distress in affected patients.[3,4] Perivaginal skin infiltrated by dense fibrotic tissue has been described in a patient with dSSc,[3] but no studies addressing the frequency of direct fibrotic involvement of the genital tract exist. This manifestation may benefit from the use of vaginal dilators. A small uterine size has been described in some SSc patients,[4] but there are no studies analyzing the influence of this finding on pregnancy and labor. Two studies have compared histopathological findings in cervicovaginal tissue of SSc patients with those of healthy controls, with controversial results. In one, vascular and connective tissue abnormalities typical of SSc (fibrosis, adventitial changes, medial hypertrophy or intimal proliferation) were collectively more frequent in five patients than in 26 age-matched controls, but individually every feature was observed also in the control group.[14] The authors suggest that such vascular alterations may be related not only to SSc, but at least in part also to other factors such as aging or hypertension.[14]

The other study, performed on cervical tissue of ten SSc patients and 20 age-matched controls, found that vascular medial hypertrophy, intimal thickening, and especially fibrosis were all seen significantly more often in patients than in controls.[15]

A decrease in the number and intensity of orgasms has also been described in SSc patients, which is not present in other rheumatic diseases.[4] A vascular compromise has been suggested as the most probable cause of this finding.[1,4] Nevertheless, other mechanisms involving neurogenic or hormonal factors, as suggested for erectile dysfunction in male scleroderma patients, may also be involved.[2]

Raynaud's phenomenon, fatigue, body pain, limited mobility, and heartburn are all reported by SSc patients as factors negatively influencing their sexual function.[4,5] Fatigue is a common symptom, usually more frequent and intense in the early phases of dSSc. Fatigue and chronic pain may greatly influence sexual activity, as demonstrated in patients with rheumatoid arthritis[16] or other chronic rheumatic diseases.[2] Limited mobility and tightness, especially affecting the hip and pelvic girdle, joint contractures, and muscle weakness, all may interfere with normal sexual relationship. In addition, skin thickness may result in decreased skin sensitivity and decreased hand and mouth functioning. Ischemic digital ulcers and calcinosis may be very painful if touched, preventing patients from having enjoyable sexuality. Raynaud's phenomenon, causing pain and many times a burning feeling, is most frequently found in the fingers and toes, but may also affect other parts of the body, such as the nipples.[17] The presence of Raynaud's phenomenon may make undressing very uncomfortable. Esophageal dysfunction, a very frequent symptom in SSc patients, can induce reflux and heartburn, usually more prominent in a supine position. Intestinal involvement resulting in abdominal pain, diarrhea, constipation, or fecal incontinence may also interfere with regular sexual activity. Some medications frequently used to treat SSc, such as antidepressants or antihypertensive drugs, may also produce or worsen sexual dysfunction. Some patients may also have significant limitation on exercise capacity from cough and shortness of breath secondary to lung involvement or pulmonary hypertension, which can also interfere with certain sexual behaviors. Changes in appearance from tightness of the face and body skin or development of telangiectasia may become a very important problem, especially for young women, causing a feeling of unattractiveness and lack of self-confidence, which also might interfere with normal sexuality.

Emotional health is also known to play an important role in sexual functioning. Depressive symptoms[18] and impaired psychological functioning[19] are frequent in SSc, and have important impact on the quality of life. Sexual dysfunction has also been associated with depressive symptoms and marital distress in scleroderma patients,[6] as also happens in other chronic rheumatic conditions.[2,16] Pain is an antiaphrodisiac and sexual satisfaction seems difficult when high levels of pain are being experienced.[2] Pain may also negatively influence sexual desire and correlates with depressive symptoms. Sexual desire and satisfaction seem not to be impaired in scleroderma patients compared to healthy controls in a cross-sectional study.[6] Another study found a decreased desire for intercourse in 57% of patients following disease onset; since the results were based on the responses to a self-provided questionnaire comparing sexual impairment before and after disease onset, potential bias related to ability to recall past events make such data difficult to interpret.[4] The rate of sexual inactivity was higher in female SSc patients than in healthy controls in one study, but only 17% of patients listed scleroderma as their primary reason for sexual inactivity.[5] The Female Sexual Functioning Index, which quantitatively assesses six domains of sexual functioning (desire, subjective arousal, lubrication, orgasm, pain, and satisfaction), is significantly lower in scleroderma patients than in healthy controls, and correlates with the Mental Component of the SF-36, but surprisingly not with the Physical Component.[5]

Many of the problems identified by scleroderma patients as factors contributing to sexual distress and sexual dissatisfaction could be easily ameliorated with simple health interventions. These include using vaginal lubricants, providing a warm environment, avoiding meals prior to sexual activity, taking analgesics, and exploring alternative sexual positions to minimize musculoskeletal or body pain. Depressive symptoms should be evaluated in every patient (see Chap. 24). Alleviating pain and controlling depression could help to restore normal sexual function in female scleroderma patients. In some cases, referral to the gynecology department for a complete gynecological examination might be considered.

The impact of scleroderma on sexuality seems to be a problem that is hard to address, both for patients and for health professionals. Owing to the sensitive nature of the topic, health care providers generally tend to avoid talking about sexual issues with their patients, fearing that it might lead to embarrassment or discomfort.[8] Many do not feel properly trained or competent enough to address sexual problems adequately, even if they believe it would be important.[7] On the other hand, only a small proportion of female scleroderma patients felt the need to talk to somebody about their sexual problems and, if they wanted to talk to somebody, they preferred someone who was not a health professional.[6] In order to improve communication about sexuality, offering of information in non-threatening formats, such as pamphlets describing symptoms typically associated with scleroderma, including sexual problems, has been suggested.[7,8]

In summary, sexual dysfunction may be an important problem for many scleroderma patients. Psychological health and depressive symptoms are important risk factors for decreased sexual functioning, but physical difficulties secondary to the disease also have an important impact on sexuality. Although patients and health care providers seem to be reticent about discussing sexual issues, this subject should be addressed as part of routine clinical care. The identification of specific sexual problems may afford an opportunity for new interventions, such as referring patients to appropriate counseling or therapy, which in turn might lead to an improvement in sexuality. Improving sexual function will greatly improve the quality of life for those female scleroderma patients suffering from sexual impairment.

References

1. Saad SC, Behrendt AE. Scleroderma and sexuality. *J Sex Res*. 1996;33:215-220.
2. Tristano AG. The impact of rheumatic diseases on sexual function. *Rheumatol Int*. 2009;29: 853-860.

3. Wilson D, Goerzen J, Frtzler MJ. Treatment of sexual dysfunction in a patient with systemic sclerosis. *J Rheumatol.* 1993;20:1446-1447.
4. Bhadauria S, Moser DK, Clements PJ, et al. Genital tract abnormalities and female sexual function impairment in systemic sclerosis. *Am J Obstet Gynecol.* 1995;172:580-587.
5. Impens AJ, Rothman J, Schiopu E, et al. Sexual activity and functioning in female scleroderma patients. *Clin Exp Rheumatol.* 2009;27(suppl 54):S38-S43.
6. Schouffoer AA, van der Marel J, ter Kuile MM, et al. Impaired sexual function in women with systemic sclerosis: a cross sectional study. *Arthritis Care Res.* 2009;61:1601-1608.
7. Knafo R, Thombs BD, Jewett L, Hudson M, Wigley F, Haythornthwaite JA. (Not) talking about sex: a systematic comparison of sexual impairment in women with systemic sclerosis and other chronic disease samples. *Rheumatology.* 2009;48:1300-1303.
8. Anderson E, Triplett LM, Nietert PJ, Brown AN. Sexual dysfunction among women with connective tissue disease. *Curr Rheumatol Rev.* 2009;5:126-132.
9. Sampaio-Barros PD, Samara AM, Marques-Neto JF. Gynaecologic history in systemic sclerosis. *Clin Rheumatol.* 2000;19:184-187.
10. Skopouli FN, Papanikolaou S, Malmou-Mitsi V, Papanikolaou H, Moutsopoulos M. Obstetric and gynaecological profile in patients with primary Sjögren's syndrome. *Ann Rheum Dis.* 1994;53:569-573.
11. Avouac J, Sordet C, Depinay C, et al. Systemic sclerosis-associated Sjögren's syndrome and relationship to the limited cutaneous subtype. Results of a prospective study of sicca syndrome in 133 consecutive patients. *Arthritis Rheum.* 2006;54:2243-2249.
12. Swaminathan S, Goldblatt F, Dugar M, Gordon TP, Roberts-Thomson PJ. Prevalence of sicca symptoms in a South Australian cohort with systemic sclerosis. *Intern Med J.* 2008;38:897-903.
13. Mulherin DM, Sheeran TP, Kumararatne DS, Speculand B, Luesley D, Situnayake RD. Sjögren's syndrome in women presenting with chronic dyspareunia. *Br J Obstet Gynecol.* 1997;104:1019-1023.
14. Doss BJ, Quereshi F, Mayes MD, Jacques SM. Vascular and connective tissue histopathologic alterations of the female lower genital tract in scleroderma. *J Rheumatol.* 2002;29:1384-1387.
15. Evruke C, Ertunc D, Doran F, Ozbek S, Kadayifci O. Histopathological changes of cervical tissue in women with systemic sclerosis. *Pathol Int.* 2004;54:759-764.
16. Abdel-Nasser AM, Ali EI. Determinants of sexual disability and dissatisfaction in female with rheumatoid arthritis. *Clin Rheumatol.* 2006;25:822-830.
17. Anderson JE, Held N, Wright K. Raynaud's phenomenon of the nipple: a treatable cause of painful breastfeeding. *Pediatrics.* 2004;113:e360-e364.
18. Thombs BD, Hudson M, Taillefer SS, Baron M, Canadian Scleroderma Research Group. Prevalence and clinical correlates of symptoms of depression in patients with systemic sclerosis. *Arthritis Rheum.* 2008;59:504-509.
19. Hyphantis TN, Tsifetaki N, Siafaka V, et al. The impact of psychological functioning upon systemic sclerosis patients' quality of life. *Semin Arthritis Rheum.* 2007;37:81-92.

Chapter 24
A 38-Year-Old Woman with Elevated Muscle Enzymes, Raynaud's Phenomenon, and Positive Anti-Topoisomerase I Antibody: Is She Depressed?

Lisa R. Jewett, Marie Hudson, and Brett D. Thombs

Keywords Behavioral health • Depression • Psychosocial and psychological problems • Quality of life (QOL) • Systemic sclerosis

Case Study

A 38-year-old woman presented to her family doctor with fatigue and generally feeling unwell. She was a busy family doctor who had recently resumed her full workload despite being a mother of four children, including a 7-month-old infant. She tended to downplay her symptoms, and her general assessment was rather unremarkable except for the presence of mild carpal tunnel syndrome and Raynaud's phenomenon, which she reported having developed approximately 2 years previously. Routine blood tests were conducted, with the aim of eliminating common problems such as anemia and thyroid dysfunction. However, the results were remarkable for elevated creatine kinase (CK) in the range of 2,000 U/L, and the patient was referred to the emergency room for further investigations, at which time, a rheumatologist was consulted. The rheumatologist noted early signs of scleroderma and requested a variety of serological tests. Antinuclear antibodies (ANA) by indirect immunofluorescence were positive (titer 1:160), and antibodies to topoisomerase I (Scl-70) were detected. The patient was diagnosed with early systemic sclerosis (SSc).

Over the next 4 years, the patient developed progressive skin tightening for which she was started on methotrexate (MTX). She also developed severe finger ulcerations requiring digital sympathectomy and intermittent prostacyclin infusions. Thereafter, she was noted to have falling forced vital capacity (FVC) and

B.D. Thombs (✉)
Lady Davis Institute for Medical Research, Jewish General Hospital,
4333 Cote Ste Catherine Road, Montreal, QC H3T 1E4, Canada

R.M. Silver and C.P. Denton (eds.), *Case Studies in Systemic Sclerosis*,
DOI: 10.1007/978-0-85729-641-2_24, © Springer-Verlag London Limited 2011

diffusion capacity for carbon monoxide (DLco), as well as alveolitis revealed by high resolution computed tomography of the chest, and for which she was treated with mycophenolate mofetil (MMF). Subsequently, she developed palpitations associated with pre-syncopal symptoms, for which she had an implantable cardiac defibrillator placed. In the last 2 years, she has felt better overall. No new symptoms have appeared, her skin has softened to some degree, and her lung function stabilized.

At a personal level, the patient reported that the first few years of the disease were marked by a general sense of worry. She rapidly realized that there was tremendous uncertainty about the evolution of her disease and her overall prognosis. Although she initially continued to work, she began to worry that she was not able to function competently as a physician, for example, being unable to palpate adequately or to perform gynecological exams. She therefore reluctantly stopped working. She identified numerous other worries: each time she developed a new manifestation of the disease, she worried about what was to happen next; if she were to die, she would be unable to take care of her children; whether and how to discuss her disease with her children; and how her disability would affect her husband. Nevertheless, although she recalled feeling particularly low on a few occasions, she never remained "down" for periods beyond a few hours or, at most, days, and she remained active and optimistic most of the time. She attributed that to her own personality as well as to the consistently strong support she received, mostly from her husband.

The recent years have been marked by a new and disturbing problem associated with the physical changes brought on by the disease. She noticed that her face was different, with her features more strained, her lips and eyes becoming smaller, and prominent telangiectasias appearing. She also developed severe contractures of both hands. She was quite affected on several occasions when she ran across friends she had not seen in a few years who did not recognize her. Given both the external and internal changes brought on by her disease, she felt an overwhelming sense of loss of identity and described the need to mourn this loss.

Discussion

Living with a chronic medical condition, such as SSc, often results in significant disruptions to activities of daily living (ADL) and can negatively affect quality of life (QOL) and emotional functioning.[1,2] There is little research, however, on outcomes related to QOL in SSc, and this has posed a significant clinical challenge to addressing the psychosocial needs of persons living with SSc. Recently, an international panel of experts in behavioral and psychological health and well-being in SSc, including patients and patient advocates, published a consensus statement[1] that highlighted important patient-reported problems associated with QOL and well-being in SSc. This agenda identified a number of areas that appear to be common problems with potentially important influences on QOL for many people living with scleroderma, including depression, fatigue, pain, pruritus (itching), body image distress, and sexual dysfunction.[1,2]

Depression

Major depressive disorder (MDD) is common among patients living with one or more chronic medical conditions, with rates often in the range of 15–20%,[3] which is substantially higher than the 5% prevalence in the general population[4] and the 5–10% in primary care settings.[5] Both MDD and non-diagnosed psychological distress are associated with significant morbidity and mortality among patients with chronic conditions and can impact physical health through biological pathways including immune system dysfunction and inflammation, as well as behavior, such as poor adherence to medical treatment regimens and a reduced likelihood of adapting health-promoting behaviors, such as exercise or smoking cessation.[1]

Only one relatively small study[6] has reported rates of MDD among patients with SSc. That study reported that 19% of 100 SSc patients met criteria for a current episode of MDD, including 10% of 51 patients from a SSc association meeting and 28% of 49 hospitalized patients. In the absence of large studies of psychiatric disorders in SSc, it is useful to assess the degree to which patients endorse symptoms of depressive symptoms or distress on self-report questionnaires. A 2007 systematic review in SSc found rates above cutoff scores on self-report measures of depressive symptoms that ranged from 36 to 65%, depending on the questionnaire and cutoff used.[7] A 2010 study of 566 patients from the Canadian Scleroderma Research Group Registry reported that 34% of patients scored above a standard cutoff on the 20-item Center for Epidemiologic Studies Depression Scale, whereas only 21% of the same patients exceeded the designated cutoff on the 9-item Patient Health Questionnaire.[8] As illustrated by this study, cutoffs on self-report questionnaires, which are often set to detect patients potentially at risk for depression, tend to generate rates of "at risk" patients that exceed MDD diagnostic rates, sometimes substantially, and rates that depend on the particular self-report instrument used.

Large cross-sectional studies have reported that both sociodemographic factors, such as being unmarried and having less education, as well as disease variables, including more tender joints, breathing problems, and gastrointestinal functioning, are associated with greater depression scores in SSc.[8,9] Other smaller studies have documented that factors such as overall disease severity, disability, body image, pain, sexual dysfunction, disease-related cognitions, social support, and resilience are related to mental health functioning in SSc.[7]

Based on initial research in SSc[6,7] and what we know from other chronic diseases, a substantial proportion of SSc patients with high scores on self-report measures of distress or depressive symptoms will not meet criteria for MDD. Nonetheless, many patients with and without MDD are likely experiencing a significant level of emotional distress that may be linked to problems, such as worry or fear, fatigue, pain, pruritus, body image distress, and sexual dysfunction.[1,2]

Anxiety

There has been very little research on symptoms of anxiety or anxiety disorders among persons living with SSc.[1] Only a handful of studies has assessed anxiety, but all were conducted with small patient samples and used self-report questionnaires that did not permit the estimation of prevalence of specific anxiety disorders.[10-12] A recent study from the Netherlands ($N = 123$) found that one of the top concerns expressed by patients was a fear of the future, including the potential for uncontrolled and unpredictable disease progression, major loss of function, inability to work, dependency on others, and mortality.[13] However, the extent to which these fears, and anxiety more generally, are present, as well as their impact on patients with SSc, needs more focused investigation.[1]

Fatigue

Fatigue is one of the most important factors that affects QOL in many chronic diseases.[14] A systematic review found that fatigue levels in SSc patients are similar to those reported by patients with other rheumatic diseases and cancer patients undergoing treatment, and higher than in the general population or among cancer patients in remission.[15] Fatigue is present in up to 75% of SSc patients and has been reported to be one of the most bothersome symptoms associated with the disease.[13] Fatigue in SSc is robustly associated with level of daily activity and work disability as well as physical function, even after controlling for education level, disease subtype, pain, sleep quality, and depressive symptoms.[16-19] A number of medical comorbidities are associated with fatigue in SSc, including breathing and gastrointestinal problems, pain, and depression.[20]

Pain

Pain levels in SSc are similar to those reported in other chronic pain and rheumatic conditions,[21-23] and pain is an important source of distress for many persons living with SSc.[1,2] Between 60% and 83% of SSc patients experience pain,[24] and pain is an independent predictor of work disability.[17] A number of potential sources of pain have been reported in SSc, including skin pain; pain associated with Raynaud's phenomenon; musculoskeletal pain; pain in distal extremities due to tightness, calcinosis, and ulcers; and gastrointestinal problems.[1,24]

Pruritus

Pruritus, or itching, is described as a "poorly localized, nonadapting, usually unpleasant sensation that provokes a desire to scratch."[25] Pruritus is a problem for many patients with SSc, although time of onset and duration varies across patients. There is relatively little research on pruritus in SSc. A 2009 study found that 45% of SSc patients 1 year or longer after the onset of first non-Raynaud's phenomenon symptoms reported pruritus on most days.[26] This rate was even higher for patients 1–2 years from disease onset although only a small number of patients in that group were assessed, and no patients 0–1 years from disease onset were included in the study. The presence of pruritus appears to be associated with skin involvement, gastrointestinal symptoms, Raynaud's phenomenon, and finger ulcers, although only gastrointestinal symptoms have been shown to be an independent correlate of pruritus.[26] A 2010 study found that pruritus was associated with significantly reduced QOL in SSc, even after controlling for standard predictors, including disease duration, skin score, number of tender joints, gastrointestinal symptoms, breathing problems, Raynaud's phenomenon, and finger ulcers.[27]

Body Image Distress

Patients with disfigurement that occurs in the context of injury or medical illness often struggle with body image and experience social anxiety and avoidance due to changes in appearance.[28] The appearance changes central to SSc commonly affect visible and socially relevant body parts (e.g., face and hands), posing potential challenges to maintaining healthy social interactions. Skin deformities have been rated by patients as one of the most significant stressors associated with the disease.[13] Furthermore, low levels of self-esteem in relation to appearance and high levels of body image dissatisfaction have been reported by SSc patients, both related to the extent of physical changes and disfigurement of the skin.[13,29]

The majority of existing research on body image has focused on eating disorders and weight-related concerns and has been based on instruments that measure these issues. These concerns may be of relatively less importance compared to disfiguring aspects of the disease for people living with SSc. However, research examining body image in SSc has been limited by the lack of measurement tools that assess issues related to body image concerns of patients with SSc. To address this shortcoming, the Brief-Satisfaction with Appearance Scale (Brief-SWAP), which can be used for both research and clinical purposes, was developed to assess appearance concerns (e.g., hands, face, arms) and social discomfort in SSc.[30] A recent study based on the Brief-SWAP identified disease factors (e.g., degree of skin involvement) and sociodemographic factors, including age, sex, and marital status, that were related to body image distress among persons living with SSc.[31]

Sexual Dysfunction

Sexual dysfunction refers to problems that may include decreased desire and enjoyment, impaired arousal, and painful sex.[32] In SSc, both physical and psychological aspects associated with the disease may lead to sexual dysfunction (discussed in detail in Chaps. 22 and 23). For instance, skin tightening and discomfort, shrinking of the mouth, joint pain, Raynaud's phenomenon, gastrointestinal symptoms, vaginal tightness and dryness in women, and reduced penile blood flow in men are some of the physical consequences of SSc that can impede sexual functioning.[33-35] Psychological aspects of SSc, including depressive symptoms and distress about physical appearance, can also impact sexual functioning. One study reported that more than half of women with SSc had impaired sexual functioning,[34] and another found that levels of sexual impairment in women with SSc are similar to or higher than levels for women with breast cancer, human immunodeficiency virus, and gynecologic cancer.[36] Vaginal discomfort and pain, fatigue, disease duration, and overall marital dissatisfaction are other factors that have been linked to poorer sexual functioning.[37]

Clinical Care

No strategies or interventions have been developed or tested to specifically address psychosocial problems and concerns associated with SSc. Consistent with this, the European League Against Rheumatism (EULAR)'s recent recommendations for treatment of SSc[38] highlighted the need for interventions to address psychosocial concerns, but did not make any recommendations for lifestyle or behavioral interventions and noted, "There are also other treatment options for the management of SSc patients, such as physiotherapy, education, new experimental therapies, etc., which…could not be included because of the lack of expert consensus." Efforts are currently underway to develop strategies that focus on the behavioral and psychosocial aspects of SSc; however, in the meantime, models and approaches from other fields can be applied to support people living with SSc. Given the wide range of problems and concerns faced by individuals with SSc, a broad approach, rather than an approach that focuses on a single disorder, such as depression, is recommended. The field of psycho-oncology provides a model for this kind of approach. Indeed, a core tenet of psycho-oncological care is a focus on supporting coping of patients and their support systems rather than focusing exclusively on the diagnosis and treatment of psychiatric disorders, such as mood or anxiety disorders. In the psycho-oncology model, psychosocial care involves providing services and interventions to patients and their families to help manage psychological, behavioral, and social aspects of living with the disease.[39]

A first step toward providing quality psychosocial care for persons living with SSc is to facilitate the provision of information to both patients and those who support them regarding issues common to people living with SSc, such as concerns related to changes in appearance or mood (e.g., body image distress and depression) as well as information regarding useful resources and services to address such problems. Self-help or self-management resources are a first step and most useful for relatively mild problems. To help patients access resources, nurses and rheumatologists should be aware of important psychosocial issues that affect quality of life in order to facilitate conversations that address concerns of individual patients.

Additionally, links to information and educational resources regarding self-help programs that are available as a first step in providing psychosocial support can be provided in clinics.

There are a number of resources that may be particularly useful for persons living with SSc. For instance, *Positive Coping with Health Conditions, A Self-Care Workbook*[40] is a self-care manual designed for individuals living with chronic health conditions, as well as for physicians, psychologists, nurses, rehabilitation professionals, and researchers. The workbook focuses on teaching skills to manage stress related to living with chronic disease. It is based on cognitive behavioral therapy models, framed in a manner that can be accessed by those who are not familiar with or trained in psychological interventions.

Changing Faces (www.changingfaces.org.uk) is another useful resource that provides information that can be made available in clinics. *Changing Faces* is a not-for-profit organization designed to provide support for individuals touched by disfigurement and to increase public awareness regarding issues related to living with a visibly different appearance. *Changing Faces* has published a range of resources in the form of booklets, pamphlets, and DVDs for individuals with disfigurements, their families, as well as employers and healthcare professionals. In addition to publications, *Changing Faces* carries out workshops and training on issues surrounding disfigurement. Their resources target social anxiety, body image distress, and adjustment to an altered appearance.

In addition to these resources, general self-management programs for living with a chronic disease may be useful for patients with SSc. The Chronic Disease Self-Management Program (CDSMP),[41] which was developed by Kate Lorig and modeled on her Arthritis Self-Management Program,[42] is designed to teach self-care techniques useful to persons with many chronic diseases. The CDSMP is delivered in small-group settings and led by persons who have a chronic disease. It is delivered through face-to-face meetings or via internet groups, although currently access to online groups is limited (http://www.ncoa.org/improving-health/chronic-disease/better-choices-better-health.html).

In addition to helping patients discuss problems they face and facilitating access to self-help material, rheumatologists should establish a relationship with a formal mental health provider, such as a psychologist, psychiatrist, or trained social worker to provide more specialized treatment to patients, as needed. Some organizations, such as the United States Preventive Services Task Force (USPSTF)[43] have recommended that physicians in primary care formally screen for depression with self-report questionnaires, such as the PHQ-9, when done in conjunction with integrated, staff-assisted programs systems for assessment and management of depression. These systems typically involve multifaceted interventions with central roles for nonmedical specialists, such as case managers, who work with the primary care physician, mental health specialists and other providers to provide depression management and treatment follow-up.[44] Other groups, including the UK National Institute for Health and Clinical Excellence, however, have argued that there is no evidence that screening would benefit patients.[45] Although it may be tempting to implement routine screening for depression and other psychological problems in rheumatology settings, the systems required, based on the USPSTF recommendation, are not likely to be present. Furthermore, there has never been a clinical trial, even in primary care, that has successfully done what is recommended by the USPSTF and that has found better depression outcomes for patients screened for depression versus those not screened when the same treatment and care resources are made available to both groups. On the other hand, there have been numerous negative trials, for example, in primary care, perinatal care, and oncological care, for depression screening without system supports. Thus, the only certainty is that screening would consume a substantial amount of resources. In addition, it might result in harm to patients due to false positive screens and side effects from medication, for instance, among other possible harms.[46,47]

In summary, persons living with SSc face a number of complex psychosocial challenges. Approaches to psychosocial care should take into account the breadth of challenges faced by patients rather than focusing only on single issues, such as depression. As a first step, care providers should become aware of problems faced by patients and their supporters, should facilitate discussions of these problems, and should help patients access self-help material. Beyond this, rheumatology clinics should develop a relationship with a competent mental health care provider to provide more focused intervention for patients, as needed.

Acknowledgments Ms. Jewett was supported by a Bourses de Formation – Formation de Maîtrise from the Fonds de la recherche en santé Québec. Drs. Thombs and Hudson are supported by New Investigator Awards from the Canadian Institutes of Health Research and Établissement de Jeunes Chercheurs awards from the Fonds de la Recherche en Santé Québec.

References

1. Thombs BD, van Lankveld W, Bassel M, et al. Psychological health and well-being in systemic sclerosis: state of the science and consensus research agenda. *Arthritis Care Res.* 2010;8:1181-1189.
2. Haythornthwaite JA, Heinberg LJ, McGuire L. Psychologic factors in scleroderma. *Rheum Dis Clin N Am.* 2003;29:427-439.
3. Evans DL, Charney DS, Lewis L, et al. Mood disorders in the medically ill: scientific review and recommendations. *Biol Psychiatry.* 2005;58:175-189.
4. Blazer DG, Kessler RC, McGonagle KA, Swartz MS. The prevalence and distribution of major depression in a national community sample: the National Comorbidity Survey. *Am J Psychiatry.* 1994;151:979-986.
5. Pignone MP, Gaynes BN, Rushton JL, et al. Screening for depression in adults: a summary of the evidence for the U.S. Preventive Services Task Force. *Ann Intern Med.* 2002;136:765-776.
6. Baubet T, Ranque B, Taïeb O, et al. Mood and anxiety disorders in systemic sclerosis patients. *Presse Méd.* 2010;40(2):e111-e119.
7. Thombs BD, Taillefer SS, Hudson M, Baron M. Depression in patients with systemic sclerosis: a systematic review of the evidence. *Arthritis Rheum.* 2007;57:1089-1097.
8. Milette K, Hudson M, Baron M, Thombs BD, Canadian Scleroderma Research Group. Comparison of the PHQ-9 and CES-D depression scales in systemic sclerosis: internal consistency reliability, convergent validity, and clinical correlates. *Rheumatology.* 2010;49:789-796.
9. Thombs BD, Hudson M, Taillefer SS, Baron M, and the Canadian Scleroderma Research Group. Prevalence and clinical correlates of symptoms of depression in patients with systemic sclerosis. *Arthritis Rheum.* 2008;59:504-509.

10. Mozzetta A, Antinone V, Alfani S, et al. Mental health in patients with systemic sclerosis: a controlled investigation. *J Eur Acad Dermatol Venereol*. 2008;22:336-340.
11. Legendre C, Allanore Y, Ferrand I, Kahan A. Evaluation of depression and anxiety in patients with systemic sclerosis. *Joint Bone Spine*. 2005;72:408-411.
12. Angelopoulos NV, Drosos AA, Moutsopoulos HM. Psychiatric symptoms associated with scleroderma. *Psychother Psychosom*. 2001;70:145-150.
13. Van Lankveld WG, Vonk MC, Teunissen H, van den Hoogen FH. Appearance self-esteem in systemic sclerosis: subjective experience of skin deformity and its relationship with physician – assessed skin involvement, disease status and psychological variables. *Rheumatology*. 2007;46:872-876.
14. Swain MG. Fatigue in chronic disease. *Clin Sci*. 2000;99:1-8.
15. Thombs BD, Bassel M, McGuire L, Smith MT, Hudson M, Haythornthwaite JA. A systematic comparison of fatigue levels in systemic sclerosis with general population, cancer and rheumatic disease samples. *Rheumatology*. 2008;47:1559-1563.
16. Hudson M, Steele R, Lu Y, Thombs BD, Baron M, Canadian Scleroderma Research Group. Work disability in systemic sclerosis. *J Rheumatol*. 2009;36:2481-2486.
17. Sandqvist G, Eklund M. Daily occupations–performance, satisfaction and time use, and relations with well-being in women with limited systemic sclerosis. *Disabil Rehabil*. 2008;30:27-35.
18. Sandqvist G, Scheja A, Eklund M. Working ability in relation to disease severity, everyday occupations and well-being in women with limited systemic sclerosis. *Rheumatology*. 2008;47:1708-1711.
19. Sandusky SB, McGuire L, Smith MT, Wigley FM, Haythornthwaite JA. Fatigue: an overlooked determinant of physical function in scleroderma. *Rheumatology*. 2009;48:165-169.
20. Thombs BD, Hudson M, Bassel M, Taillefer SS, Baron M, and the Canadian Scleroderma Research Group. Sociodemographic, disease, and symptom correlates of fatigue in systemic sclerosis: evidence from a sample of 659 Canadian Scleroderma Research Group Registry patients. *Arthritis Rheum*. 2009;61(7):966-973.
21. Benrud-Larson LM, Haythornthwaite JA, Heinberg LJ, et al. The impact of pain and symptoms of depression in scleroderma. *Pain*. 2002;95:267-275.
22. Danieli E, Airo P, Bettoni L, et al. Health-related quality of life measured by the Short Form 36 (SF-36) in systemic sclerosis: correlations with indexes of disease activity and severity, disability, and depressive symptoms. *Clin Rheumatol*. 2005;24:48-54.
23. Johnson SR, Glaman DD, Schentag CT, Lee P. Quality of life and functional status in systemic sclerosis compared to other rheumatic diseases. *J Rheumatol*. 2006;33:1117-1122.
24. Schieir O, Thombs BD, Hudson M, et al. Prevalence, severity, and clinical correlates of pain in patients with systemic sclerosis. *Arthritis Care Res*. 2010;62:409-417.
25. Weisshaar E, Kucenic MJ, Fleischer AB Jr. Pruritus: a review. *Acta Derm Venereol Suppl*. 2003;213:5-32.
26. Razykov I, Thombs BD, Hudson M, Bassel M, Baron M, and the Canadian Scleroderma Research Group. Prevalence and clinical correlates of pruritus in patients with systemic sclerosis. *Arthritis Rheum*. 2009;61:1765-1770.
27. El-Baalbaki G, Razykov I, Hudson M, et al. Association of pruritus with quality of life and disability in systemic sclerosis. *Arthritis Care Res*. 2010;62:1489-1495.
28. Pruzinsky T. Social and psychological effects of major craniofacial deformity. *Cleft Palate Craniofac J*. 1992;29:578-584.
29. Malcarne VL, Handsdottir I, Greensbergs HL, Clements PJ, Weisman MH. Appearance self-esteem in systemic sclerosis. *Cogn Ther Res*. 1999;23:197-208.
30. Jewett LR, Hudson M, Haythornthwaite JA, et al. Development and validation of the brief-satisfaction with appearance scale (Brief-SWAP) for systemic sclerosis (SSc). *Arthritis Care Res*. 2010;62(12):1779-1786.
31. Jewett LR, Hudson M, Baron, M, Thombs BD, Canadian Scleroderma Research Group. Disentangling body image dissatisfaction and social discomfort in systemic sclerosis: a structural equation modeling approach (under review).

32. Bancroft J. *Human Sexuality and Its Problems*. 3rd ed. Edinburgh: Churchill Livingstone; 2009.
33. Schover LR, Jensen SR. *Sexuality and Chronic Illness: A Comprehensive Approach*. New York: Guilford Press; 1988.
34. Saad SC, Pietrzykowski JE, Lewis SS, et al. Vaginal lubrication in women with scleroderma and Sjögren's syndrome. *Sex Disabil*. 1999;17:103-113.
35. Saad SC, Behrend AE. Scleroderma and sexuality. *J Sex Res*. 1996;33:15-20.
36. Knafo R, Thombs BD, Jewett L, Hudson M, Wigley F, Haythornthwaite JA. (Not) talking about sex: a systematic comparison of sexual impairment in women with systemic sclerosis and other chronic disease samples. *Rheumatology*. 2009;48:1300-1303.
37. Schouffoer AA, van der Marel J, ter Kuile MM, et al. Impaired sexual function in women with systemic sclerosis: a cross-sectional study. *Arthritis Rheum*. 2009;61:1601-1608.
38. Kowal-Bielecka O, Landewe R, Avouac J, et al. EULAR recommendations for the treatment of systemic sclerosis: a report from the EULAR scleroderma trials and research group (EUSTAR). *Ann Rheum Dis*. 2009;68:620-628.
39. Department of Health, Western Australia. Psycho-Oncology Model of Care. Perth: WA Cancer and Palliative Care Network, Department of Health, Western Australia; 2008.
40. Bilsker D, Samara J, Goldner E. Positive coping with health conditions: a self-care workbook. Consortium for Organizational Mental Healthcare (COMH); 2009.
41. Lorig KR, Sobel DS, Stewart AL, et al. Evidence suggesting that a chronic disease self-management program can improve health status while reducing utilization and costs: a randomized trial. *Med Care*. 1999;37:5-14.
42. Lorig K, Lubeck D, Kraines RG, Seleznick M, Holman HR. Outcomes of self-help education for patients with arthritis. *Arthritis Rheum*. 1985;28:680-685.
43. U.S. Preventive Services Task Force. Screening for depression in adults: U.S. Preventive Services Task Force recommendation statement. *Ann Intern Med*. 2009;151:784-792.
44. Katon WJ, Seelig M. Population-based care of depression: team care approaches to improving outcomes. *J Occup Environ Med*. 2008;50:459-467.
45. National Institute for Health and Clinical Excellence (NICE). Antenatal and Postnatal Mental Health: The NICE Guideline on Clinical Management and Service Guidance. UK: NICE; 2007.
46. Ziegelstein RC, Thombs BD, Coyne JC, de Jonge P. Routine screening for depression in patients with coronary heart disease: never mind. *J Am Coll Cardiol*. 2009;54:886-890.
47. Thombs BD, Jewett LR, Knafo R, Coyne JC, Ziegelstein RC. Learning from history: a commentary on the American Heart Association Science Advisory on depression screening. *Am Heart J*. 2009;158:503-505.

Chapter 25
A Scleroderma Patient with Swollen and Tender Joints of Both Hands

Gabriele Valentini, Giovanna Cuomo, Virginia D'Abrosca, and Salvatore Cappabianca

Keywords Arthritis • MRI • MSK US • Radiographs • SSc sine Scleroderma

Case Study

A 39-year-old woman was referred to the outpatient clinic of the Rheumatology Unit of the Second University of Naples because of pain and stiffness affecting her metacarpophalangeal (MCP) and knee joints.

The patient had a 2-year history of Raynaud's phenomenon and puffy hands (without sclerodactyly). One year before, systemic sclerosis (SSc) *sine* scleroderma was diagnosed following the detection of antinuclear antibodies (ANA) by IIF on Hep-2 cells (titer 1:1,280; centromere pattern), enlarged capillaries visible on wide-field nailfold capillary microscopy, and dysphagia-heartburn associated with reduced basal lower esophageal sphincter (LES) pressure (13 mmHg) with hypotonic esophageal waves in 90% of the swallows. No alteration had been detected on chest radiograph, PFTs, ECG, and B-mode Echocardiography with Doppler flow study.

Articular involvement had developed 1 month before with pain at rest and on motion and one-half hour of morning stiffness. Initially both knees were affected with subsequent, similar additive involvement of the first, second, and third MCP joints of both hands.

G. Valentini (✉)
Dipartimento di Internistica Clinica e Sperimentale
"F Magrassi-A. Lanzara" – Rheumatology Unit,
Second University of Naples, Via Pansini, 5, 80131 Naples, Italy

R.M. Silver and C.P. Denton (eds.), *Case Studies in Systemic Sclerosis*, 239
DOI: 10.1007/978-0-85729-641-2_25, © Springer-Verlag London Limited 2011

Physical Examination

On physical examination, the second and third MCP joints of each hand were found to be swollen (Fig. 25.1a, b). The same joints as well as both knees and the first MCP joints were tender and painful on motion. No other joint was involved. The Health Assessment Questionnaire Disability Index (HAQ-DI) score was 1. No skin sclerosis was detectable.

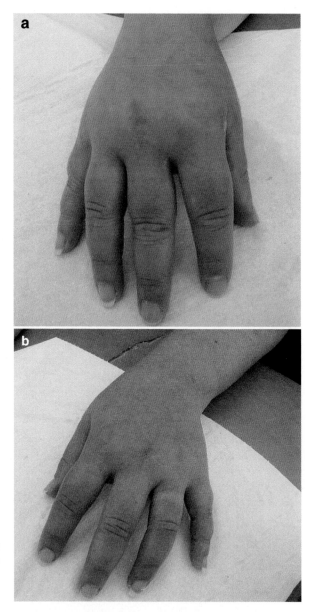

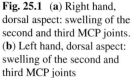

Fig. 25.1 (a) Right hand, dorsal aspect: swelling of the second and third MCP joints. (b) Left hand, dorsal aspect: swelling of the second and third MCP joints

Table 25.1 Results of main laboratory and functional tests at presentation

ESR 15 mm/h
CRP 1.5 mg/L
Hb 12.4 g/dL
WBC 5,790 cells/mm^3
PLT 307,000/mm^3
Gammaglobulins 1.17 g/dL
C3 116 mg/dL
C4 19 mg/dL (normal values 20–50)
RF 1 IU (negative)
Anti-CCP antibodies 3 IU (negative)
ANA (IIF) titer 1:1,280, centromere pattern
FVC (% predicted) 102
DLco (% predicted) 96

Laboratory and Functional Tests

Table 25.1 lists the main results of laboratory and functional tests at the time of initial consultation.

Imaging

Hand radiographs showed juxta-articular osteopenia at the MCP joints and joint space narrowing of the PIP joints without erosions (Fig. 25.2). Musculoskeletal ultrasonography (MSK US) executed with a 7–12 MHz linear array transducer, revealed synovial effusions at both first MCP joints (Fig. 25.3), and power Doppler study was consistent with synovial vascularization at second and third MCP joints of both hands.

Course

The patient was diagnosed with a symmetric seronegative polyarthritis secondary to SSc *sine* scleroderma. She was prescribed low-dose corticosteroids (prednisone 5 mg daily) plus vitamin D 5,600 U weekly. After 3 months, articular manifestations were only slightly improved, ESR was 12 mm/h; CRP 0.18 mg/L and HAQ-DI was 0.875. Prednisone dosage was increased to 7.5 mg daily. At 6 months, articular

Fig 25.2 Hand radiographs: juxta-articular osteopenia of MCP joints; joint space narrowing of PIP joints

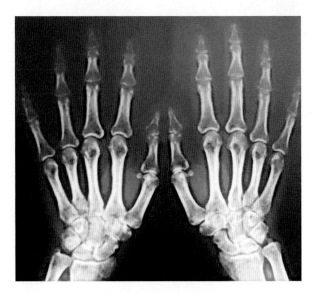

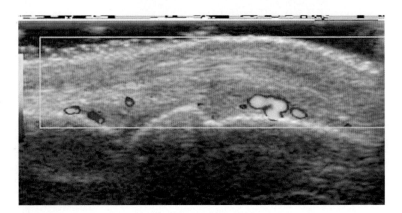

Fig 25.3 Baseline MSK US of the second MCP joint: Power Doppler positive, synovial hypertrophy plus effusion

manifestations had definitely improved, but arthritis of the second and third MCP joints was still present. The HAQ-DI was 0.75. MSK-US examination demonstrated a small intraarticular effusion at both second and third MCP joints without synovial proliferation (Fig. 25.4). Magnetic resonance imaging revealed no erosions (T1-weighted image) but confirmed the presence of small effusions (T2-weighted image) (Fig. 25.5). Methotrexate (10 mg weekly) with folic acid supplementation was added. Three months later, her arthritis was in remission and prednisone was gradually tapered.

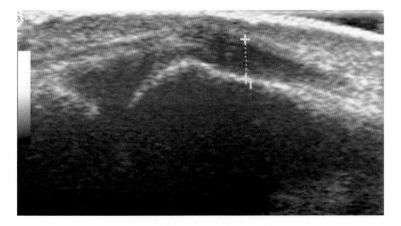

Fig 25.4 MSK US of the second MCP joint, 6 months later: small effusion

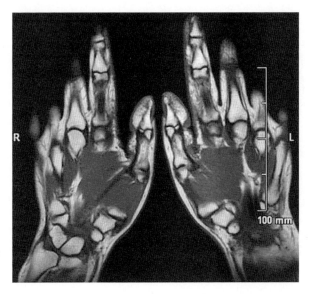

Fig 25.5 T1-weighted MRI
of MCP joints: small effusion
at second MCP joints
bilaterally

Discussion

SSc is a systemic autoimmune disorder characterized by microvascular obliterative
and small artery proliferative alterations and by deposition of collagen and other
matrix constituents affecting target organs, e.g., skin, gut, lung, heart, kidney, joint-
tendons, and muscles.[1] The diagnosis of SSc is commonly based upon the preliminary ACR (formerly ARA) criteria for the classification of SSc,[2] even though such
criteria lack sensitivity (see Chap. 1). Our patient did not satisfy such criteria but

was clinically diagnosed as having SSc based on the constellation of Raynaud's phenomenon with a distinct autoimmune profile, megacapillaries, and typical esophageal involvement. In the absence of overt skin involvement our patient was classified as SSc *sine* scleroderma, a recognized variant of limited cutaneous systemic sclerosis (lSSc).[3]

Articular Involvement in SSc

Pathologic and Clinical Features

Musculoskeletal manifestations occur in a high percentage of patients with SSc, involving joints, muscles and tendons: the most characteristic articular–periarticular manifestations being arthralgia–arthritis, joint contractures, and tendon friction rubs.[4-6]

Synovium from SSc patients may be normal or may demonstrate inflammatory and fibrotic changes of variable severity.[7,8] When involved, the synovium is infiltrated in the early stages by lymphocytes and plasma cells surrounding blood vessels and sometimes organized in small focal aggregates, and may be covered by a layer of fibrin which is thought to cause loud joint rubs detectable during joint motion. In these cases, synovial fluid analysis shows inflammatory features: it is turbid, contains an increased amount of proteins (fibrin, fibrin breakdown products, immunoglobulins) and an increased number of polymorphonuclear leukocytes. Later, as the arthritis progresses, fibrosis of the synovium ensues loss of normal villous folds and obliteration of vascular structures. Finally, the synovium is replaced by dense homogeneous, hypocellular collagenous connective tissue, analogous to what may be seen in late-stage SSc affecting the dermis. Fibrosis of tendons and periarticular structures can occur. In addition, thickening of tendon sheaths accompanied in some cases by fibrin deposition on the surface may be observed.

Clinically detectable articular involvement has been reported in up to 97% of SSc patients.[9-13] Articular manifestations can be the presenting feature of SSc, heralding the development of diffuse disease. Rodnan and Medsger[9] investigated 150 patients and reported that polyarthralgia or arthritis was the initial manifestation, or developed within 1 year from the onset of the disease in 61 patients (41%). Baron et al.[11] investigated 38 SSc patients during a 6-month period. Joint pain was present in 25 cases (66%), 5 of whom had experienced joint symptoms 1 year or more before the diagnosis of SSc, with an additional eight patients having articular symptoms during the first year after diagnosis. Arthritis, however, can develop in any disease stage and in patients with either the diffuse (dSSc) or limited (lSSc) subset.

Symmetric polyarthralgia and stiffness are the usual presentations, but frank arthritis can occur. Baron et al.[11] detected joint inflammation in 61% of their 38 patients, but it consisted in most cases of tenderness and stress pain without other signs. La Montagna et al.[12] retrospectively evaluated 100 SSc patients followed for years. They recorded arthralgia in 36% of the patients and well-defined arthritis in 25%. The same authors[13] subsequently carried out a prospective 1-year study on 76 SSc patients. They detected arthralgia in 29 (38%) and arthritis in 10 (13%). Articular involvement was associated with a significant degree of disability in some patients as measured by the Health Assessment Questionnaire Disability Index (HAQ-DI), with scores as high as 2.875 (range 0–2.875), although most patients had a HAQ-DI score that was less than the upper limit of normal (median 0.44). Recently, arthritis was reported to be present in 16% of over 7,000 patients from the EUSTAR database.[14]

In most cases SSc arthritis is a symmetric, nonerosive, and seronegative (RF and anti-CCP antibody) polyarthritis affecting small joints of the hands, wrists, knees and ankles, and is associated with morning stiffness of 30 min or greater.[11] Commonly, it has an insidious onset and runs a chronic course. Nevertheless, patients with acute disease and intermittent or rapidly progressive course as well as patients with an oligoarticular or monoarticular pattern have been reported, the monoarticular, acute pattern being characteristic of patients with arthritis–periarthritis due to hydroxyapatite crystal deposition.[9,11-13]

Tendon friction rubs (TFR) were first described by Shulman et al.[15] who detected in two patients peritendinous collagen accumulation and fibrin deposition along the surface of the tendon sheath (see Chap. 28). TFR mainly affect younger and earlier disease patients with dSSc. Patients with limited skin thickening who have TFR are apt to develop more severe disease (digital ulcers, pulmonary fibrosis, muscle weakness) and have higher frequency of antitopoisomerase-1 and anti-RNA polymerase III antibodies, which suggests that these patients may represent a subset of individuals with "subclinical" diffuse SSc.[16]

Joint contractures were detected by Baron et al.[11] in 4 out of the 38 cases, by La Montagna et al.[13] in 52.6% (finger flexion) of 76 patients, and by Avouac et al.[14] in 31% of 7,286 patients enrolled in the EUSTAR data base. Synovitis, TFR, and joint contractures frequently coexist in the same patient.[14]

In addition to the articular involvement inherent to the disease, SSc patients may be affected by an SSc-RA (rheumatoid arthritis) overlap syndrome, which has been reported by a number of authors and may be considered a distinct genetic, immunological, and clinical entity.[17-20]

Finally, SSc patients can by chance be affected by other conditions, which can be either influenced by disease (e.g., osteoporosis secondary to malabsorption) or independent of their SSc (e.g., osteoarthritis or erosive osteoarthritis).[11-13]

Laboratory Findings

Joint involvement was found to be associated with acute-phase reactants (e.g., ESR, CRP) by Avouac et al.[14] suggesting that joint disease has a role in promoting systemic inflammation in SSc. Rheumatoid factor (RF) is detected in a variable percentage of patients with SSc (4–66%)[9,11,13] with or without clinical evidence of arthritis. On the contrary, anticyclic citrullinated peptide antibodies (anti-CCP antibodies), especially when present at a high titer, can help to differentiate SSc-RA overlap from simple SSc polyarthritis.[21,22]

Clinical Associations

Joint involvement, in particular TFR and flexion contractures, has long been known to mainly affect patients with dSSc.[4,13,14,16] Analysis of the large EUSTAR database[14] pointed out that synovitis, joint contractures, and TFR are more likely to occur together and that their occurrence is significantly associated with disease activity and severe vascular, muscular, renal, and lung involvement, suggesting that rheumatic manifestations mainly occur in patients with more advanced internal organ involvement.

Imaging

Articular manifestations in SSc have long been investigated by imaging techniques. By plain radiography, Baron et al.[11] reported generalized osteopenia in 26% of their 38 patients, periarticular osteopenia in 42%, erosions in 40%, joint space narrowing in 34%, terminal phalangeal tuft resorption (i.e., acro-osteolysis) in 37%, and calcinosis in 50%. These authors pointed out that SSc erosions are generally smaller than those detectable in patients with RA, found a significant association between calcinosis and erosions, and, notably, detected erosive osteoarthritis associated with impaired finger flexion in seven patients.

In a retrospective study of 100 SSc patients, La Montagna et al.[12] compared foot and hand involvement. They found foot involvement to be less frequent, having a later onset, and being characterized by a lower prevalence of acro-osteolysis, calcinosis, and erosions, underlining the difference with respect to RA in which radiologic features occur earlier in the feet than in the hands.[23]

In a subsequent prospective study, La Montagna et al.[12] identified three radiographic patterns of articular involvement in SSc: (1) inflammatory, consisting of juxtaarticular osteopenia, erosive changes, and narrowing of proximal interphalangeal joints; (2) degenerative, characterized by narrowing of proximal and/or distal interphalangeal joints, subchondral sclerosis, and/or osteophytes; and (3) periarticular fibrotic, characterized by digital flexion and joint space narrowing. These patterns were found to be mutually exclusive in 75 out of the 76 patients investigated. These results might indicate that there are distinct phenotypes of articular involvement in SSc. However, they wait to be confirmed in a separate series.

SSc articular involvement has been recently investigated by musculoskeletal ultrasonography (MSK US) and magnetic resonance imaging (MRI). Grassi et al.[24] first assessed the distal phalanx MSK US features in patients with different rheumatic diseases including SSc. Cuomo et al.[25] investigated 45 SSc patients by clinical examination, hand and wrist radiographs, and MSK US. These authors found a high prevalence of joint alterations by ultrasonography (effusions in 49%; synovial proliferation in 42%, erosions in 11%, joint space narrowing in 18%, and osteophytes in 59%) pointing out a high sensitivity of MSK US in detecting effusions and osteophytes. These results clearly underline the existence of a subclinical SSc arthropathy.

Chitale et al.[26] investigated 17 SSc patients with arthralgia and no overt synovitis by MSK US at baseline, and then reevaluated 13 of them 6 months later by the same technique and 8 out of the 13 by MRI. MSK US demonstrated the presence of synovitis in 6% of the patients at baseline and 23% of those examined 6 months later; tenosynovitis was evident in 46% and 47%, respectively. MRI showed synovitis in 100% of the patients, tenosynovitis in 88%, and erosions in 75%. These results cannot be extrapolated to all SSc patients since only symptomatic patients were investigated. Nevertheless, the study clearly indicates the presence of an inflammatory, erosive arthritis in SSc patients who present with arthralgia only.

Course

Most patients with SSc arthralgia/arthritis have a chronic, indolent course. Disability rarely results from articular disease *per se* but is mainly the consequence of flexion contractures, particularly at the hands in patients with dSSc. Patients with a SSc-RA overlap syndrome have a disease course that reflects the evolution of both conditions. Patients with crystal deposition disease recover from the acute phase of the disease, but may experience recurrent inflammatory symptoms over time.

Pathogenesis and Treatment

The pathogenesis of articular involvement is poorly understood. The pathologic, radiographic, US and MRI features of SSc synovitis and tenosynovitis share a number of features with that of RA.[26] Increased serum concentrations of YKL-40, a glycoprotein secreted by chondrocytes and synovial fibroblasts, have been demonstrated, and the levels correlate with joint involvement and T lymphocyte activation.[27] Flexion contractures are caused by fibrotic changes of periarticular structures. Calcium deposition is a typical example of dystrophic calcification, the cause of which has not been elucidated.

Because of these limitations, there is no established treatment for SSc articular involvement.[5,6,28] Patients with tenosynovitis, arthralgia/arthritis, and stiffness are commonly treated with low-dose prednisone (7.5 mg daily) and/or nonsteroidal anti-inflammatory drugs; however, one must be mindful of the potential negative effect of prostaglandin inhibition on renal blood flow and on the integrity of the gastrointestinal tract. In addition, despite limited evidence for efficacy, other drugs such as methotrexate, azathioprine, and hydroxychloroquine may be prescribed.[29] In regard to immunosuppressive therapies, in 158 patients enrolled in the Scleroderma Lung Study no difference was noted in the musculoskeletal disease course between patients treated with cyclophosphamide and those treated with placebo.[30] In small uncontrolled series, favorable effects have been reported with anti-TNFa agents,[31] but such results await further confirmation.

Patients with acute arthritis/periarthritis caused by crystal deposition are commonly treated with colchicine,[32] while warfarin has been advocated for the prophylaxis of calcium deposition disease.[33]

Dynamic splinting has not been shown to be of any value in the treatment of flexion contractures.[34] Nevertheless, a tailored rehabilitation program has been reported to improve hand disability.[35] Surgical treatment has been successful in some cases.[36]

Our Patient

Our case study presents some peculiarities: (1) she suffered from SSc *sine* scleroderma of recent onset; (2) she had an autoantibody and capillaroscopic profile typical of lSSc; (3) nevertheless, she developed a symmetric polyarthritis similar to that encountered in SSc patients with early diffuse disease (dSSc). All of these aspects clearly underscore that there is no mutually exclusive pattern of joint involvement in patients affected by distinct SSc subsets. Moreover, from a therapeutic point of view she failed to respond to low-dose steroids and appeared to respond to MTX, which has not yet been proven to be effective in SSc arthritis.

References

1. Bolster MB, Silver RM. Clinical features of systemic sclerosis. In: Hochberg MC, Silman AJ, Smolen JS, Weinblatt ME, Weisman MH, eds. *Rheumatology*. 4th ed. Philadelphia: Mosby Elsevier; 2008:1375-1386.
2. Subcommittee for Scleroderma Criteria of the American Rheumatism Association Diagnostic and Therapeutic Criteria Committee. Preliminary criteria for classification of systemic sclerosis (scleroderma). *Arthritis Rheum*. 1980;23:581-590.
3. Poormoghim H, Lucas M, Fertig N, Medsger TA Jr. Systemic sclerosis sine scleroderma: demographic, clinical, and serologic features and survival in forty-eight patients. *Arthritis Rheum*. 2000;43:444-451.
4. Rodnan GP, Medsger TA Jr. The rheumatic manifestations of progressive systemic sclerosis (scleroderma). *Clin Orthop Relat Res*. 1968;57:81-93.
5. Pope JE. Musculoskeletal involvement in scleroderma. *Rheum Dis Clin North Am*. 2003;29: 391-408.

6. Blocka KLN. Musculoskeletal involvement in systemic sclerosis. In: Clements PJ, Furst DE, eds. *Systemic Sclerosis*. 2nd ed. Philadelphia: Lippincott Williams & Wilkins; 2004:249-260.

7. Rodnan GP. The nature of joint involvement in progressive systemic sclerosis (diffuse sclerodermia). Clinical study and pathologic examination of the synovium in 29 patients. *Ann Intern Med*. 1962;56:422-439.

8. Schumacher HR Jr. Joint involvement in progressive systemic sclerosis (scleroderma): light and electron microscopic study of synovial membrane and fluid. *Am J Clin Pathol*. 1973;60: 593-600.

9. Rodnan GP, Medsger TA Jr. Musculo-skeletal involvement in progressive systemic sclerosis (scleroderma). *Bull Rheum Dis*. 1966;17:419.

10. Lovell CR, Jayson MIV. Joint involvement in systemic sclerosis. *Scand J Rheumatol*. 1979;8:154-160.

11. Baron M, Lee P, Keistone EC. The articular manifestations of progressive systemic sclerosis (scleroderma). *Ann Rheum Dis*. 1982;41:147-152.

12. La Montagna G, Baruffo A, Tirri R, Buono G, Valentini G. Foot involvement in systemic sclerosis. *Semin Arthritis Rheum*. 2002;31:248-255.

13. La Montagna G, Sodano A, Capurro V, Malesci D, Valentini G. The arthropathy of systemic sclerosis: a 12 month prospective clinical and imaging study. *Skeletal Radiol*. 2005;34:35-41.

14. Avouac J, Walzer U, Tyndall A, Kahan A, Matucci-Cerinic M, Allanore Y. Characteristics of joint involvement and relationships with systemic inflammation in systemic sclerosis: results from the EULAR Scleroderma Trial and Research group (EUSTAR) database. *J Rheumatol*. 2010;37(7):1488-1501.

15. Shulman LE, Kurban AK, Harvey AM. Tendon friction rubs in progressive systemic sclerosis (scleroderma). *Trans Assoc Am Physician*. 1961;74:378-388.

16. Steen VD, Medsger TA. The palpable tendon friction rub. An important physical finding in patient with systemic sclerosis. *Arthritis Rheum*. 1997;40:1146-1151.

17. Horiki T, Moriuchi J, Takaya M, et al. The coexistence of systemic sclerosis and rheumatoid arthritis in five patients. Clinical and immunogenetic features suggest a distinct entity. *Arthritis Rheum*. 1996;39(1):152-156.

18. Zimmermann C, Steiner G, Skriner K, Hassfeld W, Petera P, Smolen JS. The concurrence of rheumatoid arthritis and limited systemic sclerosis: clinical and serologic characteristics of an overlap syndrome. *Arthritis Rheum*. 1998;41:1938-1945.

19. Doran M, Wordsworth P, Bresnihan B, Fitzgerald O. A distinct syndrome including features of systemic sclerosis, erosive rheumatoid arthritis, anti-topoisomerase antibody, and rheumatoid factor. *J Rheumatol*. 2001;28:921-922.

20. Szucs G, Szekanecz Z, Zilahi E, et al. Systemic sclerosis-rheumatoid arthritis overlap syndrome: a unique combination of features suggest a distinct genetic, serological and clinical entity. *Rheumatology*. 2007;46:989-993.

21. Ingegnoli F, Galbiati V, Zeni S, et al. Use of antibodies recognizing cyclic citrullinated peptide in the differential diagnosis of joint involvement in systemic sclerosis. *Clin Rheumatol*. 2007;26:510-514.

22. Morita Y, Muro Y, Sugiura K, Tomita Y. Anti-cyclic citrullinated antibody in systemic sclerosis. *Clin Exp Rheumatol*. 2008;26:524-527.

23. Brook A, Corbett M. Radiographic changes in early rheumatoid disease. *Ann Rheum Dis*. 1977;36:71-73.

24. Grassi W, Filippucci E, Farina A, Cervini C. Sonographic image of the distal phalanx. *Semin Arthritis Rheum*. 2000;29:379-384.

25. Cuomo G, Zappia M, Abignano G, Iudici M, Rotondo A, Valentini G. Ultrasonographic features of the hand and the wrist in systemic sclerosis. *Rheumatology*. 2009;48:1414-1417.

26. Chitale S, Ciapetti A, Hodgson R, et al. Magnetic resonance imaging and musculoskeletal ultrasonography detect and characterize covert inflammatory arthropathy in systemic sclerosis with arthralgia. *Rheumatology*. 2010;49(12):2357-2361.

27. La Montagna G, D'Angelo S, Valentini G. Cross-sectional evaluation of YKL-40 serum concentrations in patients with clinical and serological aspects of disease. *J Rheumatol*. 2003;30:2147-2151.

28. Denton CP, Black CM. Management of systemic sclerosis. In: Hochberg MC, Silman AJ, Smolen JS, Weinblatt ME, Weisman MH, eds. *Rheumatology*. 4th ed. Philadelphia: Mosby Elsevier; 2008:1375-1386.

29. Hunzelmann N, Moinzadeh P, Genth E, et al. High frequency of corticosteroid and immuno-suppressive therapy in patients with systemic sclerosis despite limited evidence for efficacy. *Arthritis Res Ther*. 2009;11:R30.

30. Au K, Mayes MD, Maranian P, et al. Course of dermal ulcers and musculoskeletal involvement in systemic sclerosis patients in the scleroderma lung study. *Arthritis Care Res*. 2010; 62(12):1772-1778.

31. Bosello S, De Santis M, Tolusso B, Zoli A, Ferraccioli GF. Tumour necrosis factor-alpha inhibitor therapy in erosive polyarthritis secondary to systemic sclerosis. *Ann Intern Med*. 2005;143:918-920.

32. Fuchs D, Fruchter L, Fishel B, Holtzman M, Yaron M. Colchicine suppression of local inflammation due to calcinosis in dermatomyositis and progressive systemic sclerosis. *Clin Rheumatol*. 1986;5:527-530.

33. Moore SE, Jump AA, Smiley JD. Effect of warfarin on excretion of 4-carboxy-L-glutamic acid in scleroderma, dermatomyositis and myositis ossificans progressive. *Arthritis Rheum*. 1986;29:344-351.

34. Seeger MR, Furst DE. Effects of splinting in the treatment of hand contractures in progressive systemic sclerosis. *Am J Occup Ther*. 1987;41:118-121.

35. Maddali Bongi S, Del Rosso A, Galluccio F, et al. Efficacy of a tailored rehabilitation program for systemic sclerosis. *Clin Exp Rheumatol*. 2009;27(suppl 54):44-50.

36. Norris RW, Brown HG. The proximal interphalangeal joint in systemic sclerosis and its surgical management. *Br J Plast Surg*. 1985;38:526-531.

Chapter 26
Two Scleroderma Patients with Differing Patterns of Muscle Disease

Robyn T. Domsic and Thomas A. Medsger Jr.

Keywords Muscle weakness • Myopathy • Systemic sclerosis

Patient #1

A 33-year-old woman developed symptoms of Raynaud's phenomenon and swollen fingers with sclerodactyly. The serum antinuclear antibody (ANA) was positive in a titer of 1:640 and with a nucleolar staining pattern. The diagnosis of systemic sclerosis was made 1 year later. An extensive evaluation was performed regarding internal organ involvement and she was found to have asymptomatic distal esophageal hypomotility with gastroesophageal reflux and mild bibasilar pulmonary fibrosis. The forced vital capacity (FVC) was 86% predicted and the diffusing capacity for carbon monoxide (DLco) was 78% predicted. An echocardiogram showed a left ventricular ejection fraction of 60% and no evidence of pulmonary hypertension. Prophylactic proton pump inhibitor treatment was begun, along with symptomatic therapy for Raynaud's phenomenon.

Course

Six months after her first visit the patient complained about painless proximal muscle weakness. She had difficulty raising her arms above her head and arising from a chair unassisted. She complained of difficulty swallowing which she perceived to be a problem with initiation of swallowing. She noted a scaly photosensitive rash of the face and scalp and with erythema and scaling of skin over the

T.A. Medsger Jr. (✉)
Division of Rheumatology & Clinical Immunology, Department of Medicine,
University of Pittsburgh Medical Center, 3500 Terrace Street,
Biomedical Science Tower South, 7th Floor, Room 720, Pittsburgh, PA 15261, USA

R.M. Silver and C.P. Denton (eds.), *Case Studies in Systemic Sclerosis*,
DOI: 10.1007/978-0-85729-641-2_26, © Springer-Verlag London Limited 2011

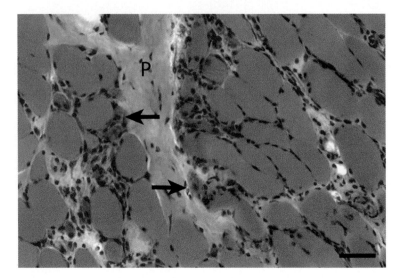

Fig. 26.1 H&E-stained cryostat section showing expansion of the perimysial connective tissue (P), regenerating basophilic fibers (see *arrows* for examples), and an endomysial mononuclear inflammatory cell infiltrate (bar = 50 μm). (Courtesy of David E. Lacomis, MD, Department of Pathology, Neuropathology Division, University of Pittsburgh)

elbows, metacarpophalangeal (MCP) and proximal interphalangeal (PIP) joints, and knees. Physical examination confirmed atrophy of the shoulder girdle muscles and weakness of the neck flexors, shoulder girdle, and hip girdle muscles. The new rash was consistent with Gottron's papules and Gottron's sign. The serum creatine phosphokinase (CPK) was elevated at 3.6 times the upper limits of normal and the serum aldolase was also elevated. Myositis was suspected. An electromyogram (EMG) of the right quadriceps muscle showed irritability on needle insertion, reduced amplitude of muscle action potentials with contraction, and a number of fibrillation potentials. A left (opposite side) vastus lateralis open muscle biopsy showed myofibril degeneration, perifascicular muscle fiber atrophy, and moderate mononuclear cell infiltrates in the perivascular and interstitial areas (Fig. 26.1).

Her physicians concluded that the patient had systemic sclerosis and dermatomyositis in overlap. Further ANA testing revealed that she had anti-PM-Scl antibody. A muscle strengthening program was begun. She was treated with a combination of low-dose prednisone and methotrexate, with normalization of the CPK and aldolase, and subsequent improvement in proximal muscle strength. Muscle strength returned to "almost normal".

Patient #2

A 44-year-old woman had the onset of Raynaud's phenomenon followed in 3 months by heartburn. Thereafter she noted swollen fingers which never again returned to normal size. The diagnosis of SSc was made 1 year after the first symptoms. The

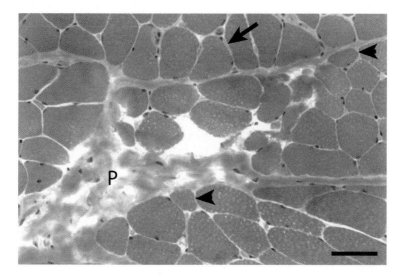

Fig. 26.2 H&E-stained cryostat section reveals a variation in myofiber sizes with some atrophic fibers (see *arrowheads* for examples). There is abnormal expansion of the perimysial connective tissue (P) and mild endomysial fibrosis (see *arrow* for example of increased endomysial connective tissue). Histochemically, most of the atrophic fibers were type 2 fibers (stain not shown). No inflammatory cells were seen (bar = 50 μm). (Courtesy of David E. Lacomis, MD, Department of Pathology, Neuropathology Division, University of Pittsburgh)

ANA was positive and anti-Scl-70 antibody was detected. Esophageal hypomotility was confirmed. Pulmonary function tests, HRCT scan of the lungs, and echocardiogram were normal. No treatment for the primary disease process was prescribed.

At 6-month follow-up evaluation, the patient complained of pain and stiffness affecting the shoulders, most prominent in the morning. She had "weakness" when she tried to elevate her arms above her shoulders and to arise from a chair. On examination the shoulder girdle motion was limited and shoulder muscles were slightly atrophic, but the strength was normal. The serum CPK was mildly elevated (232 units, normal <200 units) and the aldolase was in the normal range. Because of concern about polymyositis, an EMG was performed which showed findings consistent with a noninflammatory myopathy. A subsequent muscle biopsy was interpreted as showing an increased number of atrophic myofibers but no evidence of inflammation. Special stains did not reveal evidence of a metabolic myopathy (Fig. 26.2).

Course

The patient continued to complain about myalgia and a sense of muscle weakness. Over the next 5 years, her physicians were concerned that she had inflammatory muscle disease. However, physical examination was unchanged (no definite weakness) and the serum CPK remained either normal or minimally elevated. When she relocated to another state, her new PCP and rheumatologist decided to reinvestigate the muscle complaints. The serum CPK was at the upper limits of normal (195, normal <200 units), and a repeat EMG was essentially normal. After an additional 5 years (12 years disease duration), the patient's muscle symptoms and physical examination were unchanged. She was able to perform activities of daily living but had myalgia with activity, usually relieved by taking acetaminophen, 2–3 g daily.

Discussion

The diagnosis of myopathy can be challenging in a patient with established systemic sclerosis. Complaints of fatigue and lack of endurance are nonspecific symptoms. Dysphagia can occur with either SSc or myopathy, and detailed history to elicit the location as either proximal (myopathy), distal (SSc), or both may help. Careful attention to the physical examination is important, as myopathy patients often have atrophy and weakness of the neck flexor, shoulder girdle, and hip girdle muscles. Joint involvement, particularly of the shoulders, may result in disuse atrophy. Secondary fibromyalgia may also cause muscle pain and stiffness without objective evidence of muscle injury.[1]

The CPK is a useful screening test as it is the most sensitive and specific of the muscle enzymes. However, some SSc patients may have only an elevated serum aldolase or entirely normal serum muscle enzymes, particularly if they have decreased muscle mass as part of the disease process, or in the setting of intestinal malabsorption. Myalgia and a sensation of muscle weakness can be the presenting features of hypothyroidism, which is common in SSc. When objective weakness is present on physical examination, an EMG is the next step and if the results are suggestive of a myopathy, a muscle biopsy should be done. Magnetic resonance imaging (MRI) may demonstrate areas of edema associated with active myositis, muscle inflammation, and fibrosis, but should not replace EMG or muscle biopsy in diagnosis.

Overall, it has been estimated that approximately 10% of SSc patients develop clinical, biochemical, and histological features of an inflammatory myopathy.[1,2] Biochemical and electromyographic features in these patients are virtually indistinguishable from those of polymyositis or dermatomyositis.[3] In up to one-half of all SSc patients, mild, nonspecific abnormalities suggesting skeletal muscle involvement may occur. These include mild muscle weakness on examination, minimal CPK elevation, nonspecific EMG findings, and a muscle biopsy showing interstitial fibrosis and sparse or no mononuclear cell infiltrates. These individuals may have a normal skeletal muscle MRI.[3] Typically such patients do not have progressive muscle weakness, as demonstrated by the second case presentation.

SSc patients with an inflammatory myopathy are usually younger rather than older. Several case series have reported a higher prevalence in patients with diffuse

Table 26.1 Frequency of myositis[a] in systemic sclerosis by antibody

SSc-associated autoantibody	Percent with myositis (present/total)	Other frequent clinical features
Anti-PM-Scl	26% (12/46)	Dermatomyositis rash; ILD (mild)
Anti-Ku	25% (4/16)	"Overlap" features
Anti-U1RNP	18% (13/71)	Younger with "overlap" findings; ILD
Anti-U3RNP	18% (19/105)	Noninflammatory myopathy; cardiomyopathy; PH
Antitopoisomerase I	17% (94/551)	ILD
Anti-RNA polymerase III	12% (69/576)	Renal crisis
Anti-Th/To	5% (9/170)	PH; ILD
Anticentromere	4% (24/594)	PH
Anti-U11/U12 RNP	3% (1/35)	ILD

Based on data from University of Pittsburgh Scleroderma Database, 1972–2008
[a]Myositis defined as proximal muscle weakness plus one of the following: CPK > 2.0 times normal, EMG consistent with inflammatory myopathy, or muscle biopsy with myositis
ILD interstitial lung disease, *PH* pulmonary hypertension

cutaneous SSc compared to limited cutaneous SSc.[4,5] Overlap syndromes with inflammatory myopathy are particularly frequent in childhood-onset SSc.[6] Patients with particular serum autoantibodies are at greater risk to develop myositis, and their other clinical features are often associated with the autoantibody (Table 26.1). Patients with anti-U1RNP antibody are younger and often have features of SSc, PM/DM, and/or lupus. The ANA is positive in relatively high titer with speckled nuclear staining. Patients with anti-PM-Scl antibody, as in patient #1, may have the rash of dermatomyositis. Interstitial lung disease is common but usually is mild. These patients have the best overall survival of the SSc- and inflammatory myopathy overlap groups. Anti-U3RNP (fibrillarin) antibody-positive patients are typically African-American and frequently have a non-inflammatory myopathy.[7] They are prone to cardiomyopathy and pulmonary arterial hypertension independent of (not secondary to) pulmonary fibrosis. A subgroup of SSc patients with severe and early small intestinal involvement may have antibodies directed against neuromuscular receptors; although such patients may have intestinal smooth muscle dysfunction, they do not have a greater frequency of myositis.[8] These patients have a reduced 10-year cumulative survival. Antitopoisomerase I (Scl-70) antibody-positive SSc patients tend to have mild, easily treatable myositis. There is a high frequency of interstitial lung disease in anti-Scl-70-positive patients, which can be severe.

Rarely, patients with SSc features have anti-Jo1 antibody or one of the other antisynthetase antibodies such as anti-PL7, -PL12; -EJ; or – OJ, etc. The ANA is often negative since the synthetase antigens are located primarily in the cytoplasm. Such patients may have negative antinuclear staining with positive anticytoplasmic staining activity. Patients with antisynthetase antibodies, as well being at increased risk of inflammatory myopathy, can develop severe, progressive pulmonary fibrosis. They often have minimal or no skin thickening, but have other scleroderma features such as Raynaud's phenomenon, abnormal nailfold capillaries, and esophageal dysmotility.

We do not treat SSc patients with noninflammatory myopathy with corticosteroids or immunosuppressive drugs. These patients are referred to physical therapy for a program to maintain or improve muscle strength. When true inflammatory myositis is encountered, we typically prescribe regimens widely accepted for use in polymyositis/dermatomyositis, taking into account the individual patient's other disease manifestations and comorbidities.[9] We generally begin with prednisone 1–2 mg/kg/day in divided doses (not exceeding a total of 80 mg/day), tapering and consolidating to a single daily dose beginning after 1 month. The prednisone dose is generally tapered over 6 months. Once prednisone 5–7.5 mg daily is reached, we continue this low dose for an additional 6–12 months before attempting to discontinue the corticosteroid medication. Serum CPK and aldolase levels are monitored throughout this time period, and manual muscle strength testing is performed to help guide the steroid reduction. If difficulty in steroid reduction is encountered, then immunosuppressive therapy is initiated at that time. In cases of very active myositis with moderate to severe proximal muscle weakness, an immunosuppressive drug is prescribed at the onset with high-dose prednisone. Methotrexate is frequently the first choice in the absence of lung involvement, but other options include azathioprine, mycophenolate mofetil, cyclophosphamide, and cyclosporine. If patients have other disease manifestations requiring treatment, such as interstitial lung disease or active diffuse cutaneous scleroderma, then immunosuppressive drugs may also be started at the same time as prednisone. Patients with anti-RNA polymerase III antibody represent a special population, as these individuals are at significantly increased risk to develop "renal crisis" when receiving high doses of corticosteroids (>15 mg/day).[10] Considering this risk, in these patients we initially use only low doses of steroids at a maximum dose of 10–15 mg daily. In this circumstance, weekly blood pressure measurements should be made, as the abrupt appearance of systemic hypertension may signal the onset of scleroderma renal crisis. Immunosuppressive therapy should be started early in these patients. Osteoporosis prophylaxis should be used in all patients with scleroderma receiving steroid therapy for treatment of myositis.

References

1. Clements PJ, Furst DE, Campion DS, et al. Muscle disease in progressive systemic sclerosis: diagnostic and therapeutic considerations. *Arthritis Rheum*. 1978;21:62-71.
2. Medsger TA, Rodnan GP, Moossy J, Vester JW. The nature of skeletal muscle involvement in progressive systemic sclerosis (scleroderma). *Arthritis Rheum*. 1968;11:554-568.
3. Ranque B, Authier FJ, Le-Guern V, et al. A descriptive and prognostic study of systemic sclerosis-associated myopathies. *Ann Rheum Dis*. 2009;68:1474-1478.
4. Mimura Y et al. Clinical and laboratory features of scleroderma patients developing skeletal myopathy. *Clin Rheumatol*. 2005;24:99-102.

 5. Tager RE, Tikly M. Clinical and laboratory manifestations of systemic sclerosis (scleroderma) in Black South Africans. *Rheumatol (Oxford)*. 1999;28:297-400.
 6. Scalapino K, Arkachaisri T, Lucas M, et al. Childhood onset systemic sclerosis: classification, clinical and serologic features, and survival in comparison with adult onset disease. *J Rheumatol*. 2006;33:1004-1013.
 7. Aggarwal R, Lucas M, Fertig N, Oddis CV, Medsger TA Jr. Anti-U3RNP autoantibody in systemic sclerosis. *Arthritis Rheum*. 2009;60:1112-1118.
 8. Kawaguchi Y, Nakamura Y, Matsumoto I, et al. Muscarinic-3 acetylcholine receptor autoantibody in patients with systemic sclerosis: contribution to severe gastrointestinal tract dysmotility. *Ann Rheum Dis*. 2009;68:710-714.
 9. Catoggio LJ. Management of inflammatory muscle disease. In: Hochberg MC, Silman AJ, Smolen JS, Weinglatt ME, Weisman MH, eds. *Rheumatology*. 4th ed. Philadelphia: Mosby Elsevier; 2008:1461-1468.
10. Steen VD, Medsger TA Jr. Case-control study of corticosteroids and other drugs that either precipitate or protect from the development of scleroderma renal crisis. *Arthritis Rheum*. 1998;41:1613-1619.

Chapter 27
A Limited Cutaneous SSc Patient with Severe Calcinosis and Acro-osteolysis

Francesco Porta and Marco Matucci-Cerinic

Keywords Acro-osteolysis • Calcinosis • Limited cutaneous SSc • Scleroderma

Case Study

A 54-year-old woman presented with pain and swelling of the right elbow and arm with deformity of the distal phalanges of all the fingers. The patient had hard nodules on elbows, forearms, and legs that periodically become erythematous and painful. Nonsteroidal anti-inflammatory drugs were used to control pain.

The patient had a 6-year history of Raynaud's phenomenon (RP). In the 3 years prior to presentation, the RP had worsened and symptoms of gastroesophageal reflux had developed, partially ameliorated with proton pump inhibitor therapy together with dietary and behavioral modification.

Further review of systems revealed the recent onset of dyspnea on exertion (the patient reported shortness of breath when climbing two flights of stairs) as well as induration of the skin of the distal part of the fingers described as "stiffness and loss of sensitivity".

Physical Examination

Temperature 36.5°C, pulse 90 bpm, respiration 16/min, blood pressure 110/70 mmHg. Skin: mild thickening (score 1 of modified Rodnan Skin Score) of the skin of the middle and distal phalanges of the second to the fifth fingers of each hand. There

M. Matucci-Cerinic (✉)
Department of Medicine, University of Florence, Azienda Ospedaliero-Universitaria Careggi, c/o Villa Monna Tessa – Viale Pieraccini 18, Florence 50139, Italy

R.M. Silver and C.P. Denton (eds.), *Case Studies in Systemic Sclerosis*, DOI: 10.1007/978-0-85729-641-2_27, © Springer-Verlag London Limited 2011

Fig. 27.1 Subcutaneous nodules of the left forearm and elbow with cutaneous ulceration

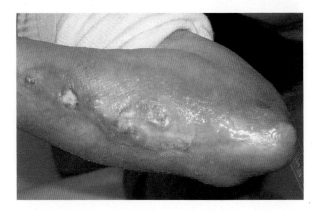

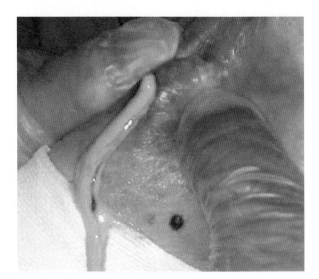

Fig. 27.2 Extrusion of purulent material from the lesion overlying the right elbow

was a pitting scar of the third fingertip of the right hand, and telangiectasias were present on the face. Musculoskeletal: shortening of all the fingers due to reduction in length of the distal phalanges. Multiple hard subcutaneous nodules of about 5 mm diameter were present on the extensor aspect of the elbows and forearms, some with ulceration (Fig. 27.1), and also on the legs and over the left iliac crest. The right elbow was erythematous, swollen, and tender with an ulcerating nodule emitting white material (Fig. 27.2). Examination of the lungs revealed bilateral lower lung crackles. The cardiac, abdominal, and neurological examination was unremarkable.

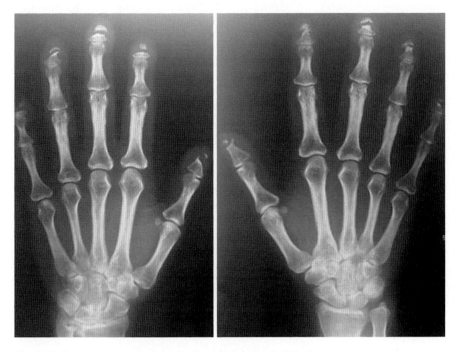

Fig. 27.3 Severe acro-osteolysis of the distal phalanges of all the fingers

Laboratory Findings

Serum electrolytes, liver and renal function tests, and urinalysis were all normal except for mild hyperuricemia. CBC: white blood cell count 16,400/mm, with neutrophilic granulocytosis (12,100/mm^2). Acute phase reactants were elevated: CRP 48 mg/dL (normal < 0.5), ESR 92 mm/h (normal 0–20), and alpha2-globulins were also increased. ANA (titer 1:640) and anticentromere antibodies: positive. Nailfold video-capillaroscopy (NVC): dilated capillary loops with megacapillaries and rare dropout (active scleroderma pattern). Hand and elbow radiographs: severe acro-osteolysis of the distal phalanges of all fingers of both hands (Fig. 27.3), with multiple calcific nodules in the subcutaneous tissue around the elbows. Leg radiographs: multiple calcific nodules in the subcutaneous tissue, notably in the distal limbs (Fig. 27.4).

Musculoskeletal ultrasound: nonhomogeneous hyperechoic material within the olecranon bursa and in the triceps muscle that was displaceable with pressure of the probe, and hyperechoic foci (Fig. 27.5a) with increased vascularization by power Doppler examination (Fig. 27.5b), compatible with a purulent collection in an area of calcinosis.

Fig. 27.4 Diffuse calcinosis of the distal legs

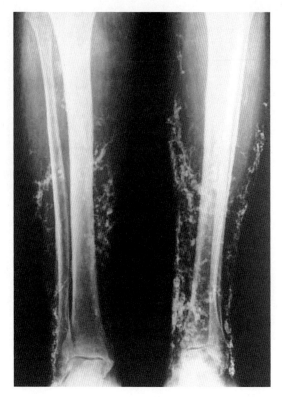

PFT: reduced FVC (55% predicted) and DLco (58% predicted). Chest HRCT: bibasilar ground glass opacities with intraparenchymal bullae. Echocardiogram: normal left ventricular function, tricuspid regurgitation with TR jet velocity of 3.4 m/s, and an estimated systolic PAP of 50 mmHg.

Gastric endoscopy and esophageal manometry: esophageal dysmotility and dilatation of the distal esophagus with gastroesophageal reflux and Grade 1 esophagitis.

Course

The patient was diagnosed with limited cutaneous systemic sclerosis (lSSc) characterized by the presence of calcinosis, Raynaud's phenomenon, sclerodactyly with acro-osteolysis, and esophageal and lung involvement. Right heart catheterization revealed a moderate increase of pulmonary arterial pressure of precapillary origin (mean PAP 39 mmHg with PCWP 11 mmHg), compatible with a diagnosis of pulmonary arterial hypertension (PAH). Significant hypoxia-related pulmonary hypertension secondary to lung fibrosis was considered unlikely due

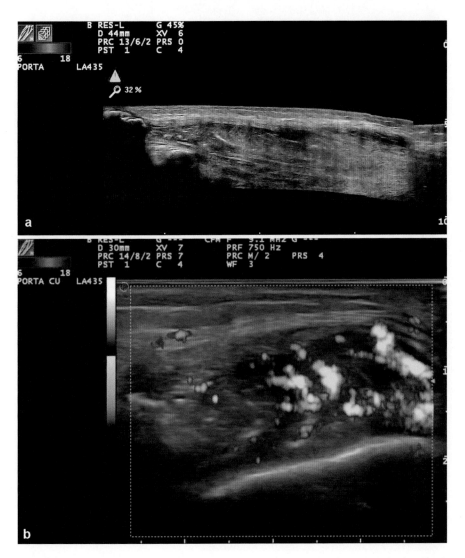

Fig. 27.5 (a) Pus and calcinosis collection of the right elbow detected with gray-scale ultrasound; (b) extensive vascularization of the abscess of the right elbow detected with power Doppler ultrasound

to the relatively high pulmonary arterial pressure and the relatively restricted distribution of the lung fibrosis.

Examination of the surgically drained fluid from the arm revealed pus and white material compatible with calcinosis. Microbiological culture grew *Staphylococcus aureus*. Treatment with parenteral antibiotics was followed by normalization of the WBC and CRP along with resolution of the local inflammatory signs. Surgical excision of the nodules at the elbows was later performed.

Discussion

Based on the distribution of skin involvement, SSc is subclassified as limited (lSSc) or diffuse (dSSc) systemic sclerosis. Usually lSSc is characterized by a slower and milder course, with less severe internal organ involvement and with PAH being the major cause of mortality.[1]

The American College of Rheumatology (ACR) preliminary criteria for the classification of SSc require the presence either of proximal skin involvement, which is the only major criterion, or the presence of two minor criteria (sclerodactyly, digital pitting scars or bibasilar pulmonary fibrosis). In these criteria there is no mention of nailfold capillary morphology or laboratory findings, e.g., ANA or scleroderma-specific autoantibodies. Although the criteria are very specific, they lack sensitivity particularly for the lSSc subset, and thus many early or mildly affected patients may go undiagnosed.[2]

Newer criteria that have been proposed for the classification of early SSc include the presence of RP, puffy fingers, abnormal nailfold capillary morphology, and SSc-specific autoantibodies.[3] (see Chap. 1).

Thus, it is important to investigate every patient who presents with RP at least with nailfold capillary microscopy and ANA, in order to ascertain if the RP is either primary or secondary and so as not to miss the opportunity of making a diagnosis of early SSc.

The patient in this case study gave a history of RP with onset during adulthood, and she was found to have digital pitting scars and gastroesophageal reflux; however, neither nailfold capillary microscopy nor ANA testing was performed at that time. Moreover, the patient had subcutaneous nodules which were not initially investigated. Actually, in this patient a diagnosis of SSc could have been made some years before with treatment started in due time.

Calcinosis is a very frequent feature of lSSc (20–60% of patients) and is localized predominantly on the extremities.[4,5] Sometimes it can affect other sites like the face or the spine.[6,7] In the literature there are several classifications of soft tissue calcifications.[4] Boulman et al. found calcinosis (dystrophic calcification) to be the most frequent type seen in rheumatic disease patients, followed by other uncommon forms such as tumoral or metastatic calcinosis.

Calcinosis consists of deposits of calcium hydroxyapatite crystals at sites of recurrent microtrauma, e.g., the fingers, elbows, and iliac crest. The pathogenesis is still under debate but seems to be promoted by tissue damage, hypoxia, mechanical trauma, or age-related tissue changes.[4]

Calcinosis is usually an incidental finding detected on radiographs, but sometimes can be painful and can ulcerate with possible secondary infection.[4,8]

Several drugs such as diltiazem,[9] warfarin,[10] colchicine,[11] probenecid,[12] bisphosphonates,[13] and minocycline[14] have been used to treat calcinosis. All have been reported to have variable degrees of success, without a clear superiority of one drug over others. A possible exception might be minocycline which, when used in a small number of patients for a long period, improvement of calcinosis and healing of the ulcers was reported. The mechanism of action is unknown but the authors suggested that matrix metalloproteinase inhibition might be the predominant mechanism.[14]

Surgical excision of calcinosis may be useful in some cases. Although the data about recurrence rates are discordant,[7] some authors consider recurrence to be related to incomplete surgical excision.[15] Indications for surgical excision would include pain, infection, ulceration, local functional impairment, and cosmetic reasons.[16]

A novel method to reduce the size of calcinosis is extracorporeal shock wave lithotripsy, which has been reported to be successful in one SSc patient.[17]

In our patient a surgical option was prompted by an abscess secondary to infection of ulcerated calcinosis.

Acro-osteolysis (AC) refers to digital tuft desorption due to bone destruction with reduction in the length of the fingers. AC has been reported to occur in 10–50% of SSc patients and is the most frequent osseous complication, involving the hands more often than the feet.[18-22] AC has been correlated with lung and esophageal involvement and with erosive arthritis. Our patient presented with both lung and esophageal involvement but had no arthritis (no erosions on radiographs).[23]

No treatment for AC is supported by the medical literature, but since chronic ischemia has been proposed as one of the main factors in its pathogenesis,[23] we initiated a trial of treatment with iloprost.

References

1. LeRoy EC, Black C, Fleischmajer R, et al. Scleroderma (systemic sclerosis): classification, subsets and pathogenesis. *J Rheumatol*. 1988;15(2):202-205.
2. Subcommittee for scleroderma criteria of the American Rheumatism Association Diagnostic and Therapeutic Criteria Committee. Preliminary criteria for the classification of systemic sclerosis (scleroderma). *Arthritis Rheum*. 1980;23(5):581-590.
3. LeRoy EC, Medsger TA. Criteria for the classification of early systemic sclerosis. *J Rheumatol*. 2001;28(7):1573-1576. Review.
4. Boulman N, Slobodin G, Rozenbaum M, Rosner I. Calcinosis in rheumatic diseases. *Semin Arthritis Rheum*. 2005;34(6):805-812.
5. Vayssairat M, Hidouche D, Abdoucheli-Baudot N, Gaitz JP. Clinical significance of subcutaneous calcinosis in patients with systemic sclerosis. Does diltiazem induce its regression? *Ann Rheum Dis*. 1998;57(4):252-254.
6. Ogawa T, Ogura T, Ogawa K, et al. Paraspinal and intraspinal calcinosis: frequent complications in patients with systemic sclerosis. *Ann Rheum Dis*. 2009;68(10):1655-1656.
7. Nestal-Zibo H, Rinne I, Glükmann M, Kaha H. Calcinosis on the face in systemic sclerosis: case report and overview of relevant literature. *J Oral Maxillofac Surg*. 2009;67(7):1530-1539.
8. Amanzi L, Braschi F, Fiori G, et al. Digital ulcers in scleroderma: staging, characteristics and sub-setting through observation of 1,614 digital lesions. *Rheumatol (Oxford)*. 2010;49(7):1374-1382.
9. Torralba TP, Li-Yu J, Navarra ST. Successful use of diltiazem in calcinosis caused by connective tissue disease. *J Clin Rheumatol*. 1999;5(2):74-78.

10. Cukierman T, Elinav E, Korem M, Chajek-Shaul T. Low dose warfarin treatment for calcinosis in patients with systemic sclerosis. *Ann Rheum Dis*. 2004;63(10):1341-1343.
11. Fuchs D, Fruchter L, Fishel B, Holtzman M, Yaron M. Colchicine suppression of local inflammation due to calcinosis in dermatomyositis and progressive systemic sclerosis. *Clin Rheumatol*. 1986;5(4):527-530.
12. Meyers D. Treatment of calcinosis circumscripta and Raynaud's phenomenon. *Med J Aust*. 1976;2(12):457.
13. Rabens SF, Bethune JE. Disodium etidronate therapy for dystrophic cutaneous calcification. *Arch Dermatol*. 1975;111(3):357-361.
14. RobertsonL P, Marshall R, Hickling P. Treatment of cutaneous calcinosis in limited systemic sclerosis with minocycline. *Ann Rheum Dis*. 2003;62:267-269.
15. Noyez JF, Murphree SM, Chen K. Tumoral calcinosis, a clinical report of eleven cases. *Acta Orthop Belg*. 1993;59(3):249-254.
16. Lipskeir E, Weizenbluth M. Calcinosis circumscripta: indications for surgery. *Bull Hosp Jt Dis Orthop Inst*. 1989;49(1):75-84.
17. Sparsa A, Lesaux N, Kessler E, et al. Treatment of cutaneous calcinosis in CREST syndrome by extracorporeal shock wave lithotripsy. *J Am Acad Dermatol*. 2005;53(5):263-265.
18. Baron M, Lee P, Keystone EC. The articular manifestations of progressive systemic sclerosis (scleroderma). *Ann Rheum Dis*. 1982;41(2):147-152.
19. La Montagna G, Sodano A, Capurro V, Malesci D, Valentini G. The arthropathy of systemic sclerosis: a 12 month prospective clinical and imaging study. *Skeletal Radiol*. 2005;34(1):35-41. Epub 2004 Sep 17.
20. Blocka KL, Bassett LW, Furst DE, Clements PJ, Paulus HE. The arthropathy of advanced progressive systemic sclerosis. A radiographic survey. *Arthritis Rheum*. 1981;24(7):874-884.
21. Avouac J, Guerini H, Wipff J, et al. Radiological hand involvement in systemic sclerosis. *Ann Rheum Dis*. 2006;65(8):1088-1092.
22. Resnick D. *Scleroderma (Progressive Systemic Sclerosis). Diagnosis of Bone and Joint Disorders*. 3rd ed. Philadelphia: Saunders; 1995:1191-1217.
23. Erre GL, Marongiu A, Fenu P, et al. The "sclerodermic hand": a radiological and clinical study. *Joint Bone Spine*. 2008;75(4):426-431.

Chapter 28
A 54-Year Old Woman with Pain and Stiffness of Hands and Tendon Friction Rubs

Dinesh Khanna and Puja P. Khanna

Keywords Diffuse cutaneous systemic sclerosis (dSSc) • Survival • Tendon friction rubs

Case Study

MW is a 54-year-old woman with generalized muscle pain and fatigue that started 2 months ago. She complained of pain and morning stiffness of her hands and feet lasting approximately 2 h. She did not complain of Raynaud's phenomenon, puffy fingers, recent upper respiratory tract infection, rash, oral ulcers, or pleuritic chest pain. On further questioning, she complained of mild heartburn consistent with gastro-esophageal reflux.

Physical Examination

Vitals: Temperature 37.6°C; pulse 88 bpm; respiration rate 14/min; blood pressure 120/80 mmHg. Musculoskeletal: Inflammatory polyarthritis of her hands, wrists, and feet. Also noted were grating, "squeaking" sensations of the extensor tendons of the wrists and ankles on active motion. Muscle strength was normal (5/5) in the proximal and distal muscle groups of all extremities. Skin: No sclerodactyly or digital pitted scars. The fingers of both hands were "puffy" and there was periungual erythema and telangiectasias on the fingers. HEENT: PERRLA, good salivary production. Chest: no adventitial breath sounds. Cardiac: regular rate and rhythm with normal S1

D. Khanna (✉)
University of Michigan, Ann Arbor, MI 48109, USA

R.M. Silver and C.P. Denton (eds.), *Case Studies in Systemic Sclerosis*,
DOI: 10.1007/978-0-85729-641-2_28, © Springer-Verlag London Limited 2011

and S2 heart sounds. Abdomen: non-distended and non-tender. Extremities: no pedal edema.

Laboratory Findings

CBC, chemistry panel, CK, and urinalysis: normal. ANA 1:1,280 with speckled pattern, negative anti-centromere antibody, positive anti-Scl-70 antibody, negative anti-CCP antibody, and negative rheumatoid factor. Barium swallow: decreased motility with spontaneous gastro-esophageal reflux. Chest radiograph: clear lung fields and normal cardiac size.

Course

The patient developed redness and pruritus of her forearms and legs and noticed skin thickening of her fingers and forearms over the following 2 months. HRCT of the chest showed minimal interstitial thickening consistent with non-specific intestinal pneumonitis. PFTs: FVC 1.90 L (75% predicted); FEV1 1.2 L (78% predicted); DLco 12.2 (68% predicted). Echocardiogram: normal LV ejection fraction, normal RA and RV dimensions, minimal tricuspid regurgitation with estimated RVSP of 30–35 mmHg. Over the next year, the patient developed skin thickening of the forearms, arms, and chest consistent with diffuse cutaneous SSc (dSSc). She developed mild hand contractures and continued to have grating sensations of the extensor tendons of fingers, wrists and ankles consistent with tendon friction rubs.

Discussion

Tendon friction rubs (TFR) were first described by Westphal in 1876, who noted coarse cracking and crepitus of the fingers and knees of a young patient with dSSc.[1] In 1961, Shulman attributed these grating sensations to the fibrinous deposits on the surface of the tendon sheaths and overlying fascia.[2] Rodnan and Medsger described this finding as a "leathery crepitus" on palpation of the knees, wrists, fingers, and ankles during motion.[3] They documented the origin of such rubs as tendons by performing sound tracings of knee joint movement in a patient with SSc and in a normal knee. Pathological examination demonstrated fibrinous deposits on the surface of the tendon sheaths and overlying fascia, but relatively little evidence of reactive inflammation.

Tendon friction rubs are common in patients with early dSSc. In two large observational studies that included both limited (lSSc) and diffuse (dSSc) patients, TFR were present in 10–28% of patients with SSc.[4,5] Importantly, TFR herald the

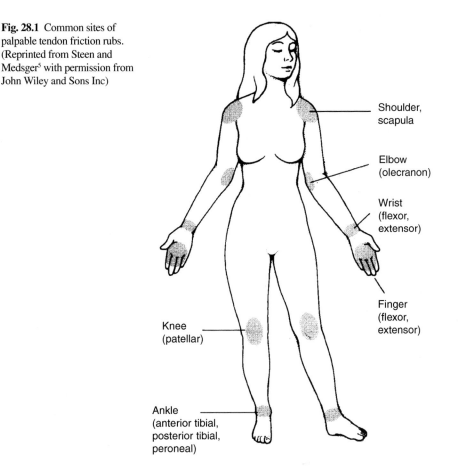

Fig. 28.1 Common sites of palpable tendon friction rubs. (Reprinted from Steen and Medsger[5] with permission from John Wiley and Sons Inc)

Shoulder, scapula

Elbow (olecranon)

Wrist (flexor, extensor)

Finger (flexor, extensor)

Knee (patellar)

Ankle (anterior tibial, posterior tibial, peroneal)

development of dSSc. In the analysis from the University of Pittsburgh database,[5] 91% of patients with early SSc who had TFR subsequently developed dSSc. When assessing patients with early dSSc (defined as within the first 5 years), TFR were prevalent in approximately 37–60% of patients.[4,5] In the Pittsburgh database, the presence of TFR had a positive predictive value of 85% for developing dSSc and a negative predictive value of 83%.[6] In other words, the presence of TFR in patients with early scleroderma predicts the development of dSSc in 85% of patients, whereas the absence of TFR portends that 83% of these patients will not develop dSSc.

Tendon friction rubs are also associated with more severe dSSc – higher skin scores, joint contractures, greater physical disability, higher prevalence of cardiac or renal involvement, and decreased survival.[4,5,7] Interestingly, patients with lSSc and TFR had greater disease severity, greater prevalence of anti-Scl-70 antibody, and poor survival suggesting "subclinical" or "aborted" dSSc.[4]

On physical examination, TFR are most commonly present in the flexor and extensor tendons of fingers and wrists and the anterior tibial and peroneal tendons (Fig. 28.1). In a randomized controlled trial (RCT) involving patients with early

Table 28.1 Locations of tendon friction rubs in the D-penicillamine study (*N*=132)

Site location	*N* (%)
Fingers	26 (20)
Wrists	18 (14)
Elbows	10 (7.6)
Knees	16 (12)
Ankles	24 (18)
Shoulders	3 (2.3)
Other areas	4 (3)

dSSc (≤18 months from first non-Raynaud's phenomenon symptom),[7] 14–20% of TFR were present in these three areas (Table 28.1). This RCT also showed the dynamic nature of TFR: only 10% of patients having TFR at baseline continued to have TFR at subsequent visits, whereas 21% developed new TFR over a 2-year follow-up period. The change in TFR (decrease or increase in the number of TFR compared with baseline) over 6 and 12 months in the D-penicillamine RCT heralded changes in skin thickening and functional disability over 12 and 24 months. In other words, an improvement/worsening of TFR at 6 and 12 months heralded an improvement/worsening in skin thickening and functional disability at 12 and 24 months.

How can these results be used in clinical practice? The presence and finding of TFR during routine examination predates and heralds development of more severe SSc. TFR are a frequent physical finding in patients with early disease that should be routinely assessed when a patient presents with a constellation of signs and symptoms that suggest SSc, including recent onset arthritis, Raynaud's phenomenon and puffy, swollen fingers. TFR produce a grating, "squeaking" sensation that is detected on passive or active motion of the affected tendon. TFR can be intermittent and may remit with repeated motion. Patients often report TFR and since they are often painless, most patients are somewhat surprised or perplexed by these "squeaky" noises. We have proposed that at least three common sites (fingers, wrists, and ankles) should be assessed for the presence of TFR during routine physical examination; improvement in the number of TFR heralds improvement in skin thickening and functional disability. Musculoskeletal ultrasound and magnetic resonance imaging (Fig. 28.2) may be helpful in the diagnosis of TFR, and these advanced imaging procedures may also demonstrate the origin of the TFR.

What should one do for patients with TFR? The presence of TFR should alert the rheumatologist to a potentially more severe SSc disease course. We recommend appropriate serological testing (anti-Scl-70 and anti-RNA polymerase III are both associated with dSSc), baseline work-up for internal organ involvement (recently detailed[8]), and an office visit at least every 3 months (preferably every 4–8 weeks) to assess progression of skin thickening and development or progression of internal organ involvement. Vigilant monitoring of blood pressure is essential and most patients can do this at home after simple instruction. They should be educated about the risks of new hypertension and the importance of seeking medical attention. We use low-dose oral prednisone (≤ 10 mg daily) since there is an increased prevalence of associated synovitis in patients with TFR. We have also used methotrexate

Fig. 28.2 Proton density fat-saturated MRI demonstrating fluid surrounding the posterior tibial and peroneal tendons (*arrows*). (Figure kindly provided by Dr. T. Pope, Medical University of South Carolina)

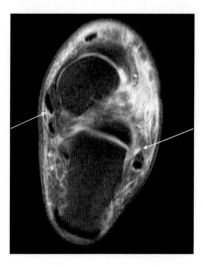

(10–25 mg weekly, administered either orally or subcutaneously) if an associated synovitis is causing moderate physical disability (defined as Health Assessment Questionnaire-Disability Index of ≥1.0). In the absence of synovitis, we treat painful TFR with non-steroidal anti-inflammatory agents, carefully monitoring renal function, and occupational/physical therapy with or without low-dose oral prednisone. Whether early treatment of SSc with immunosuppressive agents in the presence of only TFR will prevent further worsening of skin sclerosis, functional disability or internal organ involvement still needs to be addressed.

References

1. Westphal C. Zwei falle von schlerodermie. *Chariete Ann (Berlin)*. 1876;3:341-360.
2. Shulman LE, Kurban AK, Harvey AM. Tendon friction rubs in progressive system sclerosis (scleroderma). *Trans Assoc Am Physicians*. 1961;74:378-388.
3. Rodnan GP, Medsger TA. The rheumatic manifestaions of progressive systemic sclerosis (scleroderma). *Clin Orthop Relat Res*. 1968;57:81-93.
4. Avouac J, Walker U, Tyndall A, et al. Characteristics of joint involvement and relationships with systemic inflammation in systemic sclerosis: results from the EULAR Scleroderma Trial and Research Group (EUSTAR) database. *J Rheumatol*. 2010;37(7):1488-1501.
5. Steen VD, Medsger TA Jr. The palpable tendon friction rub: an important physical examination finding in patients with systemic sclerosis. *Arthritis Rheum*. 1997;40(6):1146-1151.
6. Sanchez-Guerrero J. Predictive value of the presence or absence of palpable tendon friction rubs in scleroderma: comment on the article by Steen and Medsger. *Arthritis Rheum*. 1998;41(1):186-187.
7. Khanna PP, Furst D, Clements P, Maranian P, Indulkar L, Khanna D. Tendon friction rubs in early diffuse systemic sclerosis: prevalence, characteristics and longitudinal changes in a randomized controlled trial. *Rheumatol (Oxford)*. 2010;49(5):955-959.
8. Khanna D, Denton CP. Evidence-based management of rapidly progressing systemic sclerosis. *Best Pract Res Clin Rheumatol*. 2010;24(3):387-400.

Chapter 29
A Young Diffuse Scleroderma Patient Having Difficulties with Activities of Daily Living

Janet L. Poole

Keywords Occupational therapy • Physical therapy • Activities of daily living • Exercise • Pain management • Modalities • Energy conservation

Case Study

The client is a 31-year-old woman who was diagnosed with diffuse systemic sclerosis (dSSc) 2 years ago. She is single and a student working on her master's degree in business administration at a major university. She lives by herself and enjoys hiking for leisure.

Occupational Therapy Evaluation

Client's shoulder and elbow range of motion are within normal limits. Her wrist and finger range of motion measurements are shown in Table 29.1. As part of the Occupational Therapy Evaluation, the client was interviewed using the Canadian Occupational Performance Measure in which the client identified difficulty performing the following activities of daily living: oral hygiene, manipulating fasteners on clothes, opening jars, cans, and other containers, getting on and off the sofa and toilet. She also has difficulty taking notes in class because the classroom environment is so cold and using a keyboard.

J.L. Poole
Department of Occupational Therapy Graduate Program, Pediatrics,
University of New Mexico, MSC 09 5240,
Albuquerque, NM 87131-0001, USA

R.M. Silver and C.P. Denton (eds.), *Case Studies in Systemic Sclerosis*,
DOI: 10.1007/978-0-85729-641-2_29, © Springer-Verlag London Limited 2011

Table 29.1 Hand and wrist range of motion measurements in degrees of motion

Left hand	Joint motion (norm)	Right hand
0/80	Index: MCP ext[a]/flexion (0/90)	0/80
5/95	PIP ext[a]/flex (0/100)	10/90
5/95	DIP ext[a]/flex (0/90)	5/95
0/80	Middle: MCP ext[a]/flexion (0/90)	0/80
10/95	PIP ext[a]/flex (0/100)	10/95
0/90	DIP ext[a]/flex (0/90)	0/90
0/85	Ring: MCP ext[a]/flexion (0/90)	0/85
5/100	PIP ext[a]/flex (0/100)	10/95
0/90	DIP ext[a]/flex (0/90)	0/90
0/85	Little: MCP ext[a]/flexion (0/90)	0/85
5/100	PIP ext[a]/flex (0/100)	5/100
0/90	DIP ext[a]/flex (0/90)	0/90
0/65	Wrist extension (0/70)	0/65
0/75	Wrist flexion (0/80)	0/80

MCP metacarophalangeal joint, *PIP* proximal interphangeal joint, *DIP* distal interphangeal joint, *ext* extension, *flex* flexion
[a]If the extension number is not 0, then there is a limitation in extension of the joint, that is, the joint does not extend completely

Physical Therapy Evaluation

Client has slightly decreased external rotation in her hips, extension in her knees, and dorsiflexion in her ankles. She ambulates independently without any assistive devices but fatigues easily. An evaluation of her upper and lower extremity strength revealed 3+/5 strength in the shoulder and hip muscles and 4/5 strength in the rest of her muscles.

Discussion

Occupational and physical therapists work with people who have scleroderma to maintain and/or restore maximum movement and to facilitate the performance of activities that are meaningful to them.[1,2] Around 25% of persons with SSc have arthritis; and thus, therapy along with optimal medical management is important in restoring movement. For the client described in the case study above, occupational therapy intervention would consist of instruction in range of motion exercises specifically for the hand and mouth; provision of alternative techniques and assistive devices to perform daily tasks; and instruction in energy conservation principles. Range of motion exercises are indicated to prevent further loss of motion. These should be done frequently and beyond resistance. A position of stretch should be maintained for 3–5 s even if the skin blanches. Because the client in the case has the typical contractures seen in scleroderma, i.e., decreased flexion of the metacarpo-phalangeal (MCP) joints, decreased extension of the proximal interphalangeal (PIP) joints, and decreased abduction of the thumb, the exercises would focus on increasing motion in those joints. Digital ulcers over the bony prominences, especially the dorsum of the PIP joints, make range of motion exercises particularly painful. Clients should seek immediate treatment for ulcers as cessation of the exercises may lead to further limitations in joint motion.

To increase flexion in the MCP joint, an individual makes a fist and uses the palm of the other hand to press down on the dorsum of the proximal phalanges to get more flexion. The pictures in Fig. 29.1 show exercises to increase extension in the PIP joint. Figure 29.1a shows the use of 3 points of pressure. The first point of pressure is the pulp or pad of the index finger on the volar side of the finger just distal to the joint. The second point of pressure is the third finger against the volar side of the finger just proximal to the joint, and the third point of pressure is the thumb against the dorsum of the PIP joint. The thumb pushes against the joint while the index and middle fingers apply counter pressure to attempt to straighten the joint. Figure 29.1b shows the palm of one hand pressing the fingers of the other hand flat down against the table to increase PIP extension.

Two exercises might be recommended for the thumb. For thumb abduction, the pads of the thumb and index fingers of both hands are placed together and the person attempts to push the thumbs away from the index fingers and open the web space between the fingers (Fig. 29.2a). For thumb flexion, the thumb is flexed to try to touch the base of the little finger (Fig. 29.2b).

Prior to performing the exercises, paraffin wax treatment, which delivers superficial conductive heat and softens the skin, could be used. Paraffin wax bath is a mixture of paraffin and mineral oil. The hands are dipped into the bath 1–3 times until a glove of wax forms on the hand. The limb is wrapped in a plastic bag or Saran™ wrap or between sheets of wax paper and then covered with an insulated fabric such as layers of towels. The part remains wrapped for about 20 min. Usually the temperature should be 126–130°F but may need to be lower depending on tolerance. Paraffin wax in conjunction with exercises has been shown to improve joint motion and hand function.[3-5] Massage may be indicated to increase circulation and tissue elasticity and to decrease edema. In SSc, recent studies have shown that a deep massage to the hand in conjunction with joint manipulation improved finger flexion and hand function.[6]

Oral exercises can be done to stretch the mouth to make oral hygiene and dental care easier (see Chap. 32). Three types of exercises have been shown to improve oral opening: exaggerated facial movements, manual stretching, and augmentation.[7] Exaggerated facial movements involve exaggerated smiling, pursing or puckering the lips, and opening the mouth wide. Manual stretching involves using the fingers to stretch the oral opening. The right thumb is placed in the left corner of the mouth, the left thumb in the right corner of the mouth and then the thumbs are pulled apart to the stretch the mouth laterally; the stretch is held 3–5 s and repeated. Oral augmentation exercises involve inserting tongue depressors between the teeth from the premolar area on one side of the mouth to the molar area on the other side.

Fig. 29.1 (**a**) Exercise
showing 3 points of pressure
(index and middle finger on
volar surface and thumb over
dorsum of joint) to extend
PIP joint. (**b**) Exercise using
palm of one hand to push PIP
joints on the other hand into
extension using the table
surface for counter pressure

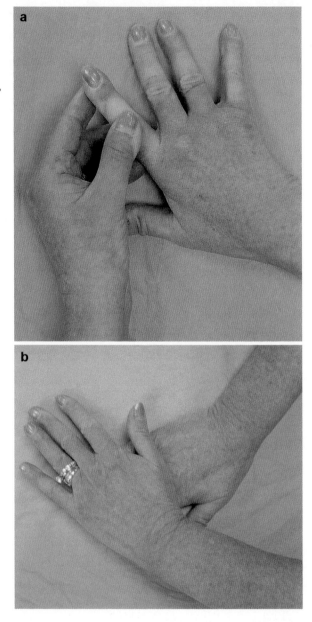

These exercises have been shown to improve oral opening and oral hygiene.[8,9] The
exercises can be done in the shower or in the dentist office before the dentist or
hygienist comes into the room.

Occupational therapists also recommend assistive devices and alternative techniques to help increase the performance of daily tasks including self care, work and

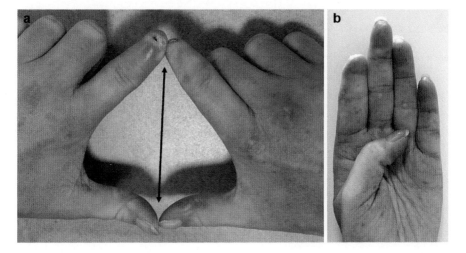

Fig. 29.2 (**a**) Exercise to increase thumb abduction; the thumbs push away from the index fingers widening the web space. (**b**) Exercise to increase thumb flexion by touching the tip of the thumb to the base of the little finger

leisure.[10] Assistive devices are items, equipment, or a system used to improve performance, reduce pain, or minimize extra stress on joints while performing activities of daily living. For a client, such as the woman described in this case study, for oral hygiene the occupational therapist would recommend electric toothbrushes, water jets or electric flossers, curved bristle brushes, or child-sized toothbrushes.

Assistive devices are also available to help compensate for deficits in hand function or object manipulation (e.g. built up utensils, button hooks, jar openers); reach (reachers, long sponges, sock aids, shoe horns), and muscle weakness (e.g. bath benches, raised toilet seats, grab bars, extenders for chair and bed legs). Alternative techniques might include wearing clothing without fasteners (pull over shirts, elastic waistbands, slip on shoes) and using electrical appliances such as can/jar openers, crock pots, and food processors. For the client in the case, who reported difficulty taking notes in a cold classroom, besides recommending wearing layers of clothes, the occupational therapist might recommend she sit in the front row of the classroom and use a tape recorder to record lectures so she could keep her hands in gloves or pockets. If the client prefers to take notes on a laptop, the OT might recommend she wear fingerless gloves to keyboard and place her hands in her pockets when not keyboarding. The client could also contact the Office of Equal Opportunity or similar unit at her university and request accommodations and ask for a note taker. Voice recognition programs could be used outside the classroom environment.

Use of energy conservation principles might be recommended for persons who complain of fatigue.[11] Clients are taught strategies to pace activities, alternate and pace heavy and light activities during the day and week, prioritize activities that

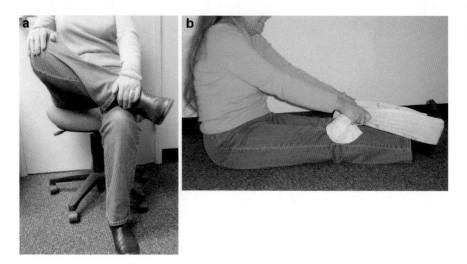

Fig. 29.3 (**a**) Exercise to increase external rotation of the hip; slight pressure on the knee to stretch the inner thigh muscles. (**b**) Exercise to stretch the hamstring muscles to increase extension of the knees by placing a towel around the bottom of the feet and pulling on the towel; exercise also increases dorsiflexion in the ankle

need to be accomplished, plan, and position the body appropriately including good posture, use of proper body mechanics, and ergonomic strategies.

For persons with scleroderma, physical therapy intervention would focus on increasing or maintaining mobility and strength and general conditioning, and pain management. Because of the decreased joint motion in the hips, knees, and ankles, the client in the case, would be encouraged to do range of motion exercise and hold the positions at the end range for 3–5 s as shown in Fig. 29.3a, b. The exercise in the picture on the left showing external rotation of the hip is stretching the inner thigh muscles and the subject pushes slightly on her knee. The picture on the right shows a stretch for the hamstring muscles. A towel is placed around the bottom of the feet and she pulls on the towel to lean forward to stretch the hamstrings; this also stretches dorsiflexion of the ankle.

Resistive exercises are often prescribed by physical therapists to strengthen weak muscles. Weight machines, resistive bands, or weight cuffs may be used depending on the strength and ability to grasp.[12] For the client described earlier, to strengthen the shoulders and hip muscles, the physical therapist might suggest using an arm ergometer and exercise bike or resistance exercises using weight cuffs or elastic material such as bands or tubing.

For general conditioning, the physical therapist might suggest a graduated cardiovascular conditioning program such as water exercise, treadmill walking or walking, biking, swimming, yoga, tai chi, etc. For a person, such as the woman described earlier, a walking program beginning 15 min once daily might be recommended. Instructions would be give to gradually increase her time, the number of days/week, and distance. Pedometers and exercise action plans such as those used in arthritis self-management programs[13] might be used to motivate and improve adherence. A recent study showed that a supervised cardiovascular exercise program of moderate intensity was safe and improved aerobic capacity and oxygen saturation in women who had SSc without pulmonary involvement.[14] Aquatic exercises such as those offered by the Arthritis Foundation can help improve cardiovascular conditioning, joint motion, and reduce pain. Since the water temperature is warm, this usually poses no problems for persons with Raynaud's phenomenon. However, the chlorine from the pool chemical can cause drying of the skin, so a shower should be taken soon after getting out of the pool followed by application of moisturizing cream.

Pain management might consist of heat modalities such as paraffin wax described earlier, hot packs, and hydrotherapy. Heat modalities deliver superficial conductive heat to relieve pain and may increase extensibility of collagen tissue. Heat modalities should be used under the direction of a therapist and with caution in the presence of Raynaud's phenomenon. Relaxation techniques such as deep breathing, guided imagery, meditation, and yoga have been recommended to release muscle tension and pain in rheumatic conditions besides SSc.[13]

In summary, referral to occupational and physical therapy should be considered as part of a comprehensive management of persons with SSc. Exercises, energy conservation, assistive devices, alternative techniques, modalities, and education have been shown to improve the performance of daily tasks and mobility in the home, work, and community environment.[15]

References

1. Standards of Practice: Occupational Therapy Competencies in Rheumatology. http://www.rheumatology.org/practice/clinical/standards/occstandards.asp. Accessed 27 Sept 2010.
2. Standards of Practice: Discipline-Specific Standards of Care: Physical Therapy Competencies in Rheumatology. http://www.rheumatology.org/practice/clinical/standards/ptstandards.asp. Accessed 27 Sept 2010.
3. Pils K, Graninger W, Sadil F. Paraffin hand bath for scleroderma. *Phys Med Rehabil*. 1991;1: 19-21.
4. Sandqvist G, Akesson A, Eklund M. Evaluation of paraffin bath treatment in patients with systemic sclerosis. *Disabil Rehabil*. 2004;26:981-987.
5. Mancuso T, Poole JL. The effect of paraffin and exercise on hand function in persons with scleroderma: a series of single case studies. *J Hand Ther*. 2009;22:71-77.
6. Maddali Bongi S, Del Rosso A, Galluccio F, et al. Efficacy of connective tissue massage and McMennel joint manipulation in the rehabilitative treatment of the hands in systemic sclerosis. *Clin Rheumatol*. 2009;28:1167-1173.
7. Naylor WP, Douglass CW, Mix E. The nonsurgical treatment of microstomia in scleroderma: a pilot study. *Oral Surg*. 1984;57:508-511.
8. Pizzo G, Scardina GA, Messina P. Effects of a nonsurgical exercise program on the decreased mouth opening in patients with systemic scleroderma. *Clin Oral Investig*. 2003;7:175-178.
9. Poole JL, Brewer C, Good C, et al. Effectiveness of customized intervention on oral hygiene in subjects with scleroderma. *Disabil Rehabil*. 2010;32:379-384.

10. Sandqvist G, Eklund M, Akesson A, Nordenskiold U. Daily activities and hand function in women with scleroderma. *Scand J Rheumatol*. 2004;33:102-107.
11. Samuelson UK, Ahlmen EM. Development and evaluation of a patient education program for persons with systemic sclerosis (scleroderma). *Arthritis Care Res*. 2000;13:141-148.
12. Antonioli CM, Bua G, Frige A, et al. An individualized rehabilitation program in patients with systemic sclerosis may improve quality of life and hand mobility. *Clin Rheumatol*. 2009;28: 159-165.
13. Lorig K, Fries JF. *The Arthritis Helpbook*. Cambridge: Perseus Books; 2000.
14. Oliveira NC, dos Santos Sabbag LM, de Sa Pinto AL, et al. Aerobic exercise is safe and effective in systemic sclerosis. *Int J Sports Med*. 2009;30:728-732.
15. Poole JL. Musculoskeletal rehabilitation in the person with scleroderma. *Curr Opin Rheumatol*. 2010;22:205-212.

Chapter 30
A Middle-Aged Male Scleroderma Patient Who Can No Longer Perform His Occupation

Janet Pope

Keywords Limited cutaneous SSc (lSSc) • Diffuse cutaneous SSc (dSSc) • Work disability (WD) • HAQ-DI (Health Assessment Questionnaire-Disability Index) • Presenteeism work questionnaires

Case Study

A 49-year-old man who works in construction has had diffuse cutaneous systemic sclerosis (dSSc) for 7 months. He has Raynaud's phenomenon, swollen hands, and tight skin on his hands, arms (upper and forearms), face, and trunk. He has had three recent digital ulcers. Other complications have included GERD, erectile dysfunction, and weakness from mild myopathy and mild dyspnea from lung involvement.

He has been struggling at work and has missed several days recently. He can no longer safely work on the current construction site as he cannot properly use the tools or lift the materials. He has thought about talking to his employer but is certain he will be fired if he does. He is now depressed and sees his doctor about applying for work disability.

His physical examination reveals a high skin score, some tendon friction rubs, multiple pits on his fingertips, an infected digital ulcer and two other healing ulcers on his fingers, some dilated nailfold capillaries, and a few telangiectasia. His Health Assessment Questionnaire Disability Index (HAQ-DI) is high (1.8). His pain is 7.5 out of 10. He appears sad and has lost interest in eating and he is not sleeping. It is determined that he is unable to work due to severe scleroderma and that he is also depressed. Forms for disability are completed and his depression is treated.

J. Pope
Division of Rheumatology, Department of Medicine, St. Joseph's Health Care,
Schulich School of Medicine & Dentistry, University of Western Ontario,
268 Grosvenor St., London, ON N6A 4V2, Canada

R.M. Silver and C.P. Denton (eds.), *Case Studies in Systemic Sclerosis*,
DOI: 10.1007/978-0-85729-641-2_30, © Springer-Verlag London Limited 2011

Discussion

Despite the poor prognosis, survival in SSc is improving.[1] Improved survival is accompanied by challenges such as loss of employment due to SSc.

There are studies of work disability (WD) in SSc, but fewer than in more common inflammatory rheumatic diseases; however, some of the findings common to other rheumatic diseases likely apply to SSc. For example, poor function, older age, physically demanding job, lower education, fatigue, pain, and depression are all related to a higher risk of WD. It is not unusual for a middle-aged man with SSc to be unable to work. Male scleroderma patients more often have dSSc, and both functional impairment and work disability are increased in this disease subset. Also, most male SSc patients have disease onset in middle-age. Disease duration is a risk for WD, but even early in the disease course some will no longer be able to work. Work disability occurs in approximately half of all people with SSc.

Definition of Work Disability (WD)

Defining Disability

Disability is difficult to define, since its characterization depends upon the viewpoint of the observer. From a medical or disease viewpoint, disability is frequently defined as the consequences or impact of a disease condition.[2] From a rehabilitation or disability perspective, the patient's health and functioning are not simply a consequence of disease, but are associated with disease itself, and are placed in the context of personal and environmental factors.[2]

Conceptual Frameworks in Disability

The most commonly used current framework of disability is the World Health Organization (WHO) International Classification of Functioning, Disability and Health (ICF).[3] Disability is an interaction between disease or illness and contextual factors that lead to impairment.[2]

Work Disability Definition

WD has been defined as the state in which the affected individual has had to leave his/her job, or forced to work fewer hours.[4] One issue that complicates the WD literature is the variable methodology used in WD studies, such as describing only those who cannot work due to their illness, using patient self-report, or using administrative databases. For WD, there is a lack of standardized terminology.

Self-Reported Function

The Health Assessment Questionnaire Disability Index (HAQ-DI) is a measure of self-reported function from a short standardized questionnaire that has been validated in SSc.[5,6] A higher HAQ is linked to WD not surprisingly, as self-reported functional problems translate into less ability to work. The HAQ is an important tool to include in the assessment of WD as it is known to correlate significantly with WD as well as other work-related measures, including work capacity, work task performance, and occupation.[7] Also, if function is preserved in early SSc, it is associated with improved disease status later. Lower scores predicted improvement in overall HAQ at 1 and 2 years of follow-up. When the HAQ improved, it was associated with improvement in physician assessment for overall SSc and most of the categories studied (subsets and early and late SSc) even at next follow-up. Thus, HAQ is a useful 'marker' of change in status in clinical practice, where an improved HAQ is associated with improved physician global assessment at the current visit and even is related to improved physician global assessment a year later.[8]

Disease Activity Versus Damage

The HAQ measures function, which has some degree of reversibility if there is active disease; however, part of the score is from damage, which is irreversible. In RA if there are swollen joints, the HAQ can be quite high and may return to a population age-matched normal score if no damage results (contractures, subluxations).[9] In SSc, hand contractures are common and occur early, and there is no major treatment to reverse these problems. Thus the HAQ often is not thought to improve a lot once the disease is established, but will worsen over time in many patients. WD can occur if there is high disease activity and/or significant impairment from damage.

Frequency of Work Disability in SSc

WD ranges from 21% to 56% among people suffering from SSc. A cross-sectional, multicenter study of patients from the Canadian Scleroderma Research Group (CSRG) Registry studied 643 patients. Twenty-one percent were work disabled.[10] This rate is likely an underestimate as this was a prevalent cohort, and many patients

Table 30.1 Work disability in diffuse SSc and limited SSc and relationships with the HAQ and pain

	Diffuse SSc	Limited SSc	OR	95% CI for OR	p-Value
N	26	35	–	–	–
Work disabled (n)	65% (17)	49% (17)	2.00	0.70–5.69	0.21
Disease duration	8.19±1.4	13.19±1.2	–	–	0.006
HAQ-DI	1.19±0.1	0.88±0.1	–	–	0.09
HAQ pain	1.31±0.2	1.39±0.1	–	–	0.72

Adapted from Ouimet et al.[11]

were beyond working age and had long-standing disease when enrolled. Another study was a single site case control study of SSc and RA patients seen at the same clinic.[11] Cross-sectional data on WD status were obtained from a questionnaire sent to all SSc (n=35 limited [lSSc], 26 diffuse [dSSc]) and RA (n=104). WD data, HAQ-DI scores, education, and disease duration were recorded. WD was found in 56% of SSc (95% CI: 43–68%); the rate was higher in dSSc than lSSc (69% vs. 49%). When WD was studied only in women with SSc in another study, WD was divided according to the degree of sick leave. Forty-four women with lSSc were included of whom 48% had no sick leave, 34% were on partial sick leave, and 18% were on full-time sick leave or had a full disability pension.[12]

Diffuse Versus Limited Cutaneous SSc

As would be expected, WD is higher in dSSc than in lSSc (65% vs. 49%) with an Odds Ratio of 2 for being work disabled when comparing dSSc to lSSc.[11] There is worse function (higher HAQ scores: 1.19 vs. 0.88) despite shorter disease duration in the dSSc subset: 8 years vs. 13 years.[11] In general, dSSc has more skin affected and complications including contractures of the hands, digital ulcers,[13] and organ involvement. Higher disease burden would increase the prevalence of WD in the dSSc subset. See Table 30.1 for comparisons of pain and function in dSSc and lSSc.

Predictors of WD in SSc

WD is multifactorial and in SSc is prevalent, occurs early but increases with disease duration, and is associated with markers of disease severity and functional status. See Table 30.2 for associations between WD and various characteristics of SSc.

In a study using patients from the Canadian Scleroderma Research Group (CSRG), WD was common, even in people with short disease duration, and increased steadily with increasing disease duration: among those who were ≤65 years and

Table 30.2 Associations with work disability in SSc

Diffuse cutaneous SSc (dSSc) subtype[a]
Longer disease duration[a]
High HAQ disability index scores[a]
Lower education[a]
More physically demanding job[a]
Also related
Higher disease severity
Higher pain
Worse hand function
Digital ulcers
More fatigue
More comorbidities

[a]Shown in more than one WD study in SSc

who reported being either disabled or working, 28% and 45% of patients with disease duration of <2 and 10–15 years, respectively, reported that they were work disabled.[10] The significant correlates of WD included comorbidities, disease duration, diffuse disease, disease severity, pain, fatigue, and physical function.

The comparative study of SSc with RA demonstrated that HAQ-DI was significantly higher in work-disabled patients (both SSc and RA) vs. those who were employed ($p<0.001$ for both). Multivariate logistic regression analysis demonstrated that higher HAQ-DI, dSSc, disease duration, and more physically demanding work were associated with WD.[11]

In a female-only SSc study, women without sick leave had less physically demanding jobs ($p=0.026$). The hypothesis that working ability reflects lower disease severity was confirmed regarding dexterity grip force and perceived fatigue and breathlessness ($p<0.05$). Greater working ability was associated with better capacity to perform activities of daily life ($p<0.01$), greater satisfaction with occupations ($p<0.01$), better well-being ($p<0.001$), and better health ($p<0.001$).[12]

Education and WD

WD occurs more if education is lower, such as not completing high school. This is the case when WD is studied in arthritis and SSc[11] (shown in Table 30.3). In SSc, patients with relatively poorer psychosocial adjustment to illness had less education and more functional disability, so this may also confound the association of WD and education.[14] Education may be a surrogate marker for type of work, income, and self-management abilities.[15]

Table 30.3 Factors associated with work disability in SSc

Systemic sclerosis	Work disabled	Not work disabled	OR	95% CI for OR	p-Value
N	34	27	–	–	–
Age (mean years ± SEM)	52.6 ± 1.72	51.3 ± 1.93	–	–	0.63
Diffuse SSc	50.0%	33.3%	2.00	0.70–5.69	0.21
Female sex	88.2%	81.5%	1.70	0.41–7.09	0.49
Disease duration (mean years ± SEM)	11.98 ± 1.29	9.85 ± 1.43	–	–	0.27
Less than high school education	26.5%	3.7%	9.36	1.10–79.37	0.03
HAQ-DI (mean ± SEM)	1.30 ± 0.10	0.66 ± 0.12	–	–	0.0001
HAQ pain (mean ± SEM)	1.49 ± 0.14	1.20 ± 0.16	–	–	0.18
Physically demanding work[a]	54.6%	31.8%	2.57	0.83–7.95	0.17

[a]This comparison is likely underpowered due to small numbers
Adapted from Ouimet et al.[11]

Effects of Age and Gender on WD in SSc

Age and female gender showed no significant association with WD status.[11] Although women are more likely to have SSc, in both subtypes, they proportionally have more lSSc, whereas men have more dSSc and the latter is a risk factor for WD. Men tend to develop SSc at a younger age than women. Disease duration but not age is a risk for WD in SSc.

Type of Employment

More physically demanding jobs are probably related to a higher chance of work disability in SSc; this is also true for arthritis (RA, OA) and SLE.[11,16]

WD in SSc Compared to Inflammatory Arthritis and Other Connective Tissue Diseases

RA has been extensively studied with respect to the prevalence and associations of WD. Five years after RA onset the prevalence of WD is at least 30%.[17] The prevalence of WD in SSc was higher than in RA (56% vs. 35%).[11] HAQ was related to WD in both groups, but the mean HAQ was lower in the RA group. A meta-analysis of studies in Ankylosing Spondylitis has shown rates of WD from 3% to 50% and many rates were approximately 20% in the papers reviewed.[18] Another meta-analysis of employment and work disability in SLE summarized that 33% have WD.[19] We can conclude that the prevalence of WD in SSc seems to be higher than in RA, AS, and SLE.

Can Work Disability be Avoided for Some Patients?

Studies of preventing WD by ergonomics, or other work interventions, are lacking.[20] One small rehabilitation program of 20 SSc patients was evaluated. In this randomized controlled trial, ten patients received hand and face-specific rehabilitation and exercise (including respiratory, hydrotherapy, and cardiovascular). The control group ($n = 10$) was provided only with educational advice and medical information. Patients were evaluated at baseline and after 9 weeks of treatment. Patients in the interventional group improved in all the parameters evaluated. At follow-up, gains in mouth mobility and global health status were partially lost, but hand mobility and function were maintained. The control group did not improve. This intervention did not examine WD but showed that some rehabilitation can improve function.[21]

In SSc, a trade-off in those who worked has been found.[12] More time spent working was related to spending less time on household chores, greater satisfaction with occupations in general, and greater well-being. Symptoms such as breathlessness, fatigue, and pain negatively influenced activities of daily living (ADL) capacity and satisfaction with occupations. The authors concluded that work is an important factor for satisfaction with occupations and well-being, emphasizing the need to detect risk factors for WD in SSc and to develop strategies for people with WD. Having a structured routine and setting goals as well as work place modification may help maintain ability to work.[22]

The work instability scale (WIS) can accurately predict arthritis-related work transitions[23,24] and may be worthwhile using in SSc, but thus far the WIS has not been validated in SSc.

The Impact of WD

Premature departure from the workforce has a multitude of outcomes, including social, psychological, and economic effects.[25]

WD Is an Important Cost in SSc

In a study of costs in SSc, disability-related productivity loss (55%) and hospitalization (28%) were the highest among the cost items. SSc-related costs were higher than in matched RA and psoriatic arthritis groups.[26]

Depression

Depression is common in any chronic disease, especially SSc where there is daily pain, problems with ADLs, changes in body image, an uncertain future, and good treatment is lacking. Depression can exacerbate WD and is an important comorbidity for quality of life in SSc.

Impact on Family

A severe disease such as SSc has a large impact on a patient's family. The patient's support group is affected and in addition to the impact on work, daily routine and socializing are all potentially affected. Depression in the SSc patient and in his/her family is not rare. Household income often decreases when someone in the family has SSc (a working patient who now cannot work or a spouse or child who has to help look after a sick family member with SSc all can occur). This often causes stress and another loss to deal with.

When Does Work Disability Occur?

WD increases with disease duration but can occur very early after onset of SSc.[10] This is true in other connective tissue diseases, e.g., SLE.[16]

Special Considerations

Surrogate outcome measures, such as days off from work, likely underestimate the full impact of disease on employment.[27]

Presenteeism

The concept of *presenteeism*, or decreased work performance due to health conditions, has emerged in the WD literature.[28] Presenteeism includes decreased productivity due to time not spent on task, decreased quality of work, decreased quantity of work, and personal factors.[28] Several self-reported workplace productivity instruments have been developed that measure elements of presenteeism.[28] A large arthritis study concluded that employed people with arthritis who continued working had reduced capacity at work.[29] This is likely also true for SSc patients remaining in the workforce, but studies are lacking. There are various questionnaires that can measure lost hours due to presenteeism, such as the Health and Labor Questionnaire (HLQ), the Work Limitations Questionnaire (WLQ), the WHO's Health and Work Performance Questionnaire (HPQ), and the Work Productivity and Activity Impairment Questionnaire (WPAI).[30]

Disclosure in the Work Place

People often have a dilemma about whether or not to inform their boss and coworkers about their disease for fear that this could lead to lack of promotion or being identified as someone who may not be able to work at usual productivity. Disclosure can help in situations where the work environment can be modified to help in retaining work, but it can also lead to potential future dismissal (although in many jurisdictions it is illegal to cease employing a person due to a disability).

Identification of Those with SSc at Risk for Job Loss Is Likely the Most Effective Way to Prevent Work Disability

It is unlikely in any chronic disease that once a person is off work they will return to work. Thus identification of at-risk patients can allow referrals to a vocational or rehabilitation specialist. Asking about employment status at each visit and if there is a problem working due to SSc can help by identifying who should have a job assessment. Some therapists and other specialists have expertise in this area and if available, their resources should be utilized.

Work transitions are changes in work pattern or job type without a necessary reduction in hours of overall employment. A recent study examined the frequency of arthritis-related work transitions made by those with inflammatory and degenerative arthritis in order to remain employed.[31] In this small interview-based study, work transitions were common, including inability to accept a promotion, inability to accept projects, change of work duties, and use of vacation time in lieu of sick leave.[31]

For patients suffering from arthritis, difficulty at work was related more to fatigue (above pain and physical limitations).[32] In RA, comprehensive occupational therapy was found to improve ability to work in a 6-month randomized trial.[33] More research is needed to determine if targeted occupational therapy can improve the ability of SSc patients to remain employed.

Measuring Limitations at Work

Workplace Activity Limitations Scale (WALS), 6-item Stanford Presenteeism Scale (SPS-6), Endicott Work Productivity Scale (EWPS), RA Work Instability Scale (WIS), and Work Limitations Questionnaire (WLQ) are self-reported measures of at-work productivity. Their reliability has been tested in OA and RA and there is no consensus on which one to choose.[34] The Work Limitations Questionnaire (WLQ) examines problems at work. It has been studied extensively in terms of reliability and validity for both OA and RA.[35,36] The RA study found that a one-unit change in WLQ corresponded to a decrease in income.[36] The WLQ was compared to similar tests of disability and found to have good construct validity for patients with RA, and it was highly reliable.[36]

Conclusions

WD is frequent in SSc and not well studied. Approximately half of all SSc patients will become work disabled, which is higher than for other rheumatic diseases. Interventions are especially needed in those with dSSc and high HAQ scores, and better research may aid in identifying successful programs that help to keep SSc patients at work.

References

1. Al-Dhaher FF, Pope JE, Ouimet JM. Determinants of morbidity and mortality of systemic sclerosis in Canada. *Semin Arthritis Rheum*. 2010;39(4):269-277.
2. Stucki G, Sigl T. Assessment of the impact of disease on the individual. *Best Pract Res Clin Rheumatol*. 2003;17(3):451-473.
3. World Health Organization. International Classification of Functioning, Disability and Health (ICF). http://www.who.int/classifications/icf/en/. Accessed September 2010.
4. Gobelet C, Luthi F, Al-Khodairy AT, Chamberlain MA. Work in inflammatory and degenerative joint diseases. *Disabil Rehabil*. 2007;29(17):1331-1339.
5. Fries JF, Spitz P, Kraines RG, Holman HR. Measurement of patient outcome in arthritis. *Arthritis Rheum*. 1980;23:137-145.
6. Poole JL, Steen VD. The use of the Health Assessment Questionnaire (HAQ) to determine physical disability in systemic sclerosis. *Arthritis Care Res*. 1991;4:27-31.
7. Bruce B, Fries JF. The Stanford Health Assessment Questionnaire: a review of its history, issues, progress, and documentation. *J Rheumatol*. 2003;30(1):167-178.
8. Lawrence L, Pope J, Al Zahraly Z, Lalani S, Baron M, The Investigators of the CSRG. The relationship between changes in self reported disability (measured by the Health Assessment Questionnaire [HAQ]) in scleroderma and improvement of disease status in clinical practice. *Clin Exp Rheumatol*. 2009;27(3 Suppl 54):32-37.
9. Aletehawa D, Smolen J, Ward MM. Measuring function in rheumatoid arthritis: identifying reversible and irreversible components. *Arthritis Rheum*. 2006;54(9):2784-2792.
10. Hudson M, Steele R, Lu Y, Thombs BD, Baron M, Canadian Scleroderma Research Group. Work disability in systemic sclerosis. *J Rheumatol*. 2009;36(11):2481-2486.
11. Ouimet JM, Pope J, Gutmanis I, Koval J. Work disability in scleroderma is greater than in rheumatoid arthritis and is predicted by high HAQ scores. *Open Rheumatol J*. 2008;2:44-52.
12. Sandqvist G, Scheja A, Eklund M. Work ability in relation to disease severity, everyday occupations and well-being in women with limited systemic sclerosis. *Rheumatology (Oxford)*. 2008;47(11):1708-1711.

13. Khimdas S, Harding S, Zummer B, Baron M, Pope J, Canadian Scleroderma Research Group. Associations with digital ulcers (DU) in a large cohort of systemic sclerosis (SSc): results from the Canadian Scleroderma Research Group Registry. *Arthritis Care Res (Hoboken)*. 2011;63(1):142-149.

14. Moser DK, Clements PJ, Brecht ML, Weiner SR. Predictors of psychosocial adjustment in systemic sclerosis. The influence of formal education level, functional ability, hardiness, uncertainty, and social support. *Arthritis Rheum*. 1993;36(10):1398-1405.

15. Mau W, Listing J, Huscher D, Zeidler H, Zink A. Employment across chronic inflammatory rheumatic diseases and comparison with the general population. *J Rheumatol*. 2005;32(4):721-728.

16. Baker K, Pope J, Fortin P, Silverman E, Peschken C, 1000 Faces of Lupus Investigators; CaNIOS (Canadian Network for Improved Outcomes in SLE). Work disability in systemic lupus erythematosus is prevalent and associated with socio-demographic and disease related factors. *Lupus*. 2009;18(14):1281-1288.

17. Allaire S, Wolfe F, Niu J, Lavalley MP. Contemporary prevalence and incidence of work disability associated with rheumatoid arthritis in the US. *Arthritis Rheum*. 2008;59(4):474-480.

18. Boonen A, Chorus A, Miedema H, van der Heijde D, van der Tempel H, van der Linden S. Employment, work disability, and work days lost in patients with ankylosing spondylitis: a cross sectional study of Dutch patients. *Ann Rheum Dis*. 2001;60(4):353-358.

19. Baker K, Pope J. Employment and work disability in systemic lupus erythematosus: a systematic review. *Rheumatology (Oxford)*. 2009;48(3):281-284.

20. Casale R, Buonocore M, Matucci-Cerinic M. Systemic sclerosis (scleroderma): an integrated challenge in rehabilitation. *Arch Phys Med Rehabil*. 1997;78(7):767-773.

21. Maddali Bongi S, Del Rosso A, Galluccio F, et al. Efficacy of a tailored rehabilitation program for systemic sclerosis. *Clin Exp Rheumatol*. 2009;27(3 Suppl 54):44-50.

22. Sandqvist G, Eklund M. Daily occupations – performance, satisfaction and time use, and relations with well-being in women with limited systemic sclerosis. *Disabil Rehabil*. 2008; 30(1):27-35.

23. Gilworth G, Chamberlain MA, Harvey A, et al. Development of a work instability scale for rheumatoid arthritis. *Arthritis Rheum*. 2003;49(3):349-354.

24. Tang K, Beaton DE, Gignac MA, et al. The work instability scale for rheumatoid arthritis (RA-WIS) predicts arthritis-related work transitions within 12 months. *Arthritis Care Res (Hoboken)*. 2010;62(11):1578-1587.

25. Lacaille D, Hogg RS. The effect of arthritis on working life expectancy. *J Rheumatol*. 2001;28(10):2315-2319.

26. Minier T, Péntek M, Brodszky V, Ecseki A, Kárpáti K, et al. Cost-of-illness of patients with systemic sclerosis in a tertiary care centre. *Rheumatology (Oxford)*. 2010;49(10):1920-1928.

27. Lacaille D. Arthritis and employment research: Where are we? Where do we need to go? *J Rheumatol Suppl*. 2005;72:42-45.

28. Schultz AB, Edington DW. Employee health and presenteeism: a systematic review. *J Occup Rehabil*. 2007;17(3):547-579.

29. Zhang W, Koehoorn M, Anis AH. Work productivity among employed Canadians with arthritis. *J Occup Environ Med*. 2010;52(9):872-877.

30. Zhang W, Gignac MA, Beaton D, Tang K, Anis AH, Canadian Arthritis Network Work Productivity Group. Productivity loss due to presenteeism among patients with arthritis: estimates from 4 instruments. *J Rheumatol*. 2010;37(9):1805-1814.

31. Gignac M, Lacaille D, Aslam A, Badley EM. Managing arthritis and employment: making arthritis-related work transitions to remain employed. *Arthritis Rheum*. 2007;56(9):S771; (Abstract 2026).

32. Lacaille D, White MA, Backman CL, Gignac MA. Problems faced at work due to inflammatory arthritis: new insights gained from understanding patients' perspective. *Arthritis Rheum*. 2007;57(7):1269-1279.

33. Macedo AM, Oakley SP, Panayi GS, Kirkham BW. Functional and work outcomes improve in patients with rheumatoid arthritis who receive targeted, comprehensive occupational therapy. *Arthritis Rheum*. 2009;61(11):1522-1530.

34. Beaton DE, Tang K, Gignac MA, et al. Reliability, validity, and responsiveness of five at-work productivity measures in patients with rheumatoid arthritis or osteoarthritis. *Arthritis Care Res (Hoboken)*. 2010;62(1):28-37.
35. Lerner D, Reed JI, Massarotti E, Wester LM, Burke TA. The Work Limitations Questionnaire's validity and reliability among patients with osteoarthritis. *J Clin Epidemiol*. 2002;55(2):197-208.
36. Walker N, Michaud K, Wolfe F. Work limitations among working persons with rheumatoid arthritis: results, reliability, and validity of the work limitations questionnaire in 836 patients. *J Rheumatol*. 2005;32(6):1006-1012.

Chapter 31
A Scleroderma Patient Presenting with Facial Pain

David Launay, Hélène Zephir, and Pierre-Yves Hatron

Keywords Trigeminal neuropathy • Cranial neuropathies • Peripheral nervous system • Facial numbness

Case Study

A 52-year-old woman was referred to our clinic for Raynaud's phenomenon. Her past medical history included hysterectomy for a fibroma and she was receiving statin treatment for hypercholesterolemia.

Some 7 years earlier, she had started to experience a sensation of numbness in her left lower lip. The sensation progressively spread, first on the left side of her face and then on the right. She also described a wooden sensation of the buccal mucous membrane and gums. These symptoms persisted and she was examined by a neurologist, who found a loss of pinprick and temperature sensitivity on both sides of the face, along the distribution of the three branches of the trigeminal nerve. There was no corneal anesthesia but sensory and taste disturbances were noted in the anterior two-thirds of the tongue and in the buccal mucosa. The ENT examination and sinus scan performed at that time did not reveal any anomalies. Brain magnetic resonance imaging (MRI) showed some nonspecific hyperintensities of the periventricular white matter but no abnormalities on the cranial nerves. Visual evoked potentials were normal, as were the brainstem potentials. The blink reflex was absent bilaterally. Cerebrospinal fluid analysis was normal without any meningitis or oligoclonal IgG bands. Serological testing for Lyme borreliosis was negative in blood and cerebrospinal fluid. On this basis the neurologist diagnosed idiopathic trigeminal neuropathy. Corticosteroid treatment with 30 mg of prednisone daily was introduced but was rapidly withdrawn due to a lack of efficacy.

P.-Y. Hatron (✉)
Department of Internal Medicine, Claude-Huriez Hospital,
rue Michel Polnovski, Lille 59037, France

R.M. Silver and C.P. Denton (eds.), *Case Studies in Systemic Sclerosis*,
DOI: 10.1007/978-0-85729-641-2_31, © Springer-Verlag London Limited 2011

At admission, the patient described Raynaud's phenomenon that had developed over the previous 18 months and was characterized by a blanching phase on exposure to cold. The thumb was affected. The Raynaud's phenomenon had worsened during the past few months, with several attacks daily. On examination, the skin of the fingers was found to be taut, and a pitting scar was observed on the third finger of the right hand. Giant capillaries were visible without magnification at the nailfold margin of several fingers. There were cutaneous telangiectasia mainly found on the face and chest.

The patient complained of occasional arthralgia of the proximal interphalangeal joints, with morning stiffness lasting about half an hour. There was no sign of synovitis. She reported a retrosternal burning sensation, accentuated in the decubitus position, which suggested gastroesophageal reflux. Further questioning elicited dyspnea when climbing stairs or walking fast. Pulmonary auscultation revealed the presence of crackles at both lung bases. Neurological examination demonstrated the persistence of bilateral facial hypoesthesia, identical to the earlier neurological findings. She had no sicca syndrome.

Nailfold capillaroscopy confirmed numerous giant capillaries, suggesting organic microangiopathy. Laboratory findings were as follows: normal complete blood count; CRP less than 5 mg/L; serum protein electrophoresis: gammaglobulin 18 g/L (normal: 7–13.5); absence of rheumatoid factor and anti-CCP antibodies; positive antinuclear antibodies (ANA) at a titer of 1:1280 and with a speckled immunofluorescence pattern; presence of anti-RNP antibodies detected using the Ouchterlony technique.

Pulmonary function tests revealed a mild restrictive syndrome with a forced vital capacity of 1.80 L (70% of predicted) and a low DLco (62% of predicted). The chest CT-scan revealed a ground-glass pattern involving the subpleural regions of both lower lobes, associated with traction bronchiectasis.

Limited cutaneous systemic sclerosis (lSSc) was diagnosed on the basis of the association of Raynaud's phenomenon with sclerodactyly, giant capillaries on capillaroscopy, digital pitting scar, telangiectasia, pyrosis, and interstitial lung disease, with an associated bilateral trigeminal neuropathy.

Discussion

Peripheral nervous system involvement is rare in SSc.[1] However, while peripheral neuropathy is very seldom described, carpal tunnel syndrome is quite common especially in the early, puffy phase of diffuse SSc, and trigeminal neuropathy (TN) as well as other cranial nerve involvement seem more frequent in SSc.[2] Senseman[3] first drew attention to the association between TN and SSc in 1957. Later, Farrell and Medsger[2] identified 16 patients with TN in a population of 442 consecutive SSc patients, which gives a prevalence of 4%. Medsger and Masi[4] found 13 (2.5%) patients with TN out of a population of 504 male US veterans with SSc. TN would therefore appear to be the most common peripheral nervous system manifestation in SSc.

Table 31.1 Diagnostic tests useful to exclude other causes of trigeminal neuropathy in patients with systemic sclerosis

Diagnostic tests	Differential diagnosis
CSF analysis	Multiple sclerosis, Lyme borreliosis, meningitis
Brain MRI	Tumors, multiple sclerosis
Serological testing for Lyme borreliosis	Lyme borreliosis
Facial electroneuromyography with blink reflex	
Panoramic radiographs	Mandible resorption if unilateral third division of the trigeminal nerve is involved

Usually, the sensory complaints in TN are numbness, paresthesias, and either constant or lancinating pain. Objective hypoesthesia was detected in almost all SSc patients in the literature.[2,4] Conversely, motor dysfunction of the fifth cranial nerve appears very rare in SSc.[5] TN is nearly always associated with an intact corneal reflex, though it can sometimes be depressed or absent.[2,4] The natural history of TN is variable in SSc. Occasionally the problem is transient, whereas in most instances the complaint is more persistent. The maximal sensory deficit is usually reached after 6–24 months.[2,4]

When compared with SSc patients without TN, SSc patients with TN appear to be more frequently young women with SSc associated with other connective tissue diseases (overlap), such as mixed connective tissue disease with myositis or Sjögren's syndrome, anti-RNP antibodies, and hypergammaglobulinemia (as in our patient).[2] Indeed, 34% of SSc patients with TN had overlap connective tissue disease vs. 5% of patients without ($p<0.05$) in Farrell's study.[2] TN most frequently occurs in a patient with known SSc. More rarely, TN precedes SSc from several months to years in 17% of cases and can be the initial symptom as in our patient.[2] Teasdall et al.[6] reported ten SSc patients with cranial nerve involvement, including the trigeminal nerve in all patients and the facial nerve in five patients: TN was the presenting feature in five patients and preceded the disease in two patients, by 6 months and 1 year, respectively. Beighton[7] was the first to describe TN in a patient who subsequently developed SSc, as in our patient.

TN in patients with SSc is bilateral in two-thirds of cases. A trigger point is found in 20% of patients. The second and third divisions of the nerve are involved together in the majority of SSc patients with TN (~80%). A review of the literature reported that all three divisions of the trigeminal nerve were affected in nearly half of all patients.[2] Other cranial neuropathies have been described in SSc, such as facial palsy,[6] glossopharyngeal neuropathy, audiovestibular impairment, and optic neuropathy.[8]

When evaluating SSc patients with TN, clinicians should always consider other possible causes in a differential diagnosis of TN. Table 31.1 summarizes the diagnostic tests to exclude other causes for TN. Clinical investigations should be directed toward discerning a central or peripheral origin of the neuropathy. Central lesions are often associated with involvement of multiple dermatomes and other neurologic findings, such as limb numbness and weakness, hearing loss and otalgia (vestibular schwannoma). If there is pain, local growth, or a positive panoramic examination, a peripheral origin is likely. However, in some conditions like SSc, a peripheral and/ or central origin can be associated. Cerebral CT scan and MRI can be used to rule out a central origin of TN. The 2008 AAN/EFNS study identified five studies that addressed the accuracy of trigeminal reflex testing in the evaluation of TN.[9] The pooled sensitivity and specificity of trigeminal reflex testing for distinguishing secondary and classic TN was 94% and 87%, respectively. Based on the high sensitivity and specificity, the AAN/EFNS concluded that abnormal trigeminal reflexes are associated with an increased risk of secondary TN.

Central causes of TN include primary and metastatic cerebral tumors and other cerebral conditions, such as demyelinating diseases and stroke. In terms of peripheral origin, iatrogenic causes (postinjection, postsurgery, etc.), infections, primary or secondary tumors of the jaw, perineural spread of squamous cell carcinoma, and peripheral neuropathy should be considered. A number of conditions are associated with a central and/or peripheral origin, such as sarcoidoisis, Lyme disease, sickle cell anemia, and vasculitis. Conditions associated with a central and/or peripheral origin of TN include connective tissue diseases, such as lupus and Sjögren's syndrome, and mixed connective tissue disease. SSc is also a possible cause. When TN occurs in a patient with known SSc, it is important to rule out other central and peripheral causes before attributing the TN to SSc, especially with a brain MRI and a cerebrospinal fluid analysis.

The pathophysiology of TN in SSc is not yet fully understood. Among the proposed mechanisms are microangiopathy and fibrosis, or a combination of both, in the trigeminal ganglion or root.[10] In clinical neurophysiology, the blink reflex is the standard test to assess trigeminal function. An electrical stimulus to the supraorbital nerves elicits two responses in the orbicularis oculi muscles: the early (R1) component in the ipsilateral muscle and the late (R2) component bilaterally. Casale et al. studied the blink reflex in 35 SSc patients without TN.[11] All patients had normal R1; however, 18% had a delayed R2. The mean blink reflex latency values were similar in SSc patients when compared to healthy controls. Facial cutaneous thickening was not more frequent in patients with TN. The findings of that study suggest that direct extension of cutaneous or subcutaneous facial fibrosis to the trigeminal nerve does not play a role in the pathophysiology of TN in SSc.[11] R2 is predominantly conveyed by the nociceptive, thin myelinated A-delta fibers. The sparing of R1 in that study suggests a central lesion, either at medullary or brain level. Microangiopathy in the central nervous system is highly probable in SSc, as suggested by many studies.[12,13] Cerebral hypoperfusion has been shown in SSc.[12] It has been suggested that the neuropathy in SSc results from ischemic lesions of the peripheral nerves through involvement of the vasa nervorum.[14] Another hypothesis is that TN could be an entrapment neuropathy in some patients because of the inflammatory reaction with edema as reflected on MRI by abnormal contrast uptake and a slight enlargement of the preganglionic segment, located between its emergence from the anterior aspect of the pons to its entrance through the porus trigeminus into Meckel's cave. Another important possible mechanism in SSc is mandibular resorption and nerve compression. In this case, the TN involves the unilateral third division of the trigeminal nerve. Mandibular resorption is thought to be related to pressure ischemia by extrinsic pressure from the tight sclerotic facial skin.[15] This resorption can be associated with the other classical orofacial manifestations of SSc: peribuccal rhagades, telangiectasia, decreased mouth opening, xerostomia, and widening of the periodontal ligament space (see Chap. 32). The angles of the mandibles are involved most often followed by the condyle, the coronoid process, and the posterior border of the ascending ramus. Mandibular resorption can lead to TN by lesion of the inferior alveolar nerve. In patients with unilateral involvement of the third division of the trigeminal nerve, pathologic conditions such as mandibular metastasis, osteomyelitis, etc. directly involving the mandible cause the condition known as mental nerve neuropathy.

Treating TN in SSc is challenging. Glucocorticoids do not seem to be beneficial and should be used with caution because of the subsequent risk of scleroderma renal crisis. Chronic pain may require the use of analgesics, antidepressants, and/or anticonvulsants, as in patients with chronic neuropathic pain due to other etiologies.

In summary, TN is the most common peripheral nervous system manifestation in SSc. In a patient without known SSc, TN can precede or be diagnosed simultaneously with SSc. In a patient with known SSc, the occurrence of TN requires differential diagnosis to rule out other possible causes, especially tumors and demyelinating diseases.

References

1. Launay D, Baubet T, Cottencin O, et al. Neuropsychiatric manifestations in systemic sclerosis. *Presse Méd*. 2010;39:539-547.
2. Farrell DA, Medsger TA Jr. Trigeminal neuropathy in progressive systemic sclerosis. *Am J Med*. 1982;73:57-62.
3. Senseman L. Scleroderma associated with neurological and psychogenic symptoms; with four case reports. *Med Health R I*. 1957;40:684.
4. Medsger TA Jr, Masi AT. The epidemiology of systemic sclerosis (scleroderma) among male U.S. veterans. *J Chron Dis*. 1978;31:73-85.
5. Varga E, Field EA, Tyldesley WR. Orofacial manifestations of mixed connective tissue disease. *Br Dent J*. 1990;168:330-331.
6. Teasdall RD, Frayha RA, Shulman LE. Cranial nerve involvement in systemic sclerosis (scleroderma): a report of 10 cases. *Medicine (Baltimore)*. 1980;59:149-159.
7. Beighton P, Gumpel JM, Cornes NG. Prodromal trigeminal sensory neuropathy in progressive systemic sclerosis. *Ann Rheum Dis*. 1969;27:367-369.
8. Hietaharju A, Jaaskelainen SK, Kalimo H, Hietarinta M. Peripheral neuromuscular manifestations in systemic sclerosis (scleroderma). *Muscle Nerve*. 1993;16:1204-1212.
9. Kimura J. Clinical uses of the electrically elicited blink reflex. *Adv Neurol*. 1983;39:773-786.
10. Lecky BR, Hughes RA, Murray NM. Trigeminal sensory neuropathy. A study of 22 cases. *Brain*. 1987;110:1463-1485.
11. Casale R, Frazzitta G, Fundaro C, et al. Blink reflex discloses CNS dysfunction in neurologically asymptomatic patients with systemic sclerosis. *Clin Neurophysiol*. 2004;115:1917-1920.

12. Cutolo M, Nobili F, Sulli A, et al. Evidence of cerebral hypoperfusion in scleroderma patients. *Rheumatology (Oxford)*. 2000;39:1366-1373.
13. Terrier B, Charbonneau F, Touze E, et al. Cerebral vasculopathy is associated with severe vascular manifestations in systemic sclerosis. *J Rheumatol*. 2009;36:1486-1494.
14. Lee P, Bruni J, Sukenik S. Neurological manifestations in systemic sclerosis (scleroderma). *J Rheumatol*. 1984;11:480-483.
15. Haers PE, Sailer HF. Mandibular resorption due to systemic sclerosis. Case report of surgical correction of a secondary open bite deformity. *Int J Oral Maxillofac Surg*. 1995;24:261-267.

Chapter 32
A Dentist Inquires About His Patient with Systemic Sclerosis

Faye N. Hant and Michele C. Ravenel

Keywords Systemic sclerosis • Sjogren's syndrome • Xerostomia • Microstomia • Osteonecrosis of the jaw • Dental care

Case Study

A 66-year-old woman with a history of limited cutaneous systemic sclerosis (lSSc) presents with a 9 month history of pain in the left posterior aspect of her mouth. She reports pain with brushing her teeth in this area as well as a sensation that she is unable to open her mouth as she had before, beyond that due to the chronic reduction in her oral aperture distance. She has chronic xerostomia as a result of secondary Sjogren's syndrome (SS), which has been minimally responsive to a variety of secretagogue agents in the past. She has generalized recession of her gingivae and multiple, painful cavities.

Physical Examination

Temperature 36.8°C; pulse 76 bpm, respirations 16/min; blood pressure 117/62 mmHg. Skin: sclerodactyly of all fingers, telangiectasias on face, hands, and chest, digital pitted scars present on the right third and fourth digits (Figs. 32.1 and 32.2). HEENT: perioral skin furrowing with reduced oral aperture, dry mucous membranes with absent salivary pooling, noted prominence of the left pterygomandibular raphe which

F.N. Hant (✉)
Department of Medicine, Rheumatology & Immunology, Medical University of South Carolina, 96 Jonathan Lucas Street, Charleston, SC 29455, USA

R.M. Silver and C.P. Denton (eds.), *Case Studies in Systemic Sclerosis*, DOI: 10.1007/978-0-85729-641-2_32, © Springer-Verlag London Limited 2011

Fig. 32.1 Characteristic SSc
facies with pursed lips, skin
thickening, and telangiectasias

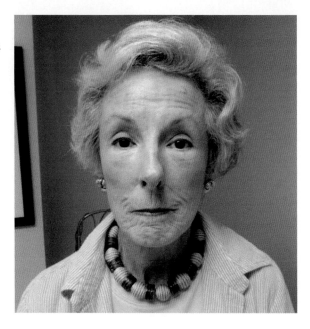

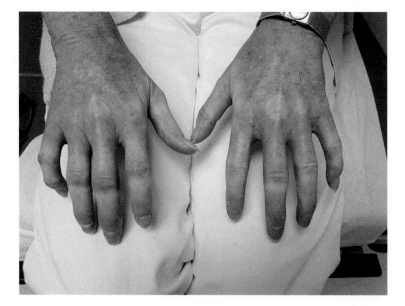

Fig. 32.2 Sclerodactyly and contractures in a patient with SSc

Fig. 32.3 Microstomia
in patient with limited
cutaneous SSc

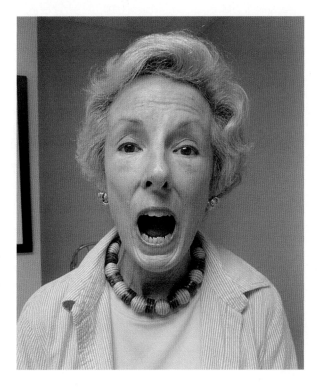

is tender to palpation and which reproduces her mouth discomfort (Figs. 32.3 and
32.4). Multiple dental fillings are noted with obvious gum recession. Prominence of
the right sublingual salivary gland is also noted with tenderness and pain to palpation.
Chest: clear to auscultation. Cardiac: regular rate and rhythm with normal S1 and S2
heart sounds. Extremities: no edema or cyanosis. Neurologic: no focal deficits.

Course

The patient has known limited cutaneous SSc and secondary SS. She has chronic
xerostomia and reduced oral aperture, as well as significant dental problems, e.g.,
dental caries and periodontal disease, noted complications of both SSc and SS. The
patient appears to have right sublingual salivary gland enlargement concerning for
a possible salivary stone, as well as prominence and tenderness of the left pterygomandibular raphe, so she was referred to her dentist for further evaluation.

The patient was found to have a right sublingual salivary gland stone which was
treated with antibiotics. She was advised on maintaining proper oral hygiene and

Fig. 32.4 Prominent left
pterygomandibular raphe,
which was tender upon
palpation

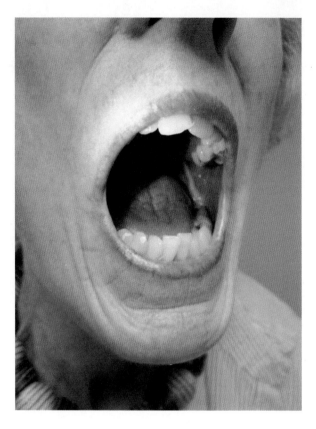

was given dental recommendations including the use of a mechanical toothbrush,
flossing aids, and stretching exercises. She was also started on a secretagogue agent.
The prominent and tender pterygomandibular raphe was felt to be related to fibrosis
from her underlying SSc and potential surgical options were discussed with her. The
patient declined surgical intervention and will be monitored closely.

Discussion

Systemic sclerosis (scleroderma, SSc) is a systemic connective tissue disease
characterized by autoantibody production, small vessel vasculopathy, and organ
fibrosis.[1] SSc commonly involves the oral and facial areas, leading to significant
morbidity in this patient population. Awareness of the potential oral manifestations
associated with SSc is important (Table 32.1). Given the importance of the mouth,
both aesthetically and functionally, repercussions of poor dental health care and
lack of proper oral health education of affected patients may have a profoundly
negative impact on their lives.

Table 32.1 Oral manifestations in patients with systemic sclerosis

Xerostomia
Enamel erosion
Microstomia
Increased risk of periodontal disease and dental caries
Mandibular resorption
Fibrosis of the soft and hard palate
Periodontal ligament space widening
Mucosal telangiectasias
Trigeminal neuralgia
Dysphagia
Osteonecrosis of the jaw (in relation to possible medication use)

Most oral clinical manifestations of SSc commence with tongue rigidity and skin hardening, leading to the characteristic facial features. In a recent study in France, the orofacial manifestations of 30 consecutive patients with SSc were characterized.[2] The authors noted the following stomatologic manifestations in their patient cohort: xerostomia ($n=20$); microstomia ($n=20$); skin atrophy ($n=28$); bone resorption ($n=2$); trigeminal neuralgia ($n=1$); periodontal ligament space widening ($n=10$); and telangiectasia ($n=21$).[2] Xerostomia was more bothersome to patients than microstomia; xerostomia was significantly associated with the lSSc phenotype ($p=0.045$) and microstomia was significantly associated with the presence of esophageal involvement ($p=0.025$).[2]

Several areas of consideration when evaluating and treating patients with dental and stomatologic complications in SSc are discussed.

Xerostomia

Xerostomia, or the complaint of dry mouth, is associated with numerous etiologic factors. In patients with SSc both the fibrotic changes of their salivary glands and the medications used to treat their disease contribute to diminished salivary flow.[3]

The importance of saliva in the maintenance of good oral health has been well documented.[4-6] In addition to providing lubrication for chewing, speaking, and swallowing, saliva plays an important role in protecting oral structures. Normal salivary flow provides mechanical cleansing of debris in the mouth. Saliva also contains a number of antimicrobial proteins important in reducing oral infections.

Treatment for dry mouth is focused on improvement of salivary gland function, management of the associated oral discomfort, and prevention of oral infections such as dental caries and candidiasis (Table 32.2). For patients with sufficient functional salivary gland tissue, the use of secretagogues may improve salivary production. Currently the US Food and Drug Administration (FDA) has approved two drugs: pilocarpine (Salagen®, MGI Pharma) and cevimiline (Evoxac®, Daiichi

Table 32.2 Management of xerostomia

Frequent sips of water
Avoidance of alcohol, caffeine
Avoidance of spicy, acidic foods
Salivary substitutes (rinses, gels, sprays)
Alcohol-free mouth rinses
Secretagogue therapy, if indicated
Increase humidity in home
Sugar free, xylitol – containing gums and mints

Sanko, INC) to increase salivary secretion in patients with Sjogren's syndrome or radiation-induced dry mouth. In randomized controlled clinical trials, both pilocarpine and cevimiline have been shown to increase salivary flow rate.[7] Unfortunately, no studies have been conducted in patients diagnosed with SSc. Side effects associated with these drugs include sweating and gastrointestinal disturbances. More serious adverse effects include cardiovascular and respiratory problems which may preclude the use of these drugs for some patients. For patients with severe glandular fibrosis or where use of a secretagogue is contraindicated, treatment of xerostomia is primarily palliative. Frequent sips of water, use of a commercially available saliva substitute, alcohol-free mouth rinses, and xylitol-containing mints or gum may be effective in alleviating the symptoms of dry mouth. Diet modifications (e.g., avoidance of sugars, alcohol, caffeine, and acidic foods), daily use of a prescription strength fluoridated dentifrice, and frequent dental evaluations are all critical in the prevention and management of the sequelae of dry mouth.[8]

Dental Caries and Other Oral Infections

Patients with SSc are at an increased risk for the development of several types of oral infections. Although different etiologies have been identified, inadequate oral hygiene due to microstomia should be considered a contributing factor in all types of oral infection in these patients. As such, improving oral hygiene at home is critical.

In the case of dental caries, a lack of saliva is thought to be the primary etiology. When left untreated, dental caries can result in significant pain, loss of teeth, and even systemic infection. Treatment for dental caries includes restoration of the carious lesion or extraction of the tooth depending upon the severity of the lesion. Prevention of dental caries includes improved oral hygiene at home and frequent professional cleanings. Aggressive management of xerostomia is critical in preventing new or recurrent dental caries.

Periodontal disease is a chronic bacterial infection of the gingiva and bone surrounding the teeth. Toxins released by bacterial dental plaque stimulate a chronic inflammatory response leading to soft tissue and bone destruction. Untreated, periodontal disease can lead to pain, difficulty eating, and tooth loss. Periodontal complications in SSc are thought primarily to be a result of an obliterative micro-vasculopathy, as seen in other tissues as well.[9] Routine dental cleanings and ade-quate oral hygiene measures (e.g., daily brushing and flossing) are critical in preventing periodontal infections. Antimicrobial rinses (e.g., chlorhexidine glu-conate) are an important part of managing periodontal disease, although alcohol-containing preparations should be avoided due to their drying effects.

Patients with hyposalivation are also at risk for oral candidiasis and related angu-lar cheilitis. This risk is increased for patients taking immunosuppressive drugs, having diabetes, smoking, or wearing dentures.[10] A number of topical (e.g., gels, rinses, creams) and systemic antifungal agents are available for treatment. To pre-vent fungal colonization, denture wearers should be instructed to remove their den-tures at bedtime and soak them overnight in a 1% sodium hypochloride or 0.12% chlorhexidine solution. Management for angular cheilitis involves treatment of the lateral commissures of the mouth with a combination anti fungal/anti-inflammatory compound (e.g., Mycologue II®).

Microstomia/Oral Fibrosis/Trismus

Subcutaneous deposition of collagen in the perioral tissues results in varying degrees of microstomia. When severe, a decreased oral aperture limits the patient's ability to perform adequate oral hygiene or to undergo professional dental therapy. Treatment for this condition consists of gentle stretching exercises, moist heat, and NSAIDs.

Stretching appliances like the *Therabite Jaw Motion®* are recommended for patients with trismus (Fig. 32.5). An economical alternative to this device is the use of stacked tongue blades to gently open the oral aperture and stretch the facial

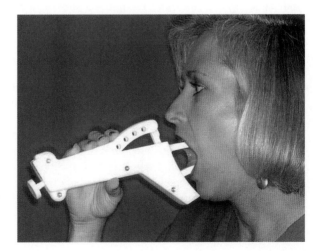

Fig. 32.5 Patient using Therabite appliance to increase the oral opening

muscles. Patients should be able to comfortably insert a stack of 15 tongue blades in between their posterior teeth. Exercise sets of ten openings four times a day is recommended to improve range of motion (see Chap. 29).[11]

Temperomandibular Disorders

The etiology of pain and dysfunction of the temperomandibular joint in SSc may be multifactorial. Osteolytic activity leads to resorption or erosion of the condylar head, coronoid process, and ramus of the mandible interrupting normal articular function. Patients may complain of facial pain, temperomandibular joint pain, and/ or difficulty opening the mouth.[12,13] Fibrosis involving the facial muscles may exacerbate these problems.[9] Treatment for temperomandibular pain is similar to that of treatment for trismus/oral fibrosis.

Implants and Dentures

For patients with an existing denture, microstomia and fibrosis of the tongue and oral vestibules may make wearing their denture difficult and painful. For some, their oral changes make fabricating a new dental prosthesis extremely difficult and, in some cases, impossible.[14] In a limited number of cases, dental specialists have successfully used custom impression trays to make a flexible or hinged prosthesis for scleroderma patients.[15,16]

Another important consideration is retention of a denture. Intraorally, fibrosis of the muco-buccal folds severely diminishes the retention and function of an existing denture. For these patients, an osseo-integrated dental implant to improve retention may be an option. A number of studies assessing implant and prosthetic treatment outcomes of patients with rheumatic disorders, including SSc, support the use of dental implants.[17-20]

Most dental implants placed today are titanium root-form endosseous implants. These root-form titanium posts are placed within the jaw bone. The bone accepts and osseointegrates with the titanium post. Osseointegration of the implant is required for the implant to function. Because the process of osseointegration is essentially a wound healing process, SSc patients should be carefully screened for conditions and medications which may impair wound healing.

As implant therapy is considered an elective treatment, selection of appropriate patients to ensure implant success is critical. Implant failure may arise from three main processes, including infection, disturbance of a weak bone to implant interface after abutment connection, and faulty host wound healing.[21] Known contraindications to dental implant include poorly controlled diabetes, immunosuppression, psychosis, drug abuse, smoking, bleeding disorders, and a history of intravenous bisphosphonate use.[22-25]

Oral surgery is contraindicated when the total white blood cell count falls below 1,500–3,000 cells/mm³, as increased risk for infection and compromised repair and regeneration may occur.[23,26] Consideration must also be taken when the total white blood cell count is normal, but the absolute neutrophil count (ANC) level is abnormal. A normal ANC level is between 3,500 and 7,000 cells/mm³. ANC levels between 1,000 and 2,000 cells/mm³ require broad-spectrum antibiotics and those with a level below 1,000 cells/mm³ require immediate medical evaluation and cannot receive dental implantation.[23,27]

A normal CD4+ T-cell level is greater than 600 cells/mm³, and values less than 500 cells/mm³ are considered immunosuppressed. There is no definitive lower limit of normal that precludes surgery; however, levels less than 400 cells/mm³ increase the risk for infection and in these cases, broad-spectrum antibiotics usage is suggested.[23]

There are no definitive guidelines on specific medications and therapies and their use during implant surgery, and only very limited investigations have been performed looking at the effects of chemotherapeutic effects on implant survival.[23]

Bisphosphonates and Implants

Bisphosphonates (BP) are an important class of drugs used in the treatment of metabolic and oncologic pathologies of the skeletal system. Since 2003, a number of cases of osteonecrosis of the jaw (ONJ) have been described in patients given intravenous bisphosphonates. In contrast, fewer cases have been reported in patients taking the oral form of such drugs. BP-related ONJ is defined as exposed, necrotic bone which persists for more than 8 weeks. Dental risk factors include surgical/invasive procedures, oral inflammation, and poor oral hygiene.[21] Suggested treatment is minor debridement, antibiotic and analgesic therapy. ONJ is extremely painful and can be refractory to treatment. Therefore, prevention of this devastating adverse effect is vital.

Dental Implants are not recommended for patients with a history of intravenous BP infusion. Ideally a thorough dental evaluation with radiographs should be conducted and dental disease treated prior to the initiation of intravenous bisphosphonate therapy.[28-30]

Currently no consensus on a maximum allowable dose of an oral BP prior to dental implant placement exists. In one published review of the literature, a total of 217 patients taking an oral BP, and who had had dental implant(s) placed, were followed for a period of 2–4 years. Implant osseointegration rates ranged between 95% and 100% and no cases of ONJ were reported. Based on this analysis, dental implant placement in patients taking an oral bisphosphonate for less than 5 years (with no other contraindications) should be considered a safe procedure, and oral BP intake does not affect short-term implant survival rates.[31] In the absence of these contraindications, a SSc patient may be referred to a dentist for a thorough implant evaluation to assess the suitability of the individual for this treatment option. It is important for the dental specialist to be experienced in dealing with the particular challenges associated with treating this patient population, the use of specific immunosuppressive therapies they may be taking for treatment of their underlying condition, and the appropriate timing for an implant surgery.

Dysphagia

Fibrotic changes to the tongue and esophagus may cause the patient to experience difficulty in swallowing. Inadequate salivary flow further exacerbates dysphagia. Esophageal dilation and efforts to increase oral lubrication, such as those recommended for treatment of xerostomia, may improve swallowing in these patients.[32]

Dental Erosion from Chronic Gastroesophageal Reflux Disease (GERD)

Normal saliva is a weak base. The amount and flow of saliva in healthy subjects helps to neutralize gastric acid reflux and to prevent the reflux of gastric fluids into the lungs, respectively.[33]

Most patients with SSc suffer from gastroesophageal reflux disease (GERD), whose pathogenesis may be related to a myriad of causes ranging from impaired esophageal clearance and gastric emptying, impaired lower esophageal pressure (LES), and transient LES relaxation.[34] Abnormal taste, mouth ulcerations and burning, and dental enamel erosions are potential extraesophageal complications of GERD.[34]

GERD-associated dental erosion is the loss of tooth structure resulting from chronic exposure to gastric secretions. Patients with dental erosion may complain of extreme dental sensitivity and are more susceptible to dental decay. Medical control of the gastric acid reflux is essential, as loss of tooth structure is irreversible (Fig. 32.6).

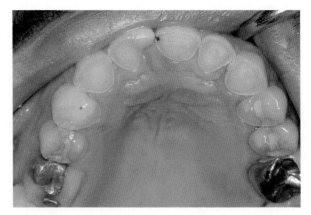

Fig. 32.6 Enamel erosion of maxillary teeth from chronic acid reflux

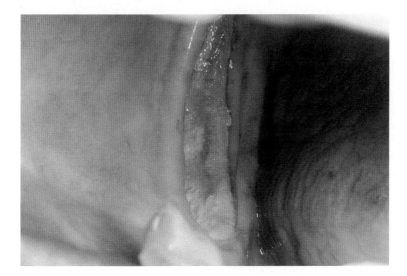

Fig. 32.7 Osteonecrosis of the mandible in patient taking a bisphosphonate

Dental management strategies include use of a soft bristle tooth brush and use of a prescription strength fluoridated, minimally abrasive dentifrice such as Prevident® 5000 Sensitive (Colgate). Since tooth brushing immediately following an acid exposure may increase the risk for erosion, patients should be encouraged to use a neutralizing agent, e.g., sugar-free antacid tablets, fresh milk, or a bicarbonate solution, prior to brushing. Avoidance of fermentable carbohydrates and acidic foods will minimize sensitivity and the risk of dental caries.[35]

Bisphosphonate-Associated Osteonecrosis of the Jaw

Bisphosphonate drugs are used for the prevention or treatment of osteopenia/ osteoporosis, for example, in patients on long-term steroid therapy, and therefore may be prescribed for some SSc patients. Recently, the FDA and the makers of these drugs issued drug precautions for health professionals regarding the occurrence of bisphosphonate-associated osteonecrosis of the jaw (BON) in these patients.

BON is a condition in which decreased metabolic support to the bony tissue results in bone necrosis. The risk for developing BON is higher in patients taking the aminobisphosphonates as compared to nonaminobisphosphonates, and for those receiving the drug intravenously.[22,36] Most reported cases have occurred following invasive dental procedures such as an extraction; however, a few cases appear to have occurred spontaneously. Patients complain of pain, ulcerations of the overlying oral tissue, and frank exposure of the jaw bone (Fig. 32.7). There is no known definitive treatment. Therapy with long-term antibiotics, hyperbaric oxygen, and surgical resection has resulted in mixed outcomes. Frequently, the disease progresses despite cessation of the bisphosphonate therapy.[36,37]

Neurological Conditions

A number of neurologic manifestations may be associated with SSc including neuropathies involving the cranial nerves, specifically the fifth and seventh cranial nerves. Rarely, involvement of the fourth, sixth, eighth, and ninth cranial nerves have been reported.[38] Patients complain of bilateral, sharp, burning, or lancinating pain of the intraoral mucosa. Others have described a sharp, stabbing sensation elicited by jaw movement, thus mimicking idiopathic trigeminal neuralgia.[9] There are reports of trigeminal neuralgia (TN) occurring in SSc patients, and these are postulated to result from mandibular resorption, nerve compression, and gasserian ganglionitis although neurologic symptoms may be iatrogenic, idiopathic, or related to the disease process itself (discussed in detail in Chap. 31).[38] In a large retrospective study, a trigeminal sensory neuropathy affected approximately 4% of SSc patients, in the form of anesthesia or paresthesias.[39] It was not felt that severe facial fibrosis played a role in the pathogenesis of TN, as the proportion of patients with and without TN was the same in that group.[39,40]

The role of TN in SSc and its possible relationship with associated autoantibodies has also been evaluated. In a study by Farrell and Medsger,[39] 467 patients with SSc and TN were compared to 426 cases of SSc patients without TN. They found that TN occurred most often in young female patients with dSSc who had an overlap syndrome with other connective tissue diseases, especially mixed connective tissue disease (MCTD) with associated myositis.[39] In these SSc patients with TN, there also appeared to be an association with Sjogren's syndrome, leukopenia, and hypothyroidism.[39] In addition, the presence of anti-U1-RNP antibodies was identified in 45% of the SSc patients with TN as compared to only 8% of SSc patients without TN.[39]

In a small prospective study of 31 SSc patients (26 with lSSc and 5 with dSSc) being evaluated for a variety of neurologic manifestations, four patients had TN which had developed within the first or second year of disease development.[41] All four patients had lSSc subset disease with three having anti-Scl-70 antibodies and one with anti-U1-RNP antibody.[41] They felt that certain subgroups of SSc patients (those with anti-U1-RNP antibody, and possibly anti-Scl-70 antibodies) may be prone to the development of neurological complications.[41] A recent study evaluated patients with idiopathic TN compared with healthy age- and sex-matched controls, to assess for the possibility of early diagnosis of a possible rheumatic disease in these patients.[42] Forty-six consecutive TN patients and 47 controls were evaluated with clinical and laboratory data. The frequency of both Raynaud's phenomenon and positive antinuclear antibodies (ANA) was significantly increased in patients with TN compared with controls ($p=0.026$ and $p=0.04$, respectively).[42] In addition, a coarse speckled nuclear immunofluorescent staining pattern was the most common pattern found in TN patients compared with controls ($p=0.013$).[42]

Therapies for this and other cranial neuropathies may involve minimally invasive neuroablative techniques and the use of membrane stabilizing medications such as gabapentin.

Poor Oral Hygiene

Extensive fibrosis of the fingers coupled with decreased oral aperture can impair a patient's ability to perform the most basic of oral hygiene measures. In advanced cases, grasping a toothbrush may be impossible. Consultation with a skilled occupational therapist may also help to find assistive devices to improve oral self-care in patients with SSc (see Chap. 29).

For patients who are unable to grasp a toothbrush handle, the use of a powered toothbrush (e.g., Sonicare®, Braun Oral B®, Interplak®) is recommended. These brushes have been shown to be clinically superior to manual brushes in removing dental plaque. Use of a compact toothbrush head and perhaps a pediatric toothbrush may perform better in some patients. Limited oral opening further complicates oral hygiene measures. A number of floss aids, such as G.U.M.'s "GO Betweens"® and DenTeks "Easy Brush"® cleaners are available from most large drug store chains. These flexible aids allow cleansing in between teeth when intraoral access and/or sclerodactyly make flossing impossible. If a SSc patient is no longer able to adequately cleanse the mouth, a caregiver should be educated in these techniques.

Oral Cancer

In a large prospective cohort, 769 patients with SSc (392 with dSSc and 377 with lSSc) were followed 16 years for the development of cancer.[43] In this cohort, comprising of a total of 3,775 patient-years of follow-up, nine SSc patients were diagnosed with oral and pharyngeal carcinoma. Of these, six had squamous cell carcinoma of the tongue, which is a 25-fold higher standardized incidence ratio than would be expected in an age-adjusted population from the SEER cancer registry.[43] All these patients had dSSc and only one patient had typical risk factors for oral cancer such as tobacco and alcohol use, raising the question of whether an environmental agent acquired by an oral route may play a role in the development of SSc and/or carcinoma of the tongue.[43] Other studies looking at populations of SSc patients have failed to find an increased association of tongue and oral cavity carcinomas; however further investigation of this relationship is warranted. Regardless, routine oral cancer examinations are critical components in the oral care regimens for SSc patients.

Radiographic Changes

There are a number of radiographic changes to the maxillofacial complex that are associated with SSc. A uniform widening of the periodontal ligament (PDL) space has been described in up to 10% of patients with SSc.[11] This widening is related to the fibrotic thickening of the periodontal ligament and is of no known clinical significance.

Resorption of the coronoid process, the condylar head, and angle of the mandible has been detected radiographically in 20% of SSc patients.[32] This resorption of bone is attributed to the increased pressure associated with abnormal collagen deposition in the surrounding oral facial tissues. Another potential etiology for bone resorption is vascular ischemia, with the obstruction of small muscular vessels leading to atrophy of musculature, which adds to the pressure of tight skin to the bone and may affect the blood supply to the bone itself.[40] Severe resorption in the area of the mandibular angle may present in the "tail of the whale" pattern. If severe enough, bone resorption places these patients at risk for pathologic fracture of the mandible.[14] A study performed in 2009 sought to investigate some clinical and radiographic orofacial alterations in SSc patients, especially in relationship to the presence or absence of mandibular osteolysis.[44] They studied 25 subjects – 15 with SSc and 10 healthy controls, and they found that mandibular osteolysis appeared to develop in SSc patients with longer disease duration, and its presence appeared to have a tendency toward having an increased mouth opening, whereas this did not occur in patients without osteolysis.[44] They found no relationship between the absence or presence of teeth and osteolysis, or that and the side of osteolysis.[44]

Other imaging modalities have been evaluated in assessing the oral health in patients with SSc. A recent study analyzed the masseter musculature in patients with SSc with the use of MRI. The study aimed to investigate the relationship between mandibular osteolysis and the T1 and T2 signal morphology and strength of the masseter muscle in 15 SSc patients compared with 10 healthy controls.[45] They found that patients with SSc had increased fat replacement, rectification, and atrophy of the masseter muscle than did controls, and that the T2 signal was significantly stronger among patients with SSc without osteolysis than among SSc patients with osteolysis and normal controls.[45]

Another study in patients with SSc used sonography to assess the ultrasonographic appearance of the oral mucosa. Twenty-megahertz sonography was performed, and patients with SSc were noted to have increased echogenicity due to fibrotic deposition, and it was proposed that ultrasound may be a useful noninvasive means to evaluate fibrosis of the oral mucosa in SSc patients.[46]

Other Considerations for the Dentist and His Office Staff

Providing empathetic care to the patient with SSc can help to facilitate a safe and effective dental visit, and a variety of recommendations can be implemented to ensure optimal oral health care in this patient population (Table 32.3). Steps such as scheduling an appointment when the patient feels well and ensuring an assistant is present to aid with retraction may be helpful.[47] The use of high-speed suction, to avoid aspiration of oral debris and mouth props to gain oral access may be necessary.[47] As Raynaud's phenomenon is active in cooler temperatures, adjustment of the room temperature to a warmer clime would make the encounter improved for this patient population, in addition to reducing drafts and providing a blanket,

Table 32.3 Dental recommendations for patients with systemic sclerosis

Regular dental evaluations at 6 month intervals (surveillance for infections)
Mechanical toothbrush
Floss aids
Caregiver trained in oral hygiene in case of inability of patients
Dietary counseling
Prescription strength fluoridated toothpaste
Stretching exercises to maintain oral opening
Manage xerostomia (Table 32.2)

gloves, or hand warmers if applicable.[47] Use of an analgesic such as acetaminophen prior to the appointment may also help facilitate a more comfortable experience.

Conclusion

SSc patients suffer a number of oral complications from their disease. Early recognition and treatment of these oral sequelae is critical in maintaining adequate oral function and an acceptable quality of life. Therefore, following the diagnosis of SSc, prompt referral to a dentist for evaluation and implementation of preventive protocols should be considered standard practice.

References

1. Mayes MD, Reveille JD. Epidemiology, demographics and genetics. In: Clements PJ, Furst DE, eds. *Systemic Sclerosis*. 2nd ed. Philadelphia: Lippincott; 2004:1-15.
2. Vincent C, Agard C, Barbarot S, et al. Orofacial manifestations of systemic sclerosis: a study of 30 consecutive patients. *Rev Méd Interne*. 2009;30(1):5-11.
3. Porter SR, Scully C, Hegarty AM. An update of the etiology and management of xerostomia. *Oral Surg Oral Med Oral Pathol Oral Radiol Endod*. 2004;97(1):28-46.
4. Dawes C. Salivary flow patterns and the health of hard and soft oral tissues. *J Am Dent Assoc*. 2008;139(suppl):18S-24S.
5. Garcia-Godoy F, Hicks MJ. Maintaining the integrity of the enamel surface: the role of dental biofilm, saliva and preventive agents in enamel demineralization and remineralization. *J Am Dent Assoc*. 2008;139(suppl):25S-34S.
6. Hicks J, Garcia-Godoy F, Flaitz C. Biological factors in dental caries: role of saliva and dental plaque in the dynamic process of demineralization and remineralization (part 1). *J Clin Pediatr Dent*. 2003;28(1):47-52.
7. Bultzinglowen V. Salivary dysfunction associated with systemic diseases: systemic review and clinical management recommendations. *Oral Surg Oral Med Oral Pathol*. 2007;103(1):1-15.
8. Napenas JJ, Brennan MT, Fox PC. Diagnosis and treatment of xerostomia (dry mouth). *Odontology*. 2009;97(2):76-83.
9. Klasser GD, Balasubramaniam R, Epstein J. Topical review-connective tissue diseases: orofacial manifestations including pain. *J Orofac Pain*. 2007;21(3):171-184.

10. Guggenheimer J, Moore PA. Xerostomia: etiology, recognition and treatment. *J Am Dent Assoc.* 2003;134(1):61-69; quiz 118-119.
11. Greenberg M, Glick M. Immunologic diseases. In: Ciarroca K, Greenberg M, eds. *Burket's Oral Medicine.* 10th ed. Hamilton: BC Decker; 2003:491-494.
12. Wood RE, Lee P. Analysis of the oral manifestations of systemic sclerosis (scleroderma). *Oral Surg Oral Med Oral Pathol.* 1988;65(2):172-178.
13. Scardina GA, Messina P. Systemic sclerosis: description and diagnostic role of the oral phenomena. *Gen Dent.* 2004;52(1):42-47.
14. Albilia JB, Lam DK, Blanas N, et al. Small mouths ... Big problems? A review of scleroderma and its oral health implications. *J Can Dent Assoc.* 2007;73(9):831-836.
15. Garnett MJ, Nohl FS, Barclay SC. Management of patients with reduced oral aperture and mandibular hypomobility (trismus) and implications for operative dentistry. *Br Dent J.* 2008;204(3):125-131.
16. Samet N, Tau S, Findler M, et al. Flexible, removable partial denture for a patient with systemic sclerosis (scleroderma) and microstomia: a clinical report and a three-year follow-up. *Gen Dent.* 2007;55(6):548-551.
17. Oczakir C, Balmer S, Mericske-Stern R. Implant-prosthodontic treatment for special care patients: a case series study. *Int J Prosthodont.* 2005;18(5):383-389.
18. Patel K, Welfare R, Coonar HS. The provision of dental implants and a fixed prosthesis in the treatment of a patient with scleroderma: a clinical report. *J Prosthet Dent.* 1998;79(6): 611-612.
19. Raviv E, Harel-Raviv M, Shatz P, et al. Implant-supported overdenture rehabilitation and progressive systemic sclerosis. *Int J Prosthodont.* 1996;9(5):440-444.
20. Weinlander M, Krennmair G, Piehslinger E. Implant prosthodontic rehabilitation of patients with rheumatic disorders: a case series report. *Int J Prosthodont.* 2010;23(1):22-28.
21. Esposito M, Thomsen P, Ericson LE, et al. Histopathologic observations on early oral implant failures. *Int J Oral Maxillofac Implants.* 1999;14(6):798-810.
22. Cartsos VM, Zhu S, Zavras AI. Bisphosphonate use and the risk of adverse jaw outcomes: a medical claims study of 714,217 people. *J Am Dent Assoc.* 2008;139(1):23-30.
23. Hwang D, Wang HL. Medical contraindications to implant therapy: part I: absolute contraindications. *Implant Dent.* 2006;15(4):353-360.
24. Hwang D, Wang HL. Medical contraindications to implant therapy: part II: relative contraindications. *Implant Dent.* 2007;16(1):13-23.
25. Elsubeihi ES, Zarb GA. Implant prosthodontics in medically challenged patients: the University of Toronto experience. *J Can Dent Assoc.* 2002;68(2):103-108.
26. Mealey BL. Periodontal implications: medically compromised patients. *Ann Periodontol.* 1996;1(1):256-321.
27. Jolly DE. Interpreting the clinical laboratory. *J Calif Dent Assoc.* 1995;23(11):32-40.
28. Javed F, Almas K. Osseointegration of dental implants in patients undergoing bisphosphonate treatment: a literature review. *J Periodontol.* 2010;81(4):479-484.
29. Khan AA, Sandor GK, Dore E, et al. Canadian consensus practice guidelines for bisphosphonate associated osteonecrosis of the jaw. *J Rheumatol.* 2008;35(7):1391-1397.
30. Lazarovici TS, Yahalom R, Taicher S, et al. Bisphosphonate-related osteonecrosis of the jaw associated with dental implants. *J Oral Maxillofac Surg.* 2010;68(4):790-796.
31. Madrid C, Sanz M. What impact do systemically administrated bisphosphonates have on oral implant therapy? A systematic review. *Clin Oral Implants Res.* 2009;20(suppl 4):87-95.
32. Neville B, Damm D, Allen C, et al. Dermatologic diseases. In: *Oral and Maxillofacial Pathology.* 1st ed. Philadelphia: Saunders; 1995:585-587.
33. Fox RI, Michelson PE. Head and neck involvement in systemic sclerosis. In: Clements PJ, Furst DE, eds. *Systemic Sclerosis.* 2nd ed. Philadelphia: Lippincott; 2004:151-161.
34. Weinstein WM, Kadell BM. The gastrointestinal tract in systemic sclerosis. In: Clements PJ, Furst DE, eds. *Systemic Sclerosis.* 2nd ed. Philadelphia: Lippincott; 2004:293-308.

35. Amaechi BT, Higham SM. Dental erosion: possible approaches to prevention and control. *J Dent*. 2005;33(3):243-252.
36. Almazrooa SA, Woo SB. Bisphosphonate and nonbisphosphonate-associated osteonecrosis of the jaw: a review. *J Am Dent Assoc*. 2009;140(7):864-875.
37. Edwards BJ, Migliorati CA. Osteoporosis and its implications for dental patients. *J Am Dent Assoc*. 2008;139(5):545-552; quiz 625–626.
38. Nadeau SE. Neurologic manifestations of connective tissue disease. *Neurol Clin*. 2002; 20(1):151-178; vi.
39. Farrell DA, Medsger TA Jr. Trigeminal neuropathy in progressive systemic sclerosis. *Am J Med*. 1982;73(1):57-62.
40. Fischoff DK, Sirois D. Painful trigeminal neuropathy caused by severe mandibular resorption and nerve compression in a patient with systemic sclerosis: case report and literature review. *Oral Surg Oral Med Oral Pathol Oral Radiol Endod*. 2000;90(4):456-459.
41. Hietarinta M, Lassila O, Hietaharju A. Association of anti-U1RNP- and anti-Scl-70-antibodies with neurological manifestations in systemic sclerosis (scleroderma). *Scand J Rheumatol*. 1994;23(2):64-67.
42. Nascimento IS, Bonfa E, de Carvalho JF, et al. Clues for previously undiagnosed connective tissue disease in patients with trigeminal neuralgia. *J Clin Rheumatol*. 2010;16(5):205-208.
43. Derk CT, Rasheed M, Spiegel JR, et al. Increased incidence of carcinoma of the tongue in patients with systemic sclerosis. *J Rheumatol*. 2005;32(4):637-641.
44. Marcucci M, Abdala N. Clinical and radiographic study of orofacial alterations in patients with systemic sclerosis. *Braz Oral Res*. 2009;23(1):82-88.
45. Marcucci M, Abdala N. Analysis of the masseter muscle in patients with systemic sclerosis: a study by magnetic resonance imaging. *Dentomaxillofac Radiol*. 2009;38(8):524-530.
46. Jackowski J, Johren P, Muller AM, et al. Imaging of fibrosis of the oral mucosa by 20 MHz sonography. *Dentomaxillofac Radiol*. 1999;28(5):290-294.
47. Tolle SL. Scleroderma: considerations for dental hygienists. *Int J Dent Hyg*. 2008;6(2):77-83.

Chapter 33
A Scleroderma Patient Complaining of Dry and Gritty Sensation of the Eyes

Rajen Tailor and Vaneeta Sood

Keywords Keratoconjunctivitis sicca • Sjogren's syndrome • Dry eyes

Case Study

A 45-year-old female was referred with a 4-month history of sore and gritty eyes. She had been diagnosed by her General Practitioner as having dry eyes and she had been treated with a carbomer-based drop (viscotears) four times daily to both eyes. This marginally improved her symptoms. More recently, the patient had noticed mild photophobia and a stringy white discharge from her left eye.

In addition, the patient reported a 6-month history of a dry mouth with difficulty initiating swallowing. There were no other physical symptoms.

The patient was known to have a history of limited cutaneous systemic sclerosis (lSSc) and was under the care of a rheumatologist.

Ocular Examination

Visual acuity was reduced to 6/9 on the right and 6/18 on the left. Lid margins showed mild meibomian gland plugging. The tear strip was reduced in height in both eyes suggesting tear deficiency. The right inferior bulbar conjunctiva and cornea showed multiple areas of punctate staining using a cobalt blue light following instillation of 2% fluorescein (Fig. 33.1). The left eye had a stringy white mucoid discharge in the medial canthal region with multiple areas of punctate staining of the conjunctiva and

R. Tailor (✉)
Department of Ophthalmology, Birmingham & Midland Eye Centre,
City Hospital, Dudley Road, Birmingham, West Midlands B187QH, UK

R.M. Silver and C.P. Denton (eds.), *Case Studies in Systemic Sclerosis,*
DOI: 10.1007/978-0-85729-641-2_33, © Springer-Verlag London Limited 2011

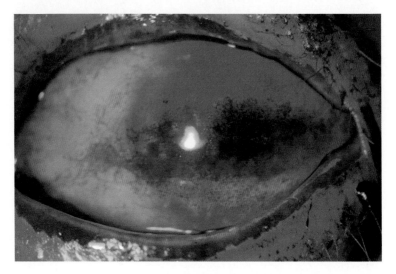

Fig. 33.1 Right cornea showing multiple yellow green areas of punctate staining following instillation of 2% fluorescein and the use of a cobalt blue light

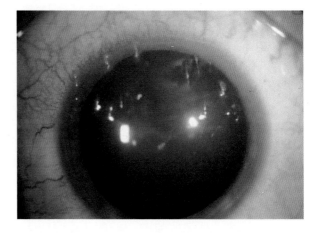

Fig. 33.2 Left cornea showing multiple white filaments adherent to the cornea

cornea following instillation of 2% fluorescein. In addition, there were multiple white "comma shaped" filaments adherent to the left cornea (Fig. 33.2). There was 2 mm of lagophthalmos (inability to completely close the eyelids).

General Physical Examination

There was asymmetric enlargement of the submandibular salivary glands. The oral mucosa appeared dry and erythematous. There was atrophy of the filiform papillae on the dorsum of the tongue. The examination also revealed sclerodactyly without proximal scleroderma, consistent with the diagnosis of limited cutaneous systemic sclerosis.

Investigations

Slit Lamp

Schirmer's test: positive. Tear film break up time (TBUT): abnormal (5 s right and left eye).

Laboratory

Erythrocyte sedimentation rate: 64 mm/h. ANA: positive by IIF. Extractable nuclear antigen antibodies (Ro/SS-A and La/SS-B): positive. Accessory salivary gland (labial) biopsy: greater than two foci of lymphocytic and histiocytic infiltration (hematoxylin–eosin stain).

Course and Management

A diagnosis of secondary Sjogren's syndrome was made based on the following clinical and laboratory findings: Severe keratoconjunctivitis sicca (KCS), history and signs of xerostomia, positive salivary gland biopsy, and previously diagnosed SSc.

Ocular surface disease severity was graded according to the dry eye severity grading scheme introduced by the Dry Eye WorkShop 2007 report.[1,2] This grading scheme is discussed in more detail in the discussion. On presentation, her left eye was graded as severity level 4 and the right eye level 3. Initial treatment consisted of lid hygiene advice, copious topical lubrication with preservative-free Carmellose 1%® hourly and Lacrilube® (a topical, preservative-free, artificial tear ointment) at night due to the risk of corneal exposure secondary to the lagophthalmos.

Preservative-free topical lubrication was continued in the long term in both eyes, though the frequency of administration was gradually reduced to four times daily over a period of 6 months. At her second outpatient appointment, the patient's left eye filamentary keratitis had not improved. Therefore, silicone punctal plugs were inserted into each lower eyelid punctum to preserve the patient's tear film, and mucolytic eyedrops (acetylcysteine) were prescribed in addition to prednisolone eyedrops 0.5%.

Discussion

The most common ocular manifestation of SSc is keratoconjunctivitis sicca (KCS) which has been found in 37–79% patients.[3-6] Depending on its severity, KCS can present with superficial punctate keratopathy, mucous strands in the precorneal tear film, or a filamentary keratitis.[3,4] As such, not all patients with SSc presenting with symptoms suggestive of KCS will require referral to an ophthalmologist or intensive treatment.

When KCS is associated with a dry mouth (xerostomia) and antibodies in the serum to Ro/SS-A or La/SS-B antigen, a diagnosis of Sjogren's syndrome (SS) must be considered. What was later to become known as Sjogren's syndrome was first described by Hadden in 1882, as a chronic disorder of exocrine glands. The defining work of the Swedish ophthalmologist Henrick Sjogren, in 1933, established the term Keratoconjunctivitis Sicca (KCS) and later documented an association between KCS, xerostomia (dry mouth), and rheumatoid arthritis (RA). Sjogren's syndrome is recognized in two forms: Primary Sjogren's syndrome characterized by KCS and xerostomia without any associated autoimmune disease and Secondary Sjogren's syndrome characterized by KCS and xerostomia with an associated autoimmune disease, such as rheumatoid arthritis, or as in this case SSc.[7] Both forms are associated with an increased incidence of lymphoma. Additionally, Sjogren's syndrome may also form part of an overlapping connective tissue disease syndrome. In the context of this case, the patient had known SSc and, therefore, secondary Sjogren's syndrome or overlap syndrome (SSc-SS) were the main differential diagnoses.

Whether Sjogren's syndrome is actually secondary to or just "associated" with SSc remains controversial.[8,9] However, of clinical significance is the fact that both subjective sicca symptoms and objective clinical signs of KCS are less frequent in secondary or associated Sjogren's syndrome than in primary Sjogren's syndrome.[8] Interestingly, patients with SSc (particularly limited cutaneous SSc) associated with SS have less severe systemic complications such as lung fibrosis and renal crisis.[8]

Investigations of Keratoconjunctivitis Sicca in Systemic Sclerosis

The purpose of investigation in cases of probable Sjogren's syndrome in patients with known SSc is two-fold: first to confirm diagnosis and second to grade the severity of KCS which will ultimately guide management. Table 33.1 provides a comprehensive list of investigations used to aid diagnosis and management of such patients. The following discussion highlights those investigations commonly used in current clinical practice with particular reference to the patient with SSc.

The principal histopathological change in the epithelial exocrine glands (lacrimal and salivary) of patients with Sjogren's syndrome is a lymphocytic (CD4+, CD8+ and CD45 Ro+cells) infiltration eventually resulting in destruction and fibrosis of

Table 33.1 Investigation of Sjogren's syndrome in the patients with known systemic sclerosis

Ocular tests	Blood tests	Histopathology and cytology	Imaging techniques
Schirmer test	ESR	Accessory salivary gland (labial) biopsy	MRI of lacrimal and parotid glands
Tear film break-up time	ANA	Impression cytology for goblet cells	Ultrasonography of salivary glands
Fluorescein test	RF		Lacrimal and
Rose Bengal test	Anti-Ro (SS-A) ab		salivary gland
Ocular feming test	Anti-La (SS-B) ab		scintigraphy
Tear lysozyme			
Tear lactoferrin			
Tear film osmolarity			

the glandular structures. The histological patterns seen in a salivary gland biopsy are similar in primary and secondary Sjogren's syndrome.[8] The severity of KCS is positively correlated with the extent of lymphocytic infiltration. Though the safety of lacrimal gland biopsy has previously been of concern, performing an exocrine gland biopsy in selected cases of suspected Sjogren's syndrome is of both diagnostic and prognostic value.[10] In cases of known SSc, there is an increased theoretical risk of exacerbation of soft tissue calcification and fibrosis following tissue biopsy, due to tissue ischemia and fibroblast stimulation resulting in accumulation of collagen.[11]

Due in part to accessibility, a biopsy of the accessory salivary glands of the lower lip is considered preferential to lacrimal or major salivary (e.g., parotid) gland biopsy. However, evidence suggests that biopsying both an accessory salivary gland and a lacrimal gland in suspected cases of Sjogren's syndrome gives much higher statistical sensitivity for accurate diagnosis.[12] Tissue sections are stained with hematoxylin–eosin stain and the presence of one or more foci of lymphocytes and histiocytes per 4 mm^2 of tissue is diagnostic of Sjogren's syndrome.

Antinuclear antibody (ANA) is positive in 70% of patients with primary Sjogren's syndrome. Antibodies to extractable nuclear antigens, anti-Ro (anti-SS-A) and anti-La (anti-SS-B), are 70–90% and 60–90% sensitive, respectively, in primary Sjogren's syndrome. They are not, however, specific to Sjogren's syndrome, as they also are present in patients with systemic lupus and inflammatory myopathy without KCS and xerostomia. The prevalence of anti-Ro (anti-SS-A) antibodies is similar in SSc associated with Sjogren's syndrome and primary Sjogren's syndrome,[8] but both anti-Ro (anti-SS-A) and anti-La (anti-SS-B) are less prevalent in patients with Sjogren's syndrome and CREST syndrome (limited cutaneous SSc) specifically.[9]

When assessing the severity of KCS, a comprehensive history and thorough assessment of ocular surface is paramount. Additional tests that may be performed in clinic or at the slit lamp to aid assessment include:

1. Schirmer test: a 35 mm by 5 mm strip of filter paper is placed in the lower eyelid fornix of both eyes and the extent of wetting is measured in mm after 5 min. The test is done under ambient light and the patient is instructed to look straight ahead and blink normally. An abnormal test result is wetting of the filter paper of

less than 10 mm at 5 min. A positive test, indicative of moderate to severe dry eyes, is wetting of the filter paper of less than 5 mm at 5 min. An important limitation is considerable variability and tendency to exhibit wide intrasubject and day-to-day variation. Hence sequential testing is of no value.

2. Tear film break up time (TBUT): a fluorescein strip is placed in the inferior fornix of the eye and then removed. The patient is asked to blink three times and then look straight ahead without blinking. The corneal surface is observed under cobalt blue light on the slit lamp. The time period from the last blink to the first break in the tear film is measured. TBUT of less than 10 s is suggestive of dry eyes.

3. Vital stainings:
   (a) Fluorescein 2%: whenever corneal surface epithelial cells are disrupted (due to dryness, degeneration, or death), fluorescein diffuses in the fluid spaces between cells and causes a green staining when viewed under cobalt blue light. The density of staining is proportional to cell disruption and hence ocular surface disease severity.
   (b) Rose Bengal 1% or Lissamine Green: when applied topically to the eye will stain devitalized cells, dead cells, and mucus. These stains are used to assess the conjunctival surface.

The Dry Eye Severity-Grading scheme[1,2] uses the above tests in addition to assessment of symptoms (discomfort levels and visual symptoms), degree of conjunctival injection, and presence or absence of meibomian gland dysfunction to ascertain the "Dry Eye Severity Level". The grading scale ranges from 1 (mild) to 4 (very severe).

Management of Keratoconjunctivitis Sicca

The medical management of KCS in the context of SSc aims to achieve three primary goals: symptomatic relief, promoting healing of the ocular surface, and preventing complications such as persistent epithelial defects and corneal ulceration.[13] To achieve these goals, tear secretion should be stimulated, inflammation should be suppressed, and tear deficiency should be treated.[14] The following discussion highlights commonly used medical, surgical, and adjunctive modalities to achieve these goals.

A more practical approach to the treatment of KCS in SSc is treatment according to disease severity. A treatment algorithm, designed by the authors and based on guidelines from DEWS 2007,[1] a Delphi approach to treatment recommendations,[2] and the Ocular Surface Workshop 2009[15] is shown in Fig. 33.3.

Stimulating Tear Secretion

Theoretically, medicinal stimulation of tear production seems a plausible option in the management of dry eyes. Unfortunately, the side effects of most such medications have limited their clinical use. Oral pilocarpine has been associated with

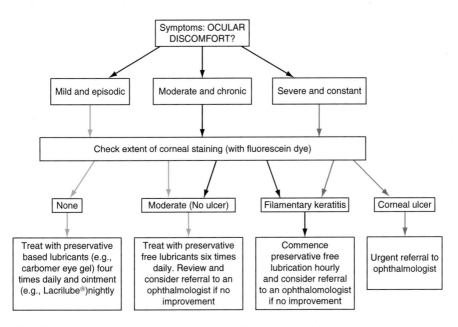

Fig. 33.3 Algorithm for the treatment of patients with systemic sclerosis who present with symptoms of dry eyes

symptomatic improvement,[16] but its poor tolerability due to profuse sweating and diarrhea has been its main downfall. Cevimeline is an oral agent approved in the United States for the treatment of dry eyes. Pharmacologically it acts by binding specifically to M3 muscarinic acetylcholine receptors in exocrine glands and has been, therefore, suggested as a targeted treatment in Sjogren's syndrome. Side effects such as sweating, nausea, and diarrhea have been reported as mild and tolerable at doses of 20 mg three times daily, with good symptomatic relief and objective improvement in Sjogren's syndrome patients.[17]

Suppressing Inflammation

Recognition of the role of inflammation of the lacrimal glands and ocular surface as integral to the cause of KCS in Sjogren's syndrome and overlap syndromes has led to the recommendation of anti-inflammatory therapy.[18] Unfortunately, the long-term side effects of topical corticosteroids, such as cataracts and glaucoma, preclude its chronic use.

Topical cyclosporine A (Restasis®, Allergan®) has a more encouraging safety profile and is, therefore, advocated for long-term use.[19,20] It is both efficacious and tolerable to the majority of patients.

Recent laboratory evidence has emerged associating decreased hormone levels with primary Sjogren's syndrome.[21-23] Specifically, dry mouth symptoms are associated with low serum androgen levels and dry eyes with low serum estrogen levels.[21] In animal models, estrogen deficiency has been shown to stimulate innate immunity resulting in autoimmune epitheliitis and lymphocytic infiltration of the salivary gland.[24] As such, the role of hormonal support therapy in the treatment of KCS appears plausible. Further in vivo studies and randomized controlled trials are awaited.

Complementary medicine may also play a role in suppressing ocular inflammation. A Scandinavian study demonstrated an improvement in the inflammatory features of Sjogren's syndrome and attributed this to oral administration of gamma-linoleic acid.[25] At a recent ocular surface workshop, supplemental nutrients, such as flaxseed oil and essential fatty acids (linoleic and linolenic acid) were also among the adjunctive treatment recommendations for dysfunctional tear syndrome.[15]

At present there is no single universally efficacious anti-inflammatory medication to treat the inflammatory component of Sjogren's syndrome. However, as this therapy evolves, we are likely to see a combination of the acute use of topical steroid for flare-ups, with long-term immunosuppression and hormonal support.

Treating Tear Deficiency

This can be done in two ways: replacing tear volume and preservation of the tear film. A combination of both is often required when symptoms or clinical signs are suggestive of moderate disease. Replacing tear film volume is achieved by the use of topical lubricants. A variety of topical artificial tear preparations with and without preservative in single use and multiuse bottles are available and continually emerging in the pharmaceutical domain. These have been extensively reviewed elsewhere.[26] The use of hypotonic solutions has also shown good patient response.

Punctal occlusion is the most common method to retain and preserve tears. The puncta can be occluded temporarily with punctual plugs and if found to be beneficial permanent closure of the puncta by thermal or electrocautery procedures may be considered. The Freeman style punctual plug, first described in 1975, remains the prototype for most styles of modern punctual plug designs. The main difference between plug types is those that are absorbable (collagen) lasting up to 3 months or permanent (silicone), which include the Freeman style plug. In Sjogren's syndrome, punctal occlusion may have a paradoxical effect due to retention of proinflammatory mediators and cytokines[27] and, therefore, may not always be beneficial.

Other Treatments

Mucolytic Agents

Ophthalmic mucolytic agents (acetylcysteine eyedrops) dissolve mucus threads and also reduce tear viscosity. Their main indication for use is in filamentary keratitis or when there is significant mucus clumping. They are rarely used in the long term and have few significant side effects.

Autologous Serum Therapy

Topical use of autologous serum is indicated when other treatments have failed. This is primarily due to the cumbersome preparation technique and unavailability of expertise. The rationale for its efficacy in KCS as well as other dry eye states is that its constituents, primarily albumin, epidermal growth factor, neurotrophic growth factor, and vitamin A, better reflect a normal tear film profile, and all of these constituents are integral to the maintenance of a healthy ocular surface.[28] Moreover, randomized controlled in vivo and in vitro studies have shown a marked suppression of apoptosis in conjunctival and corneal epithelium.[29]

Other ocular manifestations of SSc can be broadly divided into those that involve the anterior segment of the eye and those that involve the posterior segment.

Anterior Segment

Eyelid involvement can present with skin fibrosis or telangiectasia and tends to occur in patients in whom skin involvement is more extensive (i.e., diffuse cutaneous SSc).[4,6] Eyelid skin fibrosis can result in a spectrum of clinical signs, ranging from lid stiffness resulting in a "woody" texture on palpation (26–65% patients) to blepharophimosis, or bilateral ptosis with reduced lid size (3–40% patients) to lagophthalmos (rare).[4,6] It is important not to miss lagophthalmos as this can result in corneal exposure (particularly nocturnal) and exacerbation of the dry eyes. Telangiectasias are seen in 17–21% of patients and may be found on either the upper or lower lid.[4,6]

Conjunctival involvement can present with vascularization, varicosities of the conjunctival vessels, telangiectasia, vascular congestion, intravascular slugging, and shallowing of the fornices (thought to be due to subepithelial fibrosis).[5] Corneal involvement in SSc is rare, even though the rich collagen composition and vascular supply make the cornea vulnerable to damage by a number of other collagen vascular diseases. Filamentary keratitis,[4] peripheral ulcerative keratitis,[30] pellucid marginal degeneration, and keratoconus have all been described in SSc patients.[4]

Normal tension glaucoma (NTG) (glaucomatous optic nerve damage associated with a normal intraocular pressure (IOP) [less than 21 mmHg] and a visual field defect corresponding to the nerve damage) has been identified more frequently in patients with SSc compared to controls.[31] In this study, 34.4% of patients with SSc were diagnosed with NTG compared to none in the control group. The authors proposed that a lack of vascular autoregulation or dysregulation might be an etiological factor in glaucomatous optic nerve damage. However, the diagnostic criteria of NTG used in this study were questioned by Chan and Liu[32] as the intraocular pressure (IOP) was only measured once in the morning (IOP shows a diurnal variation) rather than throughout the day, and the visual field indices used to indicate significance are not wholly accepted. Allanore et al.[33] responded with the comment that their results suggested that patients with SSc have a glaucomatous propensity.

Iris transillumination defects (when a focused beam of light is shown through the pupil, defects in the iris appear bright red due to light reflecting off the retina passing through these iris defects) have been identified in many patients with SSc following exclusion of other causes.[4]

Posterior Segment

Optic disc disease in the form of bilateral optic neuropathy has been identified in a patient with CREST syndrome (limited cutaneous SSc).[34] The evidence for retinal involvement, however, in SSc is equivocal. Cotton-wool spots, retinal edema, and hemorrhages have been described in patients with SSc[35]; however, these abnormalities were mainly reported in advanced SSc (with renal involvement and hypertension). The retinal abnormalities were indistinguishable from that found in hypertensive retinopathy. In a review paper on the ocular manifestations of SSc, it was concluded that given the evidence, retinal involvement was unlikely.[36]

Parafoveal telangiectasia has been reported in association with CREST syndrome (limited cutaneous SSc). It has therefore been suggested that this condition be looked for in patients with unexplained visual loss in this group.[37]

Numerous studies have demonstrated that patients with SSc have abnormalities of the choroidal circulation and retinal pigment epithelium (RPE).[38-41] These include choroidal hypoperfusion affecting the choriocapillaries and small arterioles[38] and RPE atrophy.[40] Histological studies in patients with SSc have shown that the choroidal vessels are grossly abnormal with endothelial cell damage, basement membrane thickening, absence of pericytes, and deposition of abnormal material in and around the endothelium.[42] Similar structural alterations are known to be present in affected skin and normal appearing skin of patients with localized scleroderma and in the renal vessels in those patients suffering from SSc.[43]

Orbital involvement in SSc is very uncommon. There have been several cases of superior oblique palsy in patients with SSc.[44-46] One case resolved following the administration of oral steroids, suggesting an inflammatory etiology.[46] Brown's syndrome has been described in one case report.[47] The authors suggested it was due to deep subdermal fibrosis limiting the movement of the superior oblique tendon. Ophthalmoplegia due to orbital myositis has also been reported in patients with SSc.[48]

Orbital fat atrophy with enophthalmos has been reported in a case of linear scleroderma[49] and was shown to be due to atrophy of orbital fat, part of which was replaced by fibrosis.[49] Finally, a special mention of localized scleroderma needs to be made. In a large series of 750 patients with juvenile localized scleroderma, ocular complications was identified in 3.2% of patients, and this was almost exclusively in those patients who had the head-face subtype of linear scleroderma, i.e., the *en coup de sabre* lesion (ECDS). The most frequent ocular complications involved the adnexa, e.g., ectropion of the eyelids, loss of eyelashes, and lacrimal gland fibrosis causing aqueous-deficient dry eyes. These abnormalities may lead to lagophthalmos and exposure keratopathy. The second most frequent ocular complication involved the anterior segment (29.2% of the total cases with ocular involvement). The most important of these was anterior uveitis as it was asymptomatic in all cases and completely unrelated to the site of skin involvement (60% of cases). Hence, it is recommended that regular ophthalmic monitoring be performed to avoid complications such as secondary glaucoma and cataract which can lead to irreversible and reversible blindness, respectively. The other anterior segment complication was episcleritis (inflammation of the thin episcleral membrane overlying the sclera, causing symptoms of redness and discomfort), which is thought to be due to a subconjunctival inflammatory fibrotic lesion similar to that seen in the cutaneous lesions. Of note, episcleritis in this group of patients is often resistant to topical steroid treatment. An isolated sixth cranial nerve palsy (with a normal MRI scan of the brain) was also identified. In a small group of patients with ocular involvement (three patients – 12.5%) there were associated CNS-related abnormalities. All three patients had ECDS. One patient presented with pupil mydriasis and epilepsy, the second with pupil mydriasis, ipsilateral orbital myositis, and pseudotumor cerebri, and the third patient presented with enophthalmos, anisocoria (difference in the pupil size between the two eyes), partial iris atrophy, stellate neuroretinitis, retinal telangiectasia, and abnormalities of the brain on MRI scanning. It has therefore been recommended by the authors that neuroimaging be performed in patients with pupil and complex ocular abnormalities. In addition, the authors also recommend that patients with neurological symptoms or CNS imaging abnormalities have a complete ophthalmic examination.[50]

In summary, the commonest ocular manifestation of SSc is keratoconjunctivitis sicca (KCS), which often presents as secondary Sjogren's syndrome. Recognition of the symptoms of KCS and appropriate systematic management often result in improved symptoms, reduced ocular surface inflammation, and reduced risk of complications of dry eyes. For patients with localized scleroderma, particularly with the *en coup de sabre* lesion, physicians should consider referring all patients, even if asymptomatic, to an ophthalmologist.

References

1. Pflugfelder SC. Management and therapy of dry eye disease: report of the management and therapy subcommittee of the international dry eye workshop 2007. *Ocul Surf*. 2007;5:163-178.
2. Behrens A, Doyle JJ, Stern L, et al. Dysfunctional tear syndrome: a Delphi approach to treatment. *Cornea*. 2006;25:900-907.
3. Alarcon-Segovia D, Ibanez G, Hermandez-Ortiz J, et al. Sjogren's syndrome in progressive systemic sclerosis (scleroderma). *Am J Med*. 1974;57:78-85.
4. Horan EC. Ophthalmic manifestations of progressive systemic sclerosis. *Br J Ophthalmol*. 1969;53:388-392.
5. Kirkham TH. Scleroderma and Sjogren's syndrome. *Br J Ophthalmol*. 1969;53:131-133.
6. West RH, Barnett AJ. Ocular involvement in scleroderma. *Br J Ophthalmol*. 1979;63:845-847.
7. Vitali C, Bombardieri S, Jonsson R, et al. Classification criteria for Sjogren's syndrome: a revised version of the European criteria proposed by the American-European Consensus Group. *Ann Rheum Dis*. 2002;61:554-558.

8. Salliot C, Mouthon L, Ardizzone M, et al. Sjogren's syndrome is associated with and not secondary to systemic sclerosis. *Rheumatology.* 2007;46:321-326.

9. Doros AA, Pennec YL, Elisaf M, et al. Sjogren's syndrome in patients with CREST variant of progressive systemic scleroderma. *J Rheumatol.* 1991;18:1685-1688.

10. Tsubota K, Xu KP, et al. Decreased reflex tearing is associated with lymphocytic infiltration in lacrimal glands. *J Rheumatol.* 1996;23:313-320.

11. Caramaschi P, Baglio I, Ravagnani V, Bambara LM, Biasi D. Extensive soft tissue calcification in systemic sclerosis. *Clin Exp Rheumatol.* 2010;28(5):798-799.

12. Xu KP, Katagiri S, et al. Biopsy of labial salivary and lacrimal glands in the diagnosis of Sjogren's syndrome. *J Rheumatol.* 1996;23:76-82.

13. Tabbara K, Wagoner MD. Diagnosis and management of dry eye syndrome. New drugs in ophthalmology. Edited by Boston SG.: Little Brown and Company. Cited in *Ophthalmol Clin.* 1996;36:61-75.

14. Lemp M. New strategies in the treatment of dry eye states. *Cornea.* 1999;18:625-631.

15. Rolando M, Geerling G, Dua HS. Emerging treatment paradigms of ocular surface disease: proceedings of the ocular surface workshop. *Br J Ophthalmol.* 2010;94:i1-i9.

16. Nelson JD, Friedlander M, Yeatts RP, et al. Oral pilocarpine for symptomatic relief of keratoconjunctivitis siccain patients with Sjogren's syndrome. The MGI pharma Sjogren's syndrome study group. *Adv Exp Med Biol.* 1998;438:979-983.

17. Ono M, Takamura E, Shinozaki K, et al. Therapeutic effect of Cevimeline on dry eye in patients with Sjogren's syndrome: a randomised, double blind clinical study. *Am J Ophthalmol.* 2004;183(5):6-17.

18. Marsh P, Pflufelder SC, et al. Topical nonpreserved methylprednisolone therapy for keratoconjunctivitis sicca in Sjogren's syndrome. *Ophthalmology.* 1999;106:811-816.

19. Sall K, Stevenson OD. Two multicenter, randomized studies of the efficacy and safety of cyclosporine ophthalmic emulsion in moderate to severe dry eye disease: CsA phase III study group. *Ophthalmology.* 2000;107:631-639.

20. Donnenfield E, Pflegfelder SC. Topical ophthalmic cyclosporin: pharmacology and clinic uses. *Surv Ophthalmol.* 2009;54:321-338.

21. Forsblad-d'Elia H, Carlsten H, Labrie F, et al. Low serum levels of sex steroids are associated with disease characteristics in primary Sjogren's syndrome; supplementation with dehydroepiandrosterone restores the concentrations. *J Clin Endocrinol Metab.* 2009;94(6):2044-2051.

22. Sullivan DA, Wichkam LA, et al. Androgens and dry eyes in Sjogren's syndrome. *Ann NY Acad Sci.* 1999;876:312-324.

23. Schamberg DA, Bring JE, et al. Hormone replacement therapy and dry eye syndrome. *JAMA.* 2001;286:2114-2119.

24. Mariette X, Gottenberg JE. Pathogenesis of Sjogren's syndrome and therapeutic consequences. *Curr Opin Rheumatol.* 2010;22(5):471-477.

25. Horrobin DF. Essential fatty acid and prostaglandin metabolism in Sjogren's syndrome systemic sclerosis and rheumatoid arthritis. *Scand J Rheumatol Suppl.* 1986;6(suppl):242-245.

26. Colange M. The treatment of dry eye. *Surv Ophthalmol.* 2001;45:S227-S239.

27. Yen MT, Monroy D. Punctal occlusion decreases tear production, clearance and ocular surface sensation. *Invest Ophthalmol Vis Sci.* 1999;40:S980.

28. Tsubota K, Goto E, et al. Treatment of dry eyes by autologous serum application in Sjogren's syndrome. *Br J Ophthalmol.* 1999;83:390-395.

29. Kojima T, Higuchi A, Goto E, et al. Autologous serum eye drops for the treatment of dry eye diseases. *Cornea.* 2008;27(suppl 1):S25-S30.

30. Horie K, Nishi M, Sawa M, Mochizuki M. A case of peripheral corneal ulcer accompanied by progressive systemic sclerosis. *Acta Soc Ophthalmol Jpn.* 1992;96:922-929.

31. Allanore Y, Parc C, Monnet D, et al. Increased prevalence of ocular glaucomatous abnormalities in systemic sclerosis. *Ann Rheum Dis.* 2004;63:1276-1278.

32. Chan AYK, Liu DTL. Increased prevalence of ocular glaucomatous abnormalities in systemic sclerosis. *Ann Rheum Dis.* 2005;64:341-344.

33. Allanore Y, Kahan A, Brezin A. Authors' reply. *Ann Rheum Dis*. 2005;64:341-344.
34. Boschi A, Snyers B, Lambert M. Bilateral optic neuropathy associated with the crest variant of scleroderma. *Eur J Ophthalmol*. 1993;3:219-222.
35. Ashton N, Coomes EN, Garner A, Oliver DO. Retinopathy due to progressive systemic sclerosis. *J Pathol*. 1968;96:259-268.
36. Tailor R, Gupta A, et al. Ocular manifestations of scleroderma. *Surv Ophthalmol*. 2009;54: 292-304.
37. Proctor B, Chang T, Hay D. Parafoveal telangiectasia in association with CREST syndrome. *Arch Ophthalmol*. 1998;16:814-815.
38. Grennan DM, Forrester J. Involvement of the eye in SLE and scleroderma. A study using fluorescein angiography in addition to clinical ophthalmic assessment. *Ann Rheum Dis*. 1977;36:152-156.
39. Hesse RJ, Slagle DF. Scleroderma choroidopathy: report of an unusual case. *Ann Ophthalmol*. 1982;14:524-525.
40. Kraus A, Guerra-Bautista G, Espinoza G, et al. Defects on the retinal pigment epithelium in scleroderma. *Br J Rheumatol*. 1991;30:112-114.
41. Serup L, Serup J, Hagdrup H. Fundus fluorescein angiography in generalized scleroderma. *Ophthalmic Res*. 1987;19:303-308.
42. Farkas TG, Sylvester V, Archer D. The choroidopathy of progressive systemic sclerosis. *Am J Ophthalmol*. 1972;74:875-886.
43. MacLean H, Guthrie W. Retinopathy in scleroderma. *J Am Oph Soc*. 1969;89:209-212.
44. Mejias E. Superior oblique muscle paralysis in the CREST syndrome. *PR Health Sci J*. 1986;5:19-27.
45. Rush JA. Isolated superior oblique paralysis in progressive systemic sclerosis. *Ann Ophthalmol*. 1981;13:217-220.
46. Shimohata T, Sato T, Akaiwa Y, et al. Isolated trochlear nerve palsy in CREST syndrome. *Eur Neurol*. 2003;50:181-182.
47. Olver J, Laidler P. Acquired Brown's syndrome in a patient with combined lichen sclerosus et atrophicus and morphoea. *Br J Ophthalmol*. 1988;72:552-557.
48. Arnett FC, Michels RG. Inflammatory ocular myopathy in systemic sclerosis (scleroderma). A case report and review of the literature. *Arch Intern Med*. 1973;132(5):740-743.
49. Ramboer K, Demaerel P, Baert AL, et al. Linear scleroderma with orbital involvement: follow up and magnetic resonance imaging. *Br J Ophthalmol*. 1997;81:90-91.
50. Zannin ME et al. Ocular involvement in children with localised scleroderma – a multi-centre study. *Br J Ophthalmol*. 2007;91:1311-1314.

Chapter 34
A 34-Year-Old Woman with 2-Year History of Therapy-Resistant, Rapidly Progressive SSc Successfully Treated by Autologous Hematopoietic Stem Cell Transplantation

Alan G. Tyndall

Keywords Scleroderma • Stem cell • Transplant

Case Study

A 34-year-old woman was referred for consideration for autologous hematopoietic stem cell transplantation (HSCT) for systemic sclerosis (SSc). She had enjoyed perfect health until 2 years previously when Raynaud's phenomenon occurred, followed over weeks by puffy hands and fatigue. Within months thickened skin on face, trunk, and extremities along with digital ulcers and dysphagia led to a diagnosis of dSSc. Investigations revealed a positive ANA, positive anti-Scl-70 (topoisomerase 1) antibody, and diminished peristalsis in the lower esophagus. Otherwise there was no evidence of major organ involvement: pulmonary function tests, HRCT of the chest, echocardiogram, Holter ECG monitor, and renal function were all normal. Intravenous therapy with iloprost over 2 months was ineffective and associated with side effects, methotrexate at a maximum weekly dose of 20 mg over 9 months was ineffective, as was IVIg over the next 3 months followed by cyclophosphamide (CYC) 825 mg by monthly intravenous infusions to a total dose of 3.3 g.

Physical Examination

On examination there was hyperpigmentation and depigmentation of the skin (the patient is of Indian extraction) with loss of skin hair and sweat glands. The modified Rodnan skin score (mRSS) was 32/51. Flexion contractures were present

A.G. Tyndall
Department of Rheumatology, University Clinic, Felix Platter Spital Basel (Hospital),
Burgfelderstrasse 101, Basel CH-4012, Switzerland

R.M. Silver and C.P. Denton (eds.), *Case Studies in Systemic Sclerosis,*
DOI: 10.1007/978-0-85729-641-2_34, © Springer-Verlag London Limited 2011

at the elbows, fingers, and knees along with tendon friction rubs. Microstomia (interincisor distance 2.3 cm) was present. Pitting scars were present on several fingertips and ischemic ulceration of elbows and knuckles was noted.

The acute phase reactants were elevated (ESR 30 mm/h; CRP 15 mg/L (normal <5)) and a repeat screening revealed no internal organ involvement.

Treatment

The patient fulfilled the entry criteria for the ASTIS (Autologous Stem cell Transplantation International Scleroderma) trial (www.astistrial.com) and after extensive discussion and informed consent was randomized to the autologous hematopoietic stem cell transplant (HSCT). A pretransplant bone marrow examination (as per protocol) from the iliac crest was complicated by a retroperitoneal hemorrhage which finally resolved after 2 months. Stem cell mobilization was successful using G-CSF (filgrastim 10 mg/kg body weight/day) and CYC (2×2 g/m²) yielding a stem cell product of 16.49×10^6 CD34 cells/kg body weight. Two months later she underwent conditioning (rabbit ATG 7.5 mg/kg body weight in three divided doses and CYC 200 mg/kg body weight in four divided doses). During the ATG infusion, as per protocol, intravenous glucocorticoid was given and therapy with ACE inhibitor was commenced. On day 8 she received daily filgrastim for 4 days. Full engraftment was achieved at day 12 post conditioning and she was able to leave the isolation ward. Complications during the HSCT included nausea and vomiting with CYC; fever, chills, and pruritic skin rash with ATG; and during the aplasia, oral mucosal candida infection. All responded to standard therapy. In addition, during the aplasia, an episode of cholecystitis without gallstone was treated with piperacillin.

On discharge her medications included pantoprazole, valacyclovir, fluconazole, atovaquone, and ramipril.

Course

Within 2 months post HSCT a subjective improvement in energy and reduced fatigue was accompanied by an improved mRSS to 28/51 and increased range of movement of shoulder, elbow, and finger joints.

However, 3 months later she developed acutely a "flu-like" illness with dyspnea, fever, and diffuse pulmonary infiltrate. Blood and bronchoalveolar lavage (BAL) cultures were negative for bacteria and PCP, but contained massive lympocytosis of the NK cell type (CD56) with the morphology of large granular lymphocytes (LGL). Initially an NK cell lymphoma was considered, but subsequently a positive cytomegalovirus (CMV) infection in the lung was demonstrated. The prophylactic valacylovir was switched to valganciclovir for 15 days with satisfactory clinical response.

Over the next 12 months continuous improvement of general state, mRSS, and microvascular disturbance was observed. By 2 years post HSCT, the mRSS was 0, the pigmentation changes had reversed, normal body hair and sweat gland function

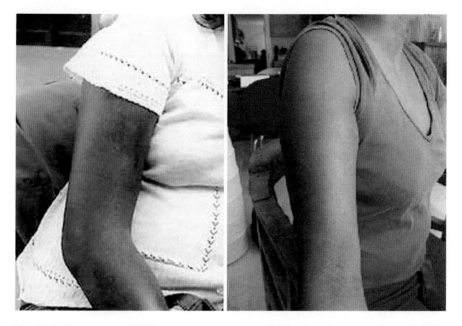

Fig. 34.1 Changes post HSCT over 4 years. Arm showing pre and 4 year post transplant skin changes. Note loss of elbow contracture and return of normal pigmentation, hair, and sweat gland function post transplant

returned, and no further episodes of Raynaud's phenomenon or digital ulcers occurred. Figure 34.1 shows the pre (2005) and 4 years post (2010) skin appearances.

She has resumed her former occupation (business woman) and married. Although the HSCT induced menopause, a known complication, she is currently exploring adoption. Her medications are pantoprazole and rimipril and the laboratory investigations demonstrate a full hematopoietic and immunological reconstitution.

Discussion

The concept of immunoablation followed by HSCT as "rescue" for severe, therapy-resistant autoimmune disease (AD) has been evolving over more than a decade and was recently reviewed.[1] Currently around 1,500 patients have received an HSCT as treatment for an AD, around 1,000 of whom are in Europe (Table 34.1). The first reported case was indeed an SSc patient with pulmonary hypertension who responded and has remained stable for 13 years.[2] An international collaboration has been proceeding since then with the aim of demonstrating through prospective controlled clinical trials associated with mechanistic studies if and how such a therapeutic strategy benefits the patients.[3]

The results of the phase I and II studies led to the development of the randomized ASTIS trial,[4] which completed recruitment in 2009. 156 patients were randomized to either HSCT or monthly IV CYC pulse therapy 750 mg/m² for 12 months.

Table 34.1 Comparison between autologous stem cell transplantation international scleroderma (ASTIS) and scleroderma cyclophosphamide or transplant (SCOT) trials

	ASTIS	SCOT
Inclusion criteria	18–60 years old	18–69 years old
	Disease duration <5 years	Disease duration ≤5 years
	Skin score >15/51	dSSc with either pulmonary disease or renal crisis
	At least one major organ	
Exclusion criteria	Defined severe organ damage	Defined severe organ damage
	Prior CYC total >5 g	Prior CYC >6 months or >3 g/m²
Mobilizing regimen	CYC + G-CSF	G-CSF
Conditioning regimen	CYC 200 mg/kg/rabbit ATG/CD34 selection	CYC 120 mg/kg/equine ATG/ TBI 800cGY/CD34 selection
Primary endpoint	Survival without organ failure at 2 years	Event-free survival without organ failure at 44 months
Control arm	CYC monthly IVI for 12 months	CYC monthly IVI for 12 months
Current status	Completed. Last patient treated mid 2009. First efficacy analysis mid 2011	Recruiting

The primary end point is event-free survival at 2 years, events being defined as death or end-stage irreversible organ failure. Although efficacy data are still outstanding, toxicity was not more than expected from previous experience. A similar study called the Scleroderma Cyclophosphamide or Transplant (SCOT) Trial is running in the US under the auspices of the NIH, the major difference being the conditioning protocol which includes total body irradiation (TBI).

Several important messages have emerged from the HSCT experience so far. First and most importantly, this treatment strategy has significant early toxicity. Transplant-related mortality (TRM) was initially 12.5%,[5] and despite better patient selection and treating center experience, remains between 8% and 10%. The patient group eligible for the ASTIS and SCOT trials has an estimated 5 year mortality from disease progression of around 50%. TRM is related to extent of major organ damage, age of patient, and intensity of the conditioning regimen.[6]

Our patient had several major infectious episodes any of which may have been fatal, especially the CMV pneumonia. This underlines the importance of the need for an experienced transplant team in continuous contact with the AD experts. SSc is associated with some special issues such as CYC cardiac toxicity[7] and ATG or TBI-associated lung toxicity.[8] In addition, fatal late toxicity in the form of fungal infections, secondary autoimmunity, for example, acquired factor VIII antibodies, and secondary leukemia have all been observed.

However, around one-third of AD patients have enjoyed a durable and often drug-free remission.[9] In some, such as the patient reported here, the response has been spectacular and beyond that to be expected from a simple cessation of inflammation. It was demonstrated that despite full return of the autologous immune repertoire, many patients with multiple sclerosis[10] and systemic lupus erythematosus[11] remained in full clinical remission, suggesting a "resetting" of autoimmunity.

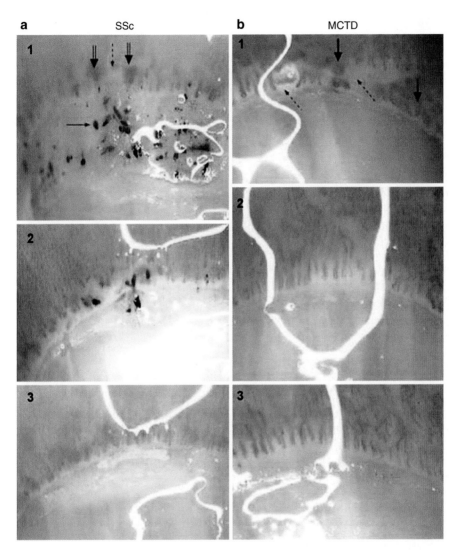

Fig. 34.2 Normalization of microvascular changes in two patients over 3 months. (**a**) Patient 1, fourth finger on the right. *Panel 1*: reduced translucency. Massive capillary bleedings (*arrow*), enlarged capillaries (*arrow*), and avascular regions (*arrow, dotted line*) before treatment. *Panel 2*: remarkable increase in capillary density and reduced bleedings but still some avascular regions after mobilization. *Panel 3*: normalized capillary number, size, and architecture with no bleedings 5 months after hematopoietic stem cell transplantation (HSCT). (**b**) Patient 2, fourth finger on the left. *Panel 1*: severe disarrangement, multiple giant capillaries (*arrow, double lined*), and large avascular fields (*arrow, dotted line*) before mobilization. *Panel 2*: increase in capillary numbers and reduced avascular areas. Loss of giant capillaries after mobilization. *Panel 3*: further increase in capillary density with only hypovascularized regions. Normalization of the capillary architecture but still many capillaries with slightly pathologic shapes. *White stripes* correspond to light reflections from the oily skin surface. (Reproduced from Aschwanden et al.[13] © 2008 with permission from BMJ Publishing Group Ltd.)

In addition, remodeling of aberrant collagen deposition[8] and microvascular changes in the nailfold (Fig. 34.2) and skin[12] suggest that some form of rebalancing of the cellular and matrix "niche" microenvironment has occurred allowing a normal return to homeostatic balance. The return of normal skin, body hair, and sweat gland function in our patient supports this, since the agents used in the initial treatment do not affect all niche cells and do not persist. Exactly which cell or cells have been positively affected by the potent but nontargeted approach of HSCT and how long the remission will last remain to be elucidated.

References

1. Tyndall A, Gratwohl A. Adult stem cell transplantation in autoimmune disease. *Curr Opin Hematol.* 2009;16(4):285-291.
2. Tamm M, Gratwohl A, Tichelli A, Perruchoud AP, Tyndall A. Autologous haemopoietic stem cell transplantation in a patient with severe pulmonary hypertension complicating connective tissue disease. *Ann Rheum Dis.* 1996;55(10):779-780.
3. Tyndall A, Gratwohl A. Blood and marrow stem cell transplants in autoimmune disease. A consensus report written on behalf of the European League Against Rheumatism (EULAR) and the European Group for Blood and Marrow Transplantation (EBMT). *Br J Rheumatol.* 1997;36(3):390-392.
4. van Laar JM, Farge D, Tyndall A. Stem cell transplantation: A treatment option for severe systemic sclerosis? *Ann Rheum Dis.* 2008;67(suppl 3):iii35-iii38.
5. Binks M, Passweg JR, Furst D, et al. Phase I/II trial of autologous stem cell transplantation in systemic sclerosis: procedure related mortality and impact on skin disease. *Ann Rheum Dis.* 2001;60(6):577-584.
6. Gratwohl A, Passweg J, Bocelli-Tyndall C, et al. Autologous hematopoietic stem cell transplantation for autoimmune diseases. *Bone Marrow Transplant.* 2005;35(9):869-879.
7. Saccardi R, Tyndall A, Coghlan G, et al. Consensus statement concerning cardiotoxicity occurring during haematopoietic stem cell transplantation in the treatment of autoimmune diseases, with special reference to systemic sclerosis and multiple sclerosis. *Bone Marrow Transplant.* 2004;34(10):877-881.
8. Nash RA, McSweeney PA, Crofford LJ, et al. High-dose immunosuppressive therapy and autologous hematopoietic cell transplantation for severe systemic sclerosis: long-term follow-up of the U.S. multicenter pilot study. *Blood.* 2007;110(4):1388-1396.
9. Farge D, Labopin M, Tyndall A, et al. Autologous hematopoietic stem cell transplantation for autoimmune diseases: an observational study on 12 years' experience from the European Group for Blood and Marrow Transplantation Working Party on Autoimmune Diseases. *Haematologica.* 2010;95(2):284-292.
10. Muraro PA, Douek DC, Packer A, et al. Thymic output generates a new and diverse TCR repertoire after autologous stem cell transplantation in multiple sclerosis patients. *J Exp Med.* 2005;201(5):805-816.
11. Alexander T, Thiel A, Rosen O, et al. Depletion of autoreactive immunologic memory followed by autologous hematopoietic stem cell transplantation in patients with refractory SLE induces long-term remission through de novo generation of a juvenile and tolerant immune system. *Blood.* 2009;113(1):214-223.

12. Fleming JN, Nash RA, McLeod DO, et al. Capillary regeneration in scleroderma: Stem cell therapy reverses phenotype? *PLoS ONE*. 2008;3(1):e1452.
13. Aschwanden M, Daikeler T, Jaeger KA, et al. Rapid improvement of nailfold capillaroscopy after intense immunosuppression for systemic sclerosis and mixed connective tissue disease. *Ann Rheum Dis*. 2008;67(7):1057-1059.

Chapter 35
Sclerodactyly and Raynaud's Phenomenon in a Patient Who Has Primary Biliary Cirrhosis

Maureen D. Mayes and Shervin Assassi

Keywords Primary biliary cirrhosis (PBC) • Cholestasis • Liver disease • Scleroderma • Antimitochondrial antibody (AMA)

History

A 55-year-old woman was referred to rheumatology because of a positive antinuclear antibody (ANA), long-standing Raynaud's phenomenon, and tender fingertips. She had been diagnosed with primary biliary cirrhosis (PBC) 10 years prior on the basis of a persistently elevated serum alkaline phosphatase associated with a positive antimitochondrial antibody (AMA), and a liver biopsy consistent with this diagnosis. She was taking ursodiol (ursodeoxycholic acid) for this with improvement but not total normalization of the alkaline phosphatase level.

She described typical color changes of Raynaud's phenomenon (consisting of cyanosis and blanching on cold exposure) involving the fingers that had been present for almost 20 years. She had developed tenderness of the fingertips more pronounced in the past 2 years but did not describe open ulcers. She also had heartburn for several years for which she was taking a proton pump inhibitor with improvement. She had no dysphagia and her weight had been stable. She had also noticed "red spots" on her face but could not recall when they first appeared.

M.D. Mayes (✉)
Department of Internal Medicine, The University of Texas-Houston Medical School, Rheumatology, 6431 Fannin Street, MSB 5.270, Houston, TX 077030, USA

R.M. Silver and C.P. Denton (eds.), *Case Studies in Systemic Sclerosis*,
DOI: 10.1007/978-0-85729-641-2_35, © Springer-Verlag London Limited 2011

Physical Exam

Vital signs: height=61 in., weight=51.4 kg; BP 102/76 mmHg; pulse 84 bpm; respirations 14 per min. She was a thin but otherwise healthy-appearing woman in good spirits. Examination of the skin showed puffy hands and mild sclerodactyly with skin thickening confined to the fingers, that is, with no other thick or tight skin elsewhere on the extremities, face, or trunk. There were tender digital pitting scars on the fingertips, most prominently noted on the index and third digits, but no open ulcers. There were multiple, prominent telangiectasias (mat-like telangiectasias that blanched with pressure) of the face and hands, particularly on the palms and also on the forearms and chest. There were no areas of clinically apparent subcutaneous calcinosis. There were mild flexion contractures of the fingers but good range of motion of other joint areas.

The physical examination was otherwise unremarkable, including pulmonary, cardiac, abdominal, neurologic, and musculoskeletal exam.

Laboratory Findings

The ANA by indirect immunofluorescence (IIF) was positive at a titer of 1:1,280 in a centromere pattern. Chemistry panel showed a mildly elevated alkaline phosphatase (at 220 with upper limits of normal being 195) but normal serum transaminases and normal renal function. A CBC and urinalysis were also normal. Antimitochondrial antibody was noted to be elevated on review of previous records.

Pulmonary function tests showed normal spirometry (FVC 90% predicted) with normal lung volumes (VC 90% predicted). However the diffusing capacity for carbon monoxide (DLco) was low (55% predicted).

An echocardiogram estimated the right ventricular systolic pressure (RVSP) to be 30 mmHg (normal <35) with a normal left ventricular ejection fraction (LVEF) of 55–60%. There was no pericardial effusion and no evidence of diastolic dysfunction.

Course

A diagnosis of limited cutaneous systemic sclerosis (lSSc) was made on the basis of sclerodactyly and digital pitting scars.[1] The presence of Raynaud's phenomenon, gastroesophageal reflux, and positive ANA in a centromere pattern are consistent with this diagnosis. There was no evidence from a clinical point of view or from radiographic studies to suggest pulmonary fibrosis. Furthermore, spirometry and lung volumes were normal. However, the isolated low DLco is unexplained. The lack of dyspnea on exertion and the normal echocardiogram with normal estimated right ventricular systolic pressure argues against pulmonary hypertension, at least currently, although she remains at risk for the development of this complication particularly as the low DLco is not explained by anemia, pulmonary fibrosis, or left ventricular systolic or diastolic dysfunction.

She was started on a calcium channel blocker for the Raynaud's phenomenon, although the dose was limited by her fairly low blood pressure. She remained on the proton pump inhibitor. She will be followed on an annual basis with PFTs and echocardiogram.

Liver function tests are being followed by her gastroenterologist on a quarterly basis.

Discussion

It is frequently difficult to determine the onset of limited cutaneous SSc (lSSc). This patient clearly had Raynaud's phenomenon prior to the diagnosis of primary biliary cirrhosis, but other manifestations of SSc (tender digital pitting, GERD, and telangiectasias) seem to postdate PBC. Although these two conditions (PBC and SSc) occur more commonly in the same individual than would be predicted by chance alone, the onset of each of these two conditions can be separated by several years. Reports of PBC preceding scleroderma tend to come from the Gastroenterology literature, while the reports of SSc predating PBC are more commonly found in the Rheumatology literature, most likely reflecting ascertainment bias. In a study conducted at a PBC tertiary care center the diagnosis of PBC occurred after SSc in 56% of cases.[2]

PBC is a chronic progressive autoimmune disease characterized by destruction of intrahepatic bile ducts causing fibrosis and eventually cirrhosis of the liver. The diagnosis of PBC is made based on the presence of two or more of the following criteria: positive antimitochondrial antibodies (AMA), increased hepatic enzymes suggesting a cholestatic pattern persisting for more than 6 months (mainly alkaline phosphatase), and a compatible or diagnostic liver biopsy.[3]

PBC is the most common liver disease associated with SSc. The prevalence of PBC among SSc patients is reported to be approximately 2%.[4,5] Considering the low prevalence of 0.04% for PBC in the general population,[6] the reported prevalence of this disease among SSc patients indicates a strong association between these two autoimmune disorders. Similarly, the prevalence of SSc among PBC is relatively high at 7.4%.[2] In contrast with PBC, autoimmune hepatitis rarely co-occurs with SSc, there being only nine reported cases of SSc with autoimmune hepatitis in the literature.[7] As shown in Table 35.1, other possible causes for liver disease in SSc include drug-induced hepatitis and viral hepatitis.

Large-scale genetic studies in SSc and PBC have provided evidence for common genetic background for these two diseases. Besides the HLA region, *IFR5-TNPO3* is identified as a susceptibility locus for SSc as well as for PBC.[8,9] Furthermore, the prevalence of PBC among first-degree relatives of SSc patients is relatively high at 0.7%, which further supports a common genetic basis for these two diseases.[10]

Table 35.1 Differential diagnoses of hepatic parameter abnormalities in SSc

	Main hepatic parameter abnormality	AMA[a] or sp100	ASMA[b] or anti-LKM-1[c]	Viral serology
Primary biliary cirrhosis	Cholestatic	+	–	–
Autoimmune hepatitis	↑ Transaminases	–	+	–
Viral hepatitis	↑ Transaminases	–	–	+
Drug-induced hepatitis	↑ Transaminases	–	–	–

[a]Antimitochondrial antibodies
[b]Antismooth muscle antibodies
[c]Antiliver kidney microsome antibodies

Table 35.2 Diagnostic accuracy of PBC-related autoantibodies in SSc

	Sensitivity %	Specificity %	LR+[a]	LR–[b]
AMA[c] by IIF[d]	43.8	98.9	39.9	0.6
AMA[c] by MIT3 ELISA	81.3	94.6	15.1	0.2
sp100	31.3	97.4	11.9	0.7
gp210	6.3	99.8	25	0.9
AMA[a] by MIT3 ELISA or sp100	100	92.6	13.6	0

[a]Positive likelihood ratio
[b]Negative likelihood ratio
[c]Antimitochondrial antibodies
[d]Indirect immunofluorescence
Adapted from Assassi et al.[5] with permission from *The Journal of Rheumatology*

PBC in SSc patients is associated with anticentromere antibodies and limited cutaneous disease type (lSSc).[2,4,11] In a large study of SSc patients, anticentromere antibody (ACA) positivity was strongly associated with PBC [$p < 0.001$, $OR = 81.82$, 95% CI 4.9-1369.4]; the association of PBC with limited cutaneous disease type did not reach statistical significance [$p = 0.12$, $OR = 2.63$, 95% CI 0.78-13.14], indicating that PBC is primarily associated with the anticentromere antibody (ACA).[5]

Antimitochondrial antibodies (AMA) are the most prominent PBC-specific autoantibody and are present in 80–96.5% of patients with PBC. Antimitochondrial antibodies can be detected by the presence of a mitochondrial staining pattern on the immunofluorescent ANA. However, not all commercial laboratories will report the pattern of non-nuclear staining when an ANA is ordered. Specific tests for antimitochondrial antibodies include M2 or a more recent test, MIT3 (commercially available and provided when "antimitochondrial antibody" testing is ordered), as well as sp100 and gp210 which are commercially available but only by specific request. The specificity and sensitivity of these autoantibodies vary and are discussed below.

In a large study of 5,805 Japanese patients with PBC, the AMA-negative patients had a higher frequency of other associated autoimmune diseases.[12] Supporting this finding, the sensitivity of AMA in a large study of 817 SSc patients using an enhanced performance MIT3 ELISA was relatively low at 81% (Table 35.2). AMA as detected by indirect immunofluorescence (IIF) on HEp-2 cell substrates had an even lower sensitivity of 44%. AMA results by these two methods were highly concordant ($p = 0.001$). Furthermore, this antibody, regardless of determination method, was highly specific for PBC (specificity by MIT3 ELISA = 95% and by IIF = 99%). The frequency of AMA (MIT3) was 7% in the overall SSc population. In this cross-sectional study, 5% of SSc patients had AMA (MIT3) antibodies without clinically apparent PBC.[5] Longitudinal studies are required to determine the risk for the future development of PBC in this group of SSc patients.

Timely diagnosis of PBC is important as introduction of treatment with ursodeoxycholic acid may improve prognosis. Especially in AMA-negative (that is M2/MIT3-NEGATIVE) PBC cases, other PBC-specific antibodies might be helpful in early detection of this disease. Sp100 and gp210 are two other highly specific PBC antibodies that are commercially available by specific request. Sp100 antibodies are directed against a nuclear protein identified as a pattern of "multiple nuclear dots" on IIF and are present in 18–44% of PBC cases.[13] Gp210 autoantibodies are directed against components of the nuclear pore complex and are present in 9–29% of PBC patients.[14] In the above-mentioned large SSc/PBC study,[5] the frequency of sp100 antibodies in SSc was approximately 3%, while the frequency of gp210 antibodies was exceedingly rare at 0.4%. The sensitivity and specificity of sp100 for PBC among SSc patients were 31% and 97%, respectively; gp100 had an even lower sensitivity of 6% for PBC in this population. However, utilizing sp100 and AMA (M2/MIT3) as a combined marker detected all PBC cases resulting in a sensitivity of 100% with an incremental decrease in specificity to 93% (Table 35.2). If confirmed in other populations, this combined marker could lead to improved detection of PBC cases among our patients with SSc. Despite the fact that sp100 had a high specificity of 97.4% for PBC, an indiscriminate use of this antibody in SSc patients will lead to a high number of false-positive results because the prevalence of PBC is only 2% in this population. Therefore, we recommend that sp100 only be ordered for AMA-negative patients with a clinical picture consistent with PBC (e.g., unexplained and persistent cholestasis).

AMA are associated with anticentromere antibodies while they do not correlate with the presence of other SSc-related antibodies such as antitopoisomerase 1 (Scl 70) or antibodies to RNA Polymerase III.[4,5] Similarly, sp100 antibodies are also associated with anticentromere antibodies and do not correlate with other SSc-related antibodies; gp210 does not correlate with any of the SSc-related antibodies.[5]

Somewhat surprisingly, patients with PBC/SSc overlap have milder liver disease than patients with PBC alone. In a prospective study, PBC/SSc overlap patients had a slower rate of bilirubin increase as well as a lower rate of liver transplantation or liver-related deaths than the PBC-alone group.[15] Supporting this finding, in another prospective study gp210 and anticentromere antibodies were associated with two different PBC progression types. In this study, while anticentromere antibodies were predictive for development of portal hypertension gp210 antibodies were associated with progression to hepatic failure; sp100 antibodies were not predictive of any investigated clinical outcomes. PBC patients with gp210 and anticentromere antibodies also differed histologically as gp210 was associated with more severe interface hepatitis and lobar inflammation.[15] The previously described low prevalence of gp210 antibodies in conjunction with the high rate of anticentromere positivity in PBC/SSc cases might partially explain the less severe course of liver disease in this group of patients.

Treatment of patients with SSc/PBC overlap should be conducted in close collaboration between rheumatologists and hepatologists. It is important to make the diagnosis in a timely fashion as treatment may delay or prevent irreversible liver damage, as noted above.

Ursodiol is the only widely accepted treatment of PBC and is considered to be a disease modifying agent. However, a group of PBC patients do not respond to this treatment and progress to advanced liver disease requiring liver transplantation. Furthermore, PBC patients may have steatorrhea secondary to malabsorption of dietary fats, confounding the diarrhea resulting from bacterial overgrowth often seen in SSc patients. Moreover, PBC patients can have deficiencies in fat soluble vitamins, including deficiencies in vitamin D detected by measuring the serum concentration of calcidiol (25-hydroxyvitamin D). Initiation of potentially hepatotoxic agents as treatment of SSc in overlap cases should occur only after consultation with the treating hepatologist and under close monitoring.

In summary, PBC is the most common liver disease in SSc patients. It is highly associated with the presence of anticentromere antibodies. The AMA are useful for early detection of SSc/PBC but have a lower sensitivity than in PBC alone. Determination of sp100 antibodies might be beneficial in AMA-negative SSc cases in which there is high clinical suspicion for PBC. The course of liver disease is less severe in SSc/PBC overlap than in PBC alone. The optimal medical management of patients with SSc/PBC overlap requires close collaboration between the treating rheumatologist and hepatologist.

References

1. Preliminary criteria for the classification of systemic sclerosis (scleroderma). Subcommittee for scleroderma criteria of the American Rheumatism Association Diagnostic and Therapeutic Criteria Committee. *Arthritis Rheum.* 1980;23(5):581-590.
2. Rigamonti C, Shand LM, Feudjo M, et al. Clinical features and prognosis of primary biliary cirrhosis associated with systemic sclerosis. *Gut.* 2006;55:388-394.
3. Kaplan MM, Gershwin ME. Primary biliary cirrhosis. *N Engl J Med.* 2005;353:1261-1273.
4. Jacobsen S, Halberg P, Ullman S, et al. Clinical features and serum antinuclear antibodies in 230 Danish patients with systemic sclerosis. *Br J Rheumatol.* 1998;37:39-45.
5. Assassi S, Fritzler MJ, Arnett FC, et al. Primary biliary cirrhosis (PBC), PBC autoantibodies, and hepatic parameter abnormalities in a large population of systemic sclerosis patients. *J Rheumatol.* 2009;36:2250-2256.
6. Feld JJ, Heathcote EJ. Epidemiology of autoimmune liver disease. *J Gastroenterol Hepatol.* 2003;18:1118-1128.
7. Efe C, Ozaslan E, Nasiroglu N, Tunca H, Purnak T, Altiparmak E. The development of autoimmune hepatitis and primary biliary cirrhosis overlap syndrome during the course of connective tissue diseases: report of three cases and review of the literature. *Dig Dis Sci.* 2010;55:2417-2421.

8. Hirschfield GM, Liu X, Han Y, et al. Variants at IRF5-TNPO3, 17q12-21 and MMEL1 are associated with primary biliary cirrhosis. *Nat Genet*. 2010;42:655-657.

9. Radstake TR, Gorlova O, Rueda B, et al. Genome-wide association study of systemic sclerosis identifies CD247 as a new susceptibility locus. *Nat Genet*. 2010;42:426-429.

10. Arora-Singh RK, Assassi S, del Junco DJ, et al. Autoimmune diseases and autoantibodies in the first degree relatives of patients with systemic sclerosis. *J Autoimmun*. 2010;35:52-57.

11. Sakauchi F, Mori M, Zeniya M, Toda G. A cross-sectional study of primary biliary cirrhosis in Japan: utilization of clinical data when patients applied to receive public financial aid. *J Epidemiol*. 2005;15:24-28.

12. Sakauchi F, Mori M, Zeniya M, Toda G. Antimitochondrial antibody negative primary biliary cirrhosis in Japan: utilization of clinical data when patients applied to receive public financial aid. *J Epidemiol*. 2006;16:30-34.

13. Zuchner D, Sternsdorf T, Szostecki C, Heathcote EJ, Cauch-Dudek K, Will H. Prevalence, kinetics, and therapeutic modulation of autoantibodies against Sp100 and promyelocytic leukemia protein in a large cohort of patients with primary biliary cirrhosis. *Hepatology*. 1997;26:1123-1130.

14. Nickowitz RE, Wozniak RW, Schaffner F, Worman HJ. Autoantibodies against integral membrane proteins of the nuclear envelope in patients with primary biliary cirrhosis. *Gastroenterology*. 1994;106:193-199.

15. Nakamura M, Kondo H, Mori T, et al. Anti-gp210 and anti-centromere antibodies are different risk factors for the progression of primary biliary cirrhosis. *Hepatology*. 2007;45:118-127.

Index

A

ACE-inhibitor therapy
  pregnancy, 206, 209, 211–212
  scleroderma renal crisis, 189–190
Acro-osteolysis (AC), 246, 261, 265
American College of Rheumatology (ACR),
  13, 264
Amlodipine, 28, 98, 101
Angiotensin receptor blockers (ARB)
  Raynaud's phenomenon, 102
  scleroderma renal crisis, 190
Angular cheilitis, 307
Antimitochondrial antibody (AMA), 344–345
Antinuclear antibody (ANA)
  calcinosis, 5
  digital pitted scars, 4, 5
  digital ulcers, 4
  dysmotility, 7
  laboratory findings, 2
  limited cutaneous SSc, 3, 8
  nailfold capillary microscopy, 3
  physical examination, 2
  proton pump inhibitor therapy, 2
  Raynaud's phenomenon, 3
  scleroderma, 3
  systemic sclerosis, 4
  telangiectasias, 5
Anxiety disorders, 232
Aquatic exercises, 281
Arthritis
  ACR criteria, 243
  arthralgia, 247
  clinical associations, 246
  corticosteroids plus vitamin D, 241
  crystal deposition disease, 247
  degenerative, 246
  effusions and osteophytes, 247
  inflammatory, 246
  laboratory and functional tests, 241
  laboratory findings, 245–246
  methotrexate with folic acid
    supplementation, 242
  MSK US, 242–243
  osteoporosis, 246
  pathogenesis and treatment, 247–248
  pathologic and clinical features, 244–245
  patient history, 239
  periarticular fibrotic, 246
  physical examination, 240
  prednisone, 241–243
  radiographs, 241, 242
  Raynaud's phenomenon, 243–244
  synovitis, 247
A Self-Care Workbook, 235
Assistive devices, 279
Autologous serum therapy, 327
Autologous stem cell transplantation
  international scleroderma (ASTIS),
    335–336
Autonomic dysfunction, 219

B

Barium esophagram, 156, 157
Bisphosphonates (BP)
  dental implants, 309–310
  osteonecrosis of the jaw, 311
Blink reflex, 298
Body image distress, 233
Bone resorption, 314
Brief-Satisfaction with Appearance Scale
  (Brief-SWAP), 233
Bronchoalveolar lavage (BAL), 120
Brown's syndrome, 328
B-type natriuretic peptide (BNP), 58

C
Calcinosis
    distal legs, 262
    drugs, 264–265
    female scleroderma, sexual
        dysfunction, 226
    late stage dSSc, 19
    limited cutaneous SSc, 5, 6
    surgical excision of, 265
Calcipotriene/betamethasone ointment, 41
Canadian Scleroderma Research Group
    (CSRG), 285, 286
Cardiac tamponade, 143
Cardiopulmonary testing, 116–117
Carpal tunnel syndrome
    ANA pattern, 18
    differential diagnosis, 14–15
    diffuse cutaneous systemic sclerosis, 12
    early diagnosis, 19–20
    immune suppressive therapy, 13
    immunosuppression, 17
    laboratory findings, 12
    monitoring lungs, 17–18
    physical examination, 12
    pregnancy, 20
    renal crisis, 16–17
    risk stratification and prognosis, 18–19
    scleroderma subsets, 14
    skin score, 15–16
    tendon friction rubs, 13
    vasodilator therapy, 13
Centrilobular fibrosis (CLF), 159–161
Cevimeline
    dry eyes, 325
    xerostomia, 305–306
Changing Faces, 235
Chronic Disease Self Management Program
    (CDSMP), 235
Cisapride, 162
Corticosteroids
    enlarged cardiac silhouette, 144
    inflammatory myopathy, 256
    KCS, 325
    localized skin sclerosis, 36
    nephrogenic systemic fibrosis, 91
    pediatric localized scleroderma, 49
    scleroderma renal crisis, 17, 188
Cranial neuropathies, 297, 312
CREST syndrome, 3, 323, 328
Cyclophosphamide, 112

D
Dental caries, 306
Dental implants

BP-related ONJ, 309–310
    contraindications, 308–309
    osseointegration, 308
    titanium root-form endosseous implants, 308
Dentures, 308
Depression
    ECDS, 44–45
    erectile dysfunction, 219
    pregnancy, 213
    sexual dysfunction, 226–227
    staff-assisted programs systems, 235–236
    work disability, 290
Dermatomyositis
    low-dose prednisone and methotrexate, 252
    patient history, 251
    physical examination, 251–252
Diffuse cutaneous systemic sclerosis
    (dSSc), 12
    aquatic exercises, 281
    arthritis, 244
    assistive devices, 279
    azotemia, 187
    bilateral hand involvement, 108
    cardiovascular conditioning program,
        280–281
    chemicals and drugs, 82
    cyclophosphamide, 112
    digital gangrene, 76
    durometers, 110
    energy conservation, 279–280
    heat modalities, 281
    heterogeneity, 112
    High-resolution CT scan, 75
    hypertension, 187
    intravenous cyclophosphamide, 74
    laboratory findings, 107, 186–187
    miscarriages, 206
    modified Rodnan skin score, 109
    motion exercises, 276–277, 280
    occupational therapy evaluation, 275–276
    oral cancer, 313
    oral exercises, 277, 278
    organic solvents, 82
    paraffin wax treatment, 277
    patient history, 185
    physical examination, 186
    physical therapy evaluation, 276
    Pittsburgh Scleroderma Databank, 111
    placebo-controlled clinical trials, 112
    pleural effusions, 187
    premature infants, 207
    pulmonary function test, 109
    pulse cyclophosphamide therapy, 74
    Raynaud's phenomenon, 73
    relaxation techniques, 281

resistive exercises, 280
scleroderma renal crisis (*see* Scleroderma
    renal crisis)
skin biopsy cores, weight of, 110
skin involvement, 77–80
skin thickening, 109
STPR, 111
tendon friction rubs, 245, 270–271
trichloroethylene, 81
work disability, 286
Digital gangrene, 76
Digital lesions, 1
D-penicillamine therapy, 200–201
Dry eyes
    carbomer-based drop, 319
    general physical examination, 320–321
    keratoconjunctivitis sicca
        (*see* Keratoconjunctivitis sicca)
    laboratory findings, 321
    ocular examination, 319–320
    ocular surface disease severity, 321
    physical symptoms, 319
    preservative-free topical lubrication, 321
    slit lamp, 321
Dry eye severity grading scheme, 321, 324
Dysfunctional tear syndrome, 326
Dyspareunia, 225
Dysphagia, 310

E
Early diffuse scleroderma
    capillaroscopy, 117
    cardiopulmonary testing, 116–117
    cyclophosphamide therapy, 117
    dyspnea, 123
    electromyography, 117
    immunosuppressive treatment, 122
    laboratory findings, 116
    organ involvement, 123
    physical examination, 116
    premature infants, 207
    shortness of breath, 117–121
Emotional distress
    anxiety, 232
    body image distress, 233
    fatigue, 232
    pain, 232
    pruritus, 232–233
    sexual dysfunction, 233–234
    worry, 230
Enamel erosion, 310
En coup de sabre lesions (ECDS), 44, 328, 329
Endicott Work Productivity Scale
    (EWPS), 291

Endothelin–1 (ET–1)
    erectile dysfunction, 219
    scleroderma renal crisis, 190
Enlarged cardiac silhouette
    cardiac tamponade, 144
    colchicine, 142
    corticosteroids, 144
    echocardiography, 142
    interstitial lung disease, 141
    laboratory findings, 140
    pericardial effusion, 141
    pericarditis, 143
    physical examination, 139–140
    renal and pulmonary involvement, 143
Eosinophilia-myalgia syndrome (EMS), 81
Eosinophilic fasciitis (EF)
    generalized morphea, 68
    groove sign, 64
    hydroxychloroquine, 69
    hypothyroidism, 67
    laboratory and pathology findings,
        65–66
    Peau d'orange, 64
    peripheral blood eosinophilia, 68
    physical examination, 64–65
    refractory skin fibrosis, 69
    skin biopsy, 67
    subcutaneous inflammation, 67
Eosinophils, 32
Episcleritis, 329
Erectile dysfunction (ED)
    abnormal nailfold capillary
        examination, 217
    autonomic dysfunction, 219
    depression, 219
    endocrinological evaluation, 218, 219
    endothelin–1, 219
    microvascular abnormalities, 218
    neurogenic dysfunction, 219
    penile fibrosis, 218, 219
    phosphodiesterase inhibitors, 219
    prevalence of, 218
    Raynaud's phenomenon, 217, 218
    rheumatoid arthritis, 218
    rheumatologic evaluation, 217
    vasodilator therapy, 219
Erythrocyte sedimentation rate (ESR), 24, 40,
        65, 174, 321
Esophageal manometry, 158
Esophageal scintigraphy, 57
Esophagogastroduodenoscopy (EGD),
        159, 166
European League Against Rheumatism
        (EULAR), 27
Eyelid skin fibrosis, 327

F
Facial pain. *See* Trigeminal neuropathy
Female scleroderma, sexual dysfunction
  depressive symptoms, 226–227
  dSSc, 223
  dyspareunia, 225
  fatigue and chronic pain, 226
  health interventions, 227
  laboratory findings, 222–223
  limited mobility, 226
  patient medical history, 221–222
  physical causes, 224
  physical changes, 225–226
  physical examination, 222
  psychological causes, 224
  Raynaud's phenomenon, 226
  secondary sicca syndrome, 223
  vaginal dryness, 225
Female Sexual Functioning Index, 227
Fertility, 204–205
Filamentary keratitis, 327
Flaxseed oil, 326
Freeman style punctual plug, 326

G
Gastric antral vascular ectasia (GAVE)
  autoimmune diseases, 168
  distalgastric mucosa, 169
  endoscopic therapy, 170
  esophagogastroduodenoscopy, 167
  histopathologic appearance, 167
  laboratory findings, 166
  physical examination, 166
  pylorus, 169
  upper gastrointestinal bleeding, 170
  watermelon stomach, 169
Gastroesophageal reflux (GER)
  anti-reflux measures, 158
  barium esophagram, 156
  cisapride, 162
  CLF, 160
  dysphagia, 158
  HRCT, 161
  laboratory findings, 157
  lung aspiration, 159
  physical examination, 156
  prokinetic medications, 162
Gastroesophageal reflux disease (GERD).
      See also Small bowel disease
  dental management strategies, 311
  enamel erosion, 310
Glomerulonephritis, 199–201
Glucocorticoids, 299
Gottron papules, 56
gp210 antibodies, 344–346

H
Health and Labor Questionnaire (HLQ), 291
Health Assessment Questionnaire Disability
      Index (HAQ-DI), 240, 245, 285
Health-related quality of life (HRQoL), 50
Hematopoietic stem cell transplantation
      (HSCT)
  ASTIS *vs.* SCOT trials, 335–336
  ATG/TBI-associated lung toxicity, 336
  autoimmune disease, 335–336
  complications, 334
  CYC cardiac toxicity, 336
  fatal late toxicity, 336
  flu-like illnes, 334
  intravenous therapy, 333
  menopause, 335
  microvascular changes, 337–338
  physical examination, 333–334
  pre and post transplant skin
      appearances, 334–335
  pretransplant bone marrow examination, 334
  pulmonary hypertension, 335
  TRM, 336
Hemolytic uremic syndrome (HUS), 188
Hemoptysis, 195
Hormonal support therapy, 325–326
Hydrogen breath tests, 177
Hydroxychloroquine, 67, 69

I
Imatinib mesylate, 87
Immunomodulator imiquimod, 41
Immunosuppression, 17
Impotence, 218
Inflammatory myopathy, 254–256
International Classification of Functioning,
      Disability and Health (ICF), 284
Interstitial lung disease (ILD)
  centrilobular fibrosis, 160, 161
  dSSc, 8, 119–120
  enlarged cardiac silhouette, 140, 141
  inflammatory myopathy, 255
  juvenile systemic scleroderma, 58
  lSSc, 8, 296
  PAH patients, 132
Iris transillumination defects, 328
6-Item Stanford Presenteeism Scale
      (SPS–6), 291

J
Joint swelling and tenderness.
      See Arthritis
Juvenile localized scleroderma

classification of, 43
mean age of, 42
ocular complications, 328
Juvenile-onset systemic sclerosis (jSSc)
anti-Scl 70 antibody, 56
esophageal scintigraphy, 57
EUSTAR/EULAR therapeutic
recommendations, 55
gottron papules, 56
laboratory findings, 55
methotrexate, 57
physical exam, 54–55
prognosis, 59
provisional classification criteria, 56
pulmonary hypertension, 58
taut skin, 54
treatment, 59

K
Keratoconjunctivitis sicca (KCS)
anterior segment, 327–329
anti-inflammatory therapy, 325–326
anti-La/SSA antibodies, 323
anti-Ro/SSA antibodies, 323
autologous serum therapy, 327
dry eye severity-grading scheme, 324
Freeman style punctual plug, 326
gamma-linoleic acid, 326
hormonal support therapy, 325–326
hypotonic solutions, 326
lacrimal gland biopsy, 323
lymphocytic infiltration, 322–323
ophthalmic mucolytic agents, 326
posterior segment, 328–329
primary Sjogren's syndrome, 322–323
punctal occlusion, 326
salivary gland biopsy, 323
Schirmer test, 323–324
secondary/associated Sjogren's syndrome,
322–323
supplemental nutrients, 326
tear film break up time, 324
tear stimulation, 324–325
topical cyclosporine A, 325
treatment algorithm, 324, 325
vital stainings, 324
xerostomia, 322
Keratoconus, 327

L
Lacrimal gland biopsy, 323
Limited cutaneous systemic sclerosis
(lSSc)

ACR criteria, 264
acro-osteolysis, 261, 265
arthritis, 244
calcinosis, 262, 264–265
dental caries, 303
D-penicillamine therapy, 200–201
glomerulonephritis, 199–201
hemoptysis and dyspnea, 195
laboratory findings, 197, 198, 261–262
microstomia, 303
miscarriages, 206
MPO-ANCA-associated vasculitis, 197,
200, 201
normotensive renal failure, 199–200
patient history, 259
periodontal disease, 303
physical examination, 196, 259–260,
301–303
proton pump inhibitor therapy, 197
pterygomandibular raphe, 304
pulmonary arterial hypertension, 262–263
pulmonary hemorrhage, 199–200
pulmonary-renal syndrome, 199–200
purpuric lesions, 196
Raynaud'sphenomenon, 264
Staphylococcus aureus, 263
tendon friction rubs, 271
trigeminal neuropathy, 296
work disability, 286
xerostomia, 303
Linear limb morphea, 44
Localized scleroderma (LSc)
abnormalities, 45
antimalarials, 36
characteristic cutaneous features, 48
circumscribed/plaque morphea, 42
classification of, 34
corticosteroids, 49
ECDS lesions, 44
extracutaneous signs and symptoms, 47
facial lesions, 46
hard skin, 42
infrared thermography, 48
pediatric population, 42
plaque morphea, 34
preliminary proposed classification, 43
seizures, 45
skin biopsies, 47
Lung fibrosis, 17, 75, 159, 263

M
Magnevist®, 85
Major depressive disorder (MDD), 231
Malabsorption

antibiotic therapy, 178
causes, 176
diagnosis of, 177–178
dietary supplements, 178
mortality rate, 176
parenteral nutrition, 178–179
probiotics, 178
Male scleroderma
    erectile dysfunction (*see* Erectile
        dysfunction)
    impotence, 218
    work disability (*see* Work disability)
Malnutrition, 176, 178
Malnutrition universal screening tool
    (MUST), 178
Mandibular osteolysis, 314
Mandibular resorption, 299
Manometry, 177
Metacarpophalangeal (MCP) joints, 100
Methotrexate (MTX), 36, 40
Microstomia, 303, 307
Mild photophobia, 319
Miscarriages, 206
Mixed connective tissue disease (MCTD),
    297, 298, 312
Modified Rodnan skin score (MRSS), 15
Morphea, 34
Motility disorders, 179
Mucolytic agents, 326
Musculoskeletal ultrasonography (MSK US),
    242–243, 247
Myalgia/myopathy
    immunosuppressive drug, 256
    inflammatory myopathy, 254–256
    methotrexate, 256
    patient history, 252–253
    physical examination, 253–254
    prednisone, 256
    steroid therapy, 256
Mycophenolate mofetil, 50
Myocardial involvement, systemic
        sclerosis
    angiotensin-converting enzyme
            inhibitors, 152
    calcium channel blockers, 152
    cardiovascular magnetic resonance
            imaging, 151
    endothelin receptor antagonist, 151
    laboratory findings, 148–149
    physical examination, 147
    thallium perfusion defect scores, 151
    tissue-Doppler echocardiography, 152
    vasospasm, 150
Myositis, 255. *See also* Dermatomyositis;
    Myalgia/myopathy

N
Neonatal deaths, 207
Nephrogenic fibrosing dermopathy, 87
Nephrogenic systemic fibrosis (NSF), 81
    chronic kidney disease, 89
    follicular dimpling, 87
    gadolinium-containing contrast agents, 90
    hemodialysis treatment, 92
    hyperpigmentation, 89
    imatinib mesylate, 87
    interstitial pulmonary fibrosis, 87
    joint contractures, 91
    laboratory findings, 86
    lipodermatosclerosis, 90
    Magnevist®, 85
    morphea, 90
    physical examination, 86
    skin induration, 91
    tyrosine kinase inhibitors, 92
Neural dysfunction, 175
New York Heart Association, 127, 128
Nicardipine, 149
Normal tension glaucoma (NTG), 327
Normotensive renal failure, 199–201

O
Occupational therapy
    assistive devices, 279
    energy conservation, 279
    evaluation, 275–276
    motion exercises, 276–277
    oral exercises, 277, 278
    paraffin wax treatment, 277
Octreotide, 174, 179
Ocular surface disease, 321
Ocular Surface Workshop 2009, 324, 326
Ophthalmic mucolytic agents, 326
Ophthalmoplegia, 328
Oral cancer, 313
Oral exercises, 277, 278
Oral fibrosis, 307–308
Oral hygiene, 313
Oral infections, 306–307
Oral pilocarpine, 324, 325
Orbital fat atrophy, 328
Osseo-integrated dental implant, 308
Osteonecrosis of the jaw (ONJ), 309, 311

P
Pansclerotic morphea, 46
Paraffin wax treatment, 277
Parafoveal telangiectasia, 328
Parry–Romberg syndrome, 35, 46

Pellucid marginal degeneration, 327
Pericarditis, 143
Periodontal disease, 306–307
Periodontal ligament (PDL), 313
Peripheral blood eosinophilia, 68
Peripheral neuropathy, 296
Peripheral ulcerative keratitis, 327
Phosphodiesterase inhibitors (PDEIs), 219
Physical therapy
    aquatic exercises, 281
    cardiovascular exercise program, 280–281
    evaluation, 276
    motion exercise, 280
    pain management, 281
    resistive exercises, 280
Pilocarpine, 305–306
Plaque morphea, 34, 44
Pneumatosis cystoides intestinalis (PCI), 176
Prednisone, 67
Pregnancy
    ACE-inhibitors, 206, 211–212
    anesthetic management, 212
    antihypertensive medications, 211–212
    blood pressure monitoring, 211
    captopril, 211–212
    cardiopulmonary problems, 208–209
    fertility, 204–205
    gastrointestinal symptoms, 208
    high-risk obstetric monitoring
        program, 213
    miscarriage, 206
    musculoskeletal complaints, 208
    negative outcomes, 206–207
    neonatal deaths, 207
    postnatal care, 213
    preeclampsia, 209–210
    premature infants, 206–207
    pulmonary arterial hypertension, 205, 209
    Raynaud's phenomenon, 208
    rheumatoid arthritis, 205
    scleroderma renal crisis, 209
    skin disease, 208
    SSc-ILD patients, 208–209
    systemic sclerosis, 207–208
    venous access, 212
Prematurity, 206–207
Presenteeism, 290–291
Primary biliary cirrhosis (PBC)
    anticentromere antibodies, 345–346
    antimitochondrial antibody, 344–346
    diagnostic accuracy of, 345
    gp210 antibodies, 344–346
    hepatic parameter abnormalities, 343–344
    laboratory findings, 342
    liver function tests, 343

    physical examination, 342
    Sp100 antibodies, 344–346
    SSc patients, 343–344
    tender fingertips, 341
    ursodiol, 346
Primary Raynaud's phenomenon (PRP), 25
Primary Sjogren's syndrome
    dyspareunia, 225
    KCS and xerostomia, 322–323
    vaginal dryness, 225
Progressive hemifacial atrophy.
        See Parry–Romberg Syndrome
Proximal interphalangeal (PIP), 100
Pruritus, 232–233
Pseudo-obstruction, 174, 176, 179
Psycho-oncology model, 234–236
Psychosocial care, systemic sclerosis, 234–236
Pulmonary arterial hypertension (PAH), 18
    algorithm for detection, 131
    cardiopulmonary hemodynamic
        abnormalities, 132
    clinical classification, 130
    endothelin receptor antagonists, 133
    heart-lung transplantation, 134
    HSCT, 335
    intravenous epoprostenol, 133
    N-TproBNP serum levels, 132
    pathogenesis of, 129
    pregnancy, 205, 209
    sildenafil, 134
    therapeutic intervention, 130
    vasodilator therapy, 133
Pulmonary hemorrhage, 199–201
Pulmonary-renal syndrome, 199–200
Punctal occlusion, 326
Purpuric lesions, 196

Q
Quality of life (QOL), 230

R
Randomized controlled trials (RCTs), 49
Raynaud's phenomenon (RP), 1
    Allen's test, 100
    amlodipine, 98
    anemia, 26
    calcium channel blockers, 28
    causes of, 26
    connective tissue disease, 26
    critical ischemia, 100
    cyanosis, 99
    cyanotic fingers, 25
    cyanotic phase, 96

digital infarct, 97
digital ulcers, 103
Doppler ultrasound, 100
drugs, 28
erectile dysfunction, 217, 218
heat modalities, 281
laboratory findings, 24, 97
magnetic resonance angiography, 100
nailfold capillaroscopy, 24, 25
nifedipine/amlodipine, 28
nonpharmacologic therapy, 100–101
pallor phase, 96
patient history, 23–24
pharmacological therapy, 101–103
physical examination, 24, 97
pregnancy, 207
scleroderma vascular disease, 99
sexual dysfunction, 226
SSc-spectrum disorder, 27
surgical interventions, 103
thermograms, 27
thermoregulation, 99
trigeminal neuropathy, 296
Retinal pigment epithelium (RPE), 328
Rheumatoid arthritis (RA)
    erectile dysfunction, 218
    pregnancy, 205
    work disability, 288–289
Rheumatoid factor (RF), 65
Right heart catheterization (RHC), 75

S
Salivary gland biopsy, 323
Schirmer test, 321, 323–324
Scleroderma cyclophosphamide or transplant
    (SCOT), 336
Scleroderma renal crisis (SRC), 16–17
    ACE-I therapy, 189–190
    amlyoidosis, 190–191
    ANCA-associated, pauci-immune
        glomerulonephritis, 188
    endothelin–1, 190
    EULAR recommendations, 192
    histopathologic finding, 188–189, 191
    mortality, 189
    pregnancy, 209
    renal biopsy, 188
    renal transplantation, 190
Secondary sicca syndrome, 223
Secondary Sjogren's syndrome, 322–323
Self-management programs, 234–236
Serum prealbumin, 178
Shortness of breath
    anemia, 121
    assessment of, SSc-PAH, 131–133

BAL fluid, 120
HRCT, 120, 129
interstitial lung disease, 119
joint contractures, 118
laboratory findings, 128
lung/heart involvement, 119
medical therapies, SSc-PAH, 133–135
physical examination, 127–128
proximal skin involvement, 118
pulmonary hypertension, 121
radiological assessment, 120
SIBO. See Small intestine bacterial overgrowth
Sjogren's syndrome (SS)
    anti-inflammatory medication, 326
    lacrimal gland biopsy, 323
    punctal occlusion, 326
    salivary gland biopsy, 323
Skin sclerosis
    antinuclear antibodies, 35
    laboratory findings, 32–33
    localized scleroderma, 33
    methotrexate, 33
    morphea, 34
    physical examination, 31–32
    ultraviolet light, 36
Skin thickness progression rate (STPR), 111
Small bowel disease
    antibiotic trial, 174
    constipation and diarrhea, 173
    malabsorption (see Malabsorption)
    malnutrition, 176, 178
    manometric study, 177
    mortality, 175
    motility disturbance, 179
    pathophysiology of, 175
    PCI, 176
    physical examination and investigations,
        173–174
    pseudo-obstruction, 174, 176, 179
    radiographic assessment, 176–177
    SIBO, 176, 177
    TPN, 174
    weight loss, 175
Small intestine bacterial overgrowth (SIBO),
    176, 177
Sp100 antibodies, 344–346
Staphylococcus aureus, 263
Superior oblique palsy, 328
Symmetric seronegative polyarthritis, 241
Sympathectomy, 103

T
Tear deficiency, 326
Tear film break up time (TBUT), 321, 324
Telangiectasias, 5, 327

Temperomandibular disorders, 308
Tendon friction rubs, 13
    Carpal tunnel syndrome, 13
Tendon friction rubs (TFR)
    dSSc, 245, 270–271
    laboratory findings, 270
    leathery crepitus, 270
    locations of, 272
    lSSc, 271
    patient history, 269
    physical examination, 269–270
    randomized controlled trial, 271–272
    serological testing, 272
    sites of, 271
    skin thickening and functional disability, 272
    squeaking sensation, 272
    treatment, 272–273
Therabite appliance, 307–308
Therabite Jaw Motion®, 307
Thermography, 24
Thrombotic thrombocytopenic purpura
        (TTP), 188
Thyroxine replacement therapy, 31
Topical cyclosporine A, 325
Total parenteral nutrition (TPN), 174
Toxic oil syndrome (TOS), 81
Transplant-related mortality (TRM), 336
Trichloroethylene (TCE), 81
Tricuspid annular systolic excursion
        (TAPSE), 133
Trigeminal neuropathy (TN)
    blink reflex, 298
    causes of, 298
    diagnostic tests, SSc patients, 297
    laboratory finding, 296
    mandibular resorption, 299
    MCTD, 297, 298, 312
    pathophysiology of, 298
    patient medical history, 295–296
    prevalence of, 296
    Raynaud's phenomenon, 296
    rheumatic disease, 312
    sensory deficit, 297
    treatment, 299
    trigeminal reflex testing, 298
Trismus, 307–308

U
Ultraviolet (UV) light therapy, 49
UnitedStates Preventive Services TaskForce
        (USPSTF), 235–236
Ursodiol, 346

V
Vasodilator therapy, 13, 133
Very Early Diagnosis of Systemic Sclerosis
        (VEDOSS), 20
Vinyl-chloride disease, 81
Viscotears, 319

W
Work disability (WD)
    age and gender, effects of, 288
    connective tissue diseases, 289
    definition, 284–285
    depression, 290
    diffuse *vs.* limited cutaneous SSc, 286
    disclosure, 291
    disease activity *vs.* damage, 285
    education, 287–288
    EWPS, 291
    frequency of, 285–286
    impact of, 289
    inflammatory arthritis, 288–289
    predictors of, 286–287
    presenteeism, 290–291
    prevention, 289
    rehabilitation, 289
    self-reported function, 285
    SPS–6, 291
    SSc patients, identification of, 291
    SSc-related costs, 289
    type of employment, 288
    WALS, 291
    WLQ, 291–292
Work instability scale (WIS), 289, 291
Work Limitations Questionnaire (WLQ),
        291–292
Workplace Activity Limitations Scale
        (WALS), 291
Work Productivity and Activity Impairment
        Questionnaire (WPAI), 291

X
Xerostomia
    etiologic factors, 305
    keratoconjunctivitis sicca, 322, 323
    management of, 306
    treatment of, 305–306

Y
Yellow scleral plaques, 89